RESEARCH in COMMUNICATION SCIENCES and DISORDERS
METHODS FOR SYSTEMATIC INQUIRY

Fifth Edition

RESEARCH in COMMUNICATION SCIENCES and DISORDERS
METHODS FOR SYSTEMATIC INQUIRY

Fifth Edition

Lauren K. Nelson, PhD, CCC-SLP
Jaimie L. Gilbert, PhD, CCC-A

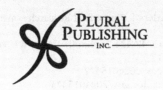

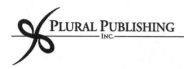

9177 Aero Drive, Suite B
San Diego, CA 92123

email: information@pluralpublishing.com
website: https://www.pluralpublishing.com

Copyright ©2026 by Plural Publishing, Inc.

Typeset in 10.5/13 Garamond by Flanagan's Publishing Services, Inc.
Printed in the United States of America by Integrated Books International

All rights, including that of translation, reserved. No part of this publication may be reproduced, stored in a retrieval system, or transmitted in any form or by any means, electronic, mechanical, recording, or otherwise, including photocopying, recording, taping, web distribution, or information storage and retrieval systems without the prior written consent of the publisher.

For permission to use material from this text, contact us by
Telephone: (866) 758-7251
Fax: (888) 758-7255
email: permissions@pluralpublishing.com

Every attempt has been made to contact the copyright holders for material originally printed in another source. If any have been inadvertently overlooked, the publisher will gladly make the necessary arrangements at the first opportunity.

NOTICE TO THE READER
Care has been taken to confirm the accuracy of the indications, procedures, drug dosages, and diagnosis and remediation protocols presented in this book and to ensure that they conform to the practices of the general medical and health services communities. However, the authors, editors, and publisher are not responsible for errors or omissions or for any consequences from application of the information in this book and make no warranty, expressed or implied, with respect to the currency, completeness, or accuracy of the contents of the publication. The diagnostic and remediation protocols and the medications described do not necessarily have specific approval by the Food and Drug administration for use in the disorders and/or diseases and dosages for which they are recommended. Application of this information in a particular situation remains the professional responsibility of the practitioner. Because standards of practice and usage change, it is the responsibility of the practitioner to keep abreast of revised recommendations, dosages, and procedures.

Library of Congress Cataloging-in-Publication Data

Names: Nelson, Lauren, author. | Gilbert, Jaimie L., author.
Title: Research in communication sciences and disorders: methods for
  systematic inquiry / Lauren K. Nelson, Jaimie L. Gilbert.
Description: Fifth edition. | San Diego, CA: Plural Publishing, Inc.,
  [2026] | Includes bibliographical references and index.
Identifiers: LCCN 2024015372 (print) | LCCN 2024015373 (ebook) | ISBN
  9781635507027 (paperback) | ISBN 1635507022 (paperback) | ISBN
  9781635504644 (ebook)
Subjects: MESH: Communication Disorders | Biomedical Research—methods |
  Research Design
Classification: LCC RC424.7 (print) | LCC RC424.7 (ebook) | NLM WL 340.2
  | DDC 616.85/5—dc23/eng/20240417
LC record available at https://lccn.loc.gov/2024015372
LC ebook record available at https://lccn.loc.gov/2024015373

CONTENTS

Preface — xi

Chapter 1. Empirical and Nonempirical Research: An Overview — 1
  Main Points — 1
  Systematic Inquiry — 2
  Some Roles for Research — 2
  Types of Research — 6
  Variables — 9
  Getting Started With Research — 9
  Summary — 11
  Review Questions — 12
  References — 13
  Appendix 1–1. Tips for Reading a Research Article — 16

Chapter 2. Ethical Considerations — 17
  Main Points — 17
  Protection of Human Participants — 18
  Special Protections — 21
  Historical Perspective — 22
  Institutional Review Boards — 26
  Current Perspective — 27
  Research Integrity — 29
  Avoiding Conflicts of Interest — 29
  Credit for Intellectual Effort — 30
  Attribution of Ideas — 31
  Accuracy in Reporting Information — 32
  Data Management — 33
  Confidentiality and Privacy — 34
  Health Insurance Portability and Accountability Act — 34
  Summary — 36
  Review Questions — 36
  Learning Activities — 37

| References | 38 |
| Appendix 2–1. Research Scenario | 42 |

Chapter 3. Identifying and Formulating Research Questions — 45
Main Points — 45
Identifying Important Questions — 46
Formulating Research Questions — 49
Ways to Formulate a Research Problem — 51
Evidence-Based Practice Questions — 55
Criteria for Well-Formed Questions — 58
Summary — 60
Review Questions — 60
Learning Activities — 61
References — 62

Chapter 4. Completing a Literature Search — 65
Main Points — 65
Purposes of a Literature Search — 66
Planning and Conducting a Search — 68
    Search Tools — 68
    Finding Information From Books — 72
Designing a Search Strategy — 73
Organizing and Documenting Your Literature Search — 75
Summary — 75
Review Questions — 76
Learning Activities — 76
References — 77
Appendix 4–1. Electronic Literature Search — 79

Chapter 5. Writing About Research: Literature Reviews and More — 87
Main Points — 87
Research Phases — 87
Purposes of a Literature Review — 88
Organization — 88
Note Taking — 91
Writing the Paper — 92
    Example of an Outline — 92
    Summary and Conclusions Section — 93
Citations and References — 94
    Example 1: Paraphrase From a Single Source — 94
    Example 2: Paraphrase From a Single Source — 94
    Example 3: Short Quote Within a Sentence — 94

Example 4: Short Quote Within Parentheses	94
Example 1: Entry for a Journal Article From a Print Source	95
Example 2: Entry for a Journal Article With a DOI Number	95
Example 3: Entry for a Journal Article Without a DOI Number	95
Example 4: Entry for a Book	95
Example 5: Entry for a Chapter in an Edited Book	95
Example 6: Entry for a Website Document	95
Literature Review Checklist	96
Types of Literature Reviews	96
Writing a Research Proposal	97
Summary	98
Review Questions	99
Learning Activities	99
References	100

Chapter 6. Nonexperimental Research Design — 103

Main Points	103
Nonexperimental Research Designs	104
Survey Research	104
Case Studies	105
Longitudinal Research	108
Correlation and Regression	109
Group Comparisons	111
Causal-Comparative Research	111
Qualitative Research	114
Sources and Analysis of Qualitative Data	116
Ethnography	117
Grounded Theory	117
Phenomenological Analysis	118
Case Study	119
Conversation Analysis	120
Scientific Rigor in Qualitative Research	122
Summary	123
Review Questions	124
Learning Activities	125
References	125
Appendix 6–1. Examples of Research Designs	133

Chapter 7. Research on Assessments and Diagnostic Approaches — 137

Main Points	137
Key Concepts in Measurement	137
Measurement Accuracy	139

Face and Content Validity ... 139
　　Criterion Validity ... 141
　　Construct Validity ... 144
　Measurement Consistency ... 146
　　Rater Reliability ... 146
　　Reliability Across Time ... 148
　　Internal Consistency Reliability ... 149
　Item Response Theory ... 150
　Summary ... 153
　Review Questions ... 155
　Learning Activities ... 156
　References ... 156

Chapter 8. Experimental Research and Levels of Evidence ... 159
　Main Points ... 159
　Experimental Research Designs ... 161
　　Posttest-Only Designs ... 161
　　Pretest-Posttest Randomized Control Group Design ... 162
　　Solomon Randomized Four-Group Design ... 163
　　Switching Replications Design ... 164
　　Factorial Designs ... 164
　Importance of Experimental Control ... 169
　　History ... 171
　　Maturation ... 171
　　Statistical Regression ... 171
　　Instrumentation ... 172
　　Selection ... 172
　　Mortality ... 173
　Quasi-Experimental Approaches ... 173
　　Nonequivalent Control Group Designs ... 174
　　Repeated Measures Group Design ... 175
　　Single-Subject Designs ... 177
　　Single-Subject Design Quality ... 184
　Experimental Designs and Levels of Evidence ... 184
　Summary ... 188
　Review Questions ... 189
　Learning Activities ... 190
　References ... 192
　Appendix 8–1. Research Scenario ... 196

Chapter 9. Research Participants and Sampling ... 199
　Main Points ... 199

Populations and Samples	200
Sample Characteristics	201
Sampling Methods	203
Simple Random Sampling	203
Systematic Sampling	203
Stratified Random Sampling	204
Cluster Sampling	205
Purposive Sampling	206
Random Assignment	206
Sample Size	207
Summary	210
Review Questions	211
Learning Activities	212
References	212

Chapter 10. Data Analysis: Tools for Describing Data   215

Main Points	215
Levels of Measurement	215
Visual Representation of Data	218
Descriptive Statistics	222
Frequencies and Percentages	222
Measures of Central Tendency	224
Measures of Variability	226
Means as Estimates	227
Shapes of Distributions	229
Summary	232
Review Questions	233
Learning Activities	234
References	234

Chapter 11. Data Analysis: Measures of Association and Difference   237

Main Points	237
Inferential Statistics	237
Measures of Association	240
Pearson Product-Moment Correlation Coefficient	240
Coefficient of Determination	245
Spearman Rank-Order Correlation	245
Chi-Square and Contingency Coefficient	246
Simple Regression and Multiple Regression	247
Testing for Differences Between Two Samples	250
Independent and Paired t-Tests	251
Confidence Intervals	254

Mann-Whitney *U* ... 256
Sign Test and Wilcoxon Matched-Pairs Signed-Ranks Test ... 257
Testing for Differences Among Three or More Samples ... 258
Statistical Analysis for Factorial Designs ... 262
Additional Tools for Analyzing Clinical Data ... 265
Caution in the Use and Reporting of Statistics ... 267
Summary ... 268
Review Questions ... 269
Learning Activities ... 270
References ... 271
Appendix 11–1. Examples of Data Analysis Procedures ... 274

Chapter 12. Research Outcomes: Clinical Guidance, Research Reports ... 277

Main Points ... 277
Knowledge Base for Evaluating Clinical Research ... 278
   Critical Appraisal ... 278
   How Applicable Are the Findings? ... 284
Reporting Research Findings ... 285
   Components of a Research Report ... 286
   Writing Guidelines and Writing Style ... 288
Disseminating Research Findings ... 289
Summary ... 291
Review Questions ... 291
Learning Activities ... 292
References ... 293

Index ... 297

PREFACE

When Dr. Lauren Nelson finished the first edition of this textbook in 2010, evidence-based practice, the use of research to inform clinical decision-making, was an emerging concept in the field of communication sciences and disorders. Currently, the situation is much different with widespread recognition of the importance of evidence to support clinical practice. Students and professionals benefit from consistent discussion of research evidence throughout the fields of audiology and speech-language pathology. If you browse current books on nearly any communication disorders topic, such as child language disorders, articulation and phonological disorders, adult neurogenic disorders, aural rehabilitation, and hearing aids, you will find a major section or chapter on research evidence. The topic of research evidence has become pervasive throughout our field of study and is a subject in many courses.

Both Dr. Nelson and Dr. Gilbert have experience teaching a research course for graduate students in communication sciences and disorders. Only a few of these students plan to pursue a career in research and/or higher education. The majority anticipate working in a clinical setting as an audiologist or speech-language pathologist, yet they nearly all express an appreciation of the role of research in the field of communication sciences and disorders. Occasionally students still worry about their motivation, expecting the topics of a research course to be less than exciting. But more often, they have already discovered that research is essential for high-quality clinical practice and that audiologists and speech-language pathologists need skills to investigate the existing research base and even to conduct their own original research. Our goal in writing this textbook is to help students and professionals develop knowledge and skills in research that will serve them throughout their professional careers.

Students frequently express concerns about the topics they expect to cover in a research methods course. Many of their concerns are similar from year to year and may be concerns you share. Students worry that they would have difficulty understanding the content of research articles, particularly the statistical information. Others describe prior frustration with their attempts to read research reports because they spent considerable time rereading material that was difficult to understand. They think that time management could be an issue, both in "keeping up" with their assigned readings and working on their own research projects. Many students are uneasy about finding a "good" topic for their own graduate research project.

If you have similar concerns, ideally this textbook will offer you some strategies for tackling those concerns. Recognizing that the way one approaches scientific inquiry is similar to the way audiologists and speech-language pathologists think about assessment and treatment of persons with communication disorders is an important first step. Our students have identified ideas for research projects by understanding that high-quality research stems from genuine curiosity and interest about a topic and that research in the field of communication sciences and disorders takes many forms. In their personal reflections, students report that repeated practice in reading research articles and a better understanding of the content and structure of those articles helped them use their study time more efficiently and effectively. The concerns our students express about research and the strategies we developed to address those concerns are the basis for this text.

This fifth edition adds a chapter on research investigating or developing assessments or diagnostic approaches. Specifically, this chapter addresses questions regarding validity and reliability. The fifth edition also updates the resources and tools available to assist us in finding and evaluating research evidence. The knowledge and skills needed to engage in empirical research and to use research in clinical practice are comparable, and that is how these topics are presented in this text. Rather than treating empirical research and searching for clinical evidence as separate topics, this text presents both as different applications of a process of scientific inquiry. The order of the chapters reflects the steps a researcher or clinician might complete when conducting an investigation. We recognize, however, that research is not a linear process and sometimes requires revisiting or revising your prior work.

Chapter 1 introduces the topic of scientific inquiry and its different applications in the field of communication sciences and disorders. Because ethical practice is a primary concern for both clinicians and researchers, Chapter 2 covers responsible conduct of research and ethical issues that affect the design and utilization of research, as well as the challenges associated with securing and using electronic records. Chapter 3 describes how researchers and clinicians might formulate questions as the starting point for their investigations. Some of these questions might be answered in the existing literature and others might be refined based on that literature. Thus, Chapter 4 addresses the information you might need to conduct a good-quality literature search. Chapter 5 provides guidance organizing and writing a literature review, and describes different types of literature reviews. Chapter 6, Chapter 7, and Chapter 8 cover the different types of research that are common in the field of communication sciences and disorders and the relationship between these types of research and the evidence audiologists and speech-language pathologists need to support their clinical endeavors. Chapter 7 is the new chapter focusing on research of assessments and diagnostic approaches. Chapter 9 reviews how researchers select persons to participate in research and issues associated with that process. Chapter 10 and Chapter 11 describe the analysis of research data using various statistical procedures. The final chapter, Chapter 12, covers how researchers and clinicians use the information gathered through their investigations. For researchers, this often involves preparation of a research report to disseminate to other professionals, and for clinicians, it usually leads to a decision about the most appropriate assessment and treatment approaches for their clients. For both clinicians and researchers, criteria for evaluating the quality of evidence are important.

Each chapter includes examples from the field of communication sciences and disorders to illustrate important concepts. New to this edition, each chapter begins with main points that the reader can use to guide their reading of the chapter. Similar to recommendations for how to read journal articles, this text and the individual chapters do not need to be read "in order." A suggestion is to first read the main points and then read the summary at the end of the chapter that often expands on the brief main points. Next, read the chapter introduction, which presents necessary background information. Finally, read the main body of the chapter, or the sections of particular interest to you. The review questions and learning activities at the end of each chapter can be used individually or in a classroom for discussion or small group activities. Two research scenarios or case studies are included in Chapter 2 and Chapter 8 to illustrate a practical application of concepts and to facilitate discussion. The online resources provide opportunities to work with examples and figures in a more dynamic way. Where appropriate, the learning activities include a list of research articles from journals in communication sciences and disorders that illustrate topics covered in the chapter. The learning activities could serve as homework assignments or, in some cases, as the focus of in-class discussions. In our own courses, we use the review questions in small group activities. Students benefit from explaining difficult questions to each other and doing so in a way that illustrates their own mastery of the concepts.

Empirical and Nonempirical Research: An Overview

Main Points

- Research is systematic inquiry that can be applied in scientific, academic, and clinical settings.
- Examples of roles for research include:
  - Gather information to answer scientific or clinical questions
  - Guide evidence-based practice
  - Evaluate programs for funding or resource allocation
- There are different categories of research relating to:
  - "Old"/new observations
  - Form of observations
  - Manipulation of variables
  - Random assignment to experimental variables
  - Manner of reporting results
- Research categories are to be used as guidelines. Research may include multiple categories/multiple methods (mixed methods).
- Research involves variables.
  - Independent ~ input
  - Dependent ~ output
- When reading research reports, you do not have to read it in order. Identify the research question and the authors' answer before reading the specific details and taking notes in your own words.

For many students, learning that they need to complete a research course is a cause of considerable anxiety. Audiologists and speech-language pathologists who are already engaged in their professional practice often recognize the importance of a strong research base in communication sciences and disorders but may view research as an activity unique to those who hold research-oriented doctoral degrees. Perhaps you are someone who views research as a requirement to endure rather than as a topic to embrace, or perhaps you acknowledge the importance of research in communication sciences and disorders but consider it something that others with unique talents undertake. One aim of this introductory chapter is to establish the fact that research encompasses many different kinds of activities, and professionals in clinical settings already engage in some of these. Furthermore, the knowledge and skills we need to be effective researchers are not necessarily unique talents but often parallel the processes and procedures employed by audiologists and speech-language pathologists.

Systematic Inquiry

One way to view research is as a process of systematic inquiry. Making an inquiry involves asking a question and then engaging in a process to determine the answer to that question. Asking and answering questions is at the heart of research endeavors. Research is systematic because the approach you use to find answers has predetermined procedures, and these procedures are carried out in a regular, orderly manner. Usually, the questions that researchers investigate are ones that are recognized as important to a field of study, such as communication sciences and disorders, and to persons in society, such as children and adults with communication disorders.

The *scientific method* is an approach to systematic inquiry. This method involves a series of steps that lead from identifying a problem and formulating a question to discovering possible answers to that question.

The generally accepted steps include the following: (1) Identify a problem and further define that problem through background research, (2) develop a specific hypothesis or question to investigate, (3) plan a set of procedures for testing the hypothesis or answering the question, (4) collect data using those procedures, (5) analyze the data, and (6) make a decision about the viability of the hypothesis or answer to the question.

You would expect to find the steps of the scientific method in a research text. However, Pindzola et al. (2016) included similar steps in their diagnosis and evaluation textbook when discussing the "science and art" of diagnosis (p. 19). These authors observed that clinicians engage in a way of thinking that parallels the method scientists employ in their experimental research. When faced with a clinical problem, such as a person referred for an evaluation, audiologists and speech-language pathologists gather and analyze data to test a hypothesis. In the case of a speech, language, or hearing evaluation, the hypotheses relate to whether or not someone has a disorder, the nature of that disorder, and how to best treat that disorder. Although the types of questions or hypotheses differ, both clinical practice and research involve ways of thinking and problem solving that are systematic in nature. When the process of inquiry is systematic, both clinicians and scientists have greater confidence that the information they provide is accurate and trustworthy, whether providing that information to individual clients and their families or to the scientific community.

Some Roles for Research

Scientific research has many roles in the fields of audiology and speech-language pathology. Perhaps the most basic role is to satisfy scientific curiosity. Researchers in communication sciences and disorders regularly participate in a process of identifying unanswered questions and designing information-gathering procedures to answer those questions. Researchers focus on questions they regard as important for understanding the nature of human communication; the underlying physiology of speaking and hearing; the causes of speech, language, and hearing disorders; and so forth. Researchers who are motivated primarily by scientific curiosity might still include persons with speech, language, or hearing disorders in their studies and conduct research that has implications for assessing and treating communication disorders. For example, researchers gained new evidence about the neurological bases of speech and language by including persons with aphasia in their studies. These types of studies provided information about the effects of brain lesions on speech and language use but did not necessarily lead directly to specific assessment or treatment recommendations.

Research is also valuable in guiding clinical practice in audiology and speech-language pathology. Scientific and clinical research follow similar processes (Figure 1–1). The two paths differ mainly in the order of gaining knowledge and identifying questions. In scientific research, knowledge is first gained in order to develop a question, with a refining process of learning more about specific topics to narrow down the research question. In clinical research, the question is often the first step, identified through a clinical concern. After identifying the question, then knowledge is gathered, again with a refining process.

Sometimes audiologists and speech-language pathologists are motivated to conduct research because of unanswered questions they encounter in their clinical practice. The term *clinician-scientist* is a way to refer to health care professionals, including audiologists and speech-language pathologists, whose primary responsibility is providing clinical services but who also engage in research in their profession (Chute, 2013). Sometime clinicians are the lead researchers on a project, but many

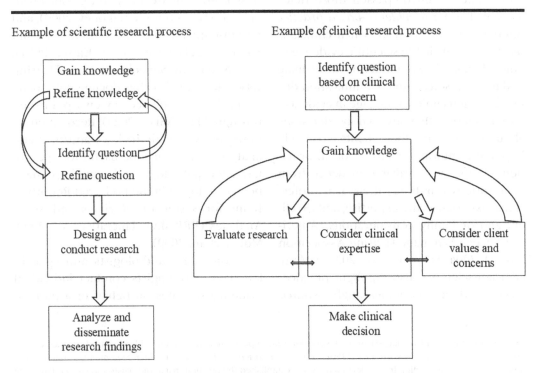

Figure 1–1. Examples of research processes.

times clinicians collaborate with a research team. Clinician-scientists are ideally positioned to conduct research that guides the way audiologists and speech-language pathologists diagnose and treat communication disorders. Clinician-scientists have firsthand knowledge regarding information that is lacking, as well as work with clients in their professional practice who would be most representative of children and adults with speech, language, and hearing disorders.

The notion of using research to guide clinical practice is important even for audiologists and speech-language pathologists who do not participate in conducting original research. A strong emphasis on using scientific evidence to guide decisions has emerged in both the fields of medicine and education. Because audiologists and speech-language pathologists are employed in medical and educational settings, this movement has encompassed those fields as well. The term *evidence-based practice* refers to an approach in which clinicians use the best available scientific evidence to guide their decisions about how to evaluate and treat persons with communication disorders. When clinicians engage in evidence-based practice, they are making decisions about how to serve their clients effectively based on multiple sources of information: (1) the best available evidence from systematic research, (2) their own professional experience and expertise, and (3) client and/or family considerations (American Speech-Language-Hearing Association [ASHA], 2004; Schmitt et al., 2021).[1] Many clinician-scientists also highlight practice-based evidence as a meaningful source of data (Dollaghan, 2007; Fissel Brannick et al., 2022).

When audiologists and speech-language pathologists participate in evidence-based practice, they might do so by consulting an existing evidence review. Usually, a panel of experts prepares such reviews. They are published in professional journals or perhaps published in electronic format on a website. When the authors of the reviews conduct a well-defined, qualitative critique of the existing research, the review is a systematic review. When the authors apply both qualitative and quantitative analysis in their review, it may be a meta-analysis. Some examples include a meta-analysis of the use of hearing aids for individuals with tinnitus (Waechter & Jönsson, 2022), a systematic review and meta-analysis of the use of nonword repetition in assessing the language of bilingual and monolingual children (Schwob et al., 2021), meta-analyses of word-finding treatment for persons with aphasia (Wisenburn & Mahoney, 2009), and parent-implemented intervention for child language delays (Roberts & Kaiser, 2011). The American Speech-Language-Hearing Association (ASHA) has documented many examples of evidence reviews published through 2024 (ASHA, 2024). Recommendations for systematic reviews and/or meta-analyses, which may be useful for speech-language pathology and audiology, have been developed in the Preferred Reporting Items for Systematic Reviews and Meta-Analyses (PRISMA) (Liberati et al., 2009; Moher et al., 2009).

Sometimes audiologists and speech-language pathologists conduct individual evidence searches on behalf of a particu-

---

[1]The American Speech-Language-Hearing Association (2005) position statement on evidence-based practice can be found in the document *Evidence-Based Practice in Communication Disorders* [Position Statement], available from http://www.asha.org/policy. In this document, ASHA established the position that audiologists and speech-language pathologists should engage in evidence-based practice to ensure provision of the highest quality clinical services.

lar client (Gallagher, 2002). Such searches begin with a client-specific question and culminate with review, evaluation, and application of existing research. Clinicians might use existing research literature when answering questions such as which of two treatment approaches produced the most improvement in the shortest time, whether a particular diagnostic procedure yields results that are accurate and reliable, or what the most effective treatment for a client with a specific diagnosis is. Evidence-based practice reflects a movement away from sole reliance on expert opinion and toward an approach that relies on careful consideration of research evidence in conjunction with clinical expertise and client/family considerations (Gallagher, 2002).

Another reason audiologists and speech-language pathologists engage in research is for program evaluation and support. This type of research is conducted at a local level sometimes in response to external requirements and sometimes due to local initiatives. For example, a medical center might evaluate the quality of its programs and services by comparing them to a set of nationally recognized standards. Professionals employed in educational settings are very much aware of the use of student achievement testing to evaluate school programs. Again, such evaluation involves comparisons to state and national standards purported to reflect the quality of school programs. At other times, program evaluation questions emerge from local rather than state or national initiatives. For example, a medical center might conduct consumer satisfaction research with the goal of improving its programs and services and increasing the likelihood that consumers choose that medical center as their health care provider. A school district might conduct program evaluation research after making changes to curriculum or teaching practices to determine if these changes led to improvements in student learning and achievement. Although professionals such as audiologists, speech-language pathologists, nurses, physicians, and teachers often debate the best approaches for program evaluation, nearly all agree that research of this type plays an important role in their professions.

Scientific research also may influence public policy, particularly policy regarding the allocation of resources. When research evidence is particularly strong, legislators and policy makers may consider this evidence in making decisions about spending public funds. An example of this is the growth of publicly funded early childhood education for all 3- and 4-year-olds. One reason for the increase in public funding is research that consistently demonstrated that children who attended good-quality preschool programs performed better in school and were more successful in their later lives. The research actually demonstrated that the funds spent early in childhood were offset by savings that occurred later through reduced educational spending on special services and reduced need for public assistance in adulthood (Barnett, 2000).

Research that demonstrates how a service or program impacts society is sometimes referred to as cost-effectiveness or cost-benefit research. Cost-effectiveness research looks at the cost of a program or service relative to the outcomes produced (Barnett, 2000). For example, if different treatment programs or different technologies varied in cost, an audiologist or speech-language pathologist would probably want confirmation that the more expensive approach produced better outcomes for their clients. Cost-benefit research looks at the cost of a program or service relative to its impact on costs that occur later in life. For preschool education, the analysis included documentation of the cost of the educational program and long-term follow-up of the children who participated. The long-term follow-up revealed actual cost benefits to society in several different ways. For example, children who received early childhood education were less likely to need special education services during the school years, were less likely to need other public services such as juvenile detention, were less likely to participate in public assistance programs as adults, and typically earned more income per year as adults (Barnett, 2000). Thus, individuals who advocated for public funding of early childhood education could point to a body of research that suggested such programs produced a net financial benefit to society that greatly offset the initial cost. Audiologists and speech-language pathologists would profit from a body of research demonstrating the benefits of our programs.

Types of Research

Taking some time to peruse published research in audiology and speech-language pathology, such as that found in our professional journals, reveals many forms of research. Generally, research studies share at least one similarity: a question that needs an answer or problem that needs a solution. How researchers formulate their questions or how they plan and conduct their studies, however, can be quite different. In this section, we consider some of the terminology researchers use to characterize these differences (Figure 1–2).

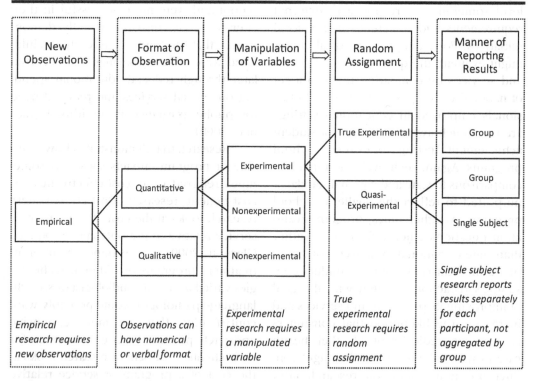

Figure 1–2. Types of research.

Most of the time when professionals in the fields of audiology and speech-language pathology use the term *research*, they are referring to *empirical* research. Empirical research involves the collection of new information or data through observation and measurement of behavior and/or physical properties (Trochim et al., 2016). Review of recent issues of professional journals in communication sciences and disorders reveals several ways that human behavior was observed as language samples (Spencer et al., 2023), survey responses (Ebert & Williams, 2023; Oliva et al., 2023), ratings of perceived effort (Cortez-Aoyagi et al., 2023), and test scores (Mues et al., 2023), as well as several ways of measuring physical properties, such as auditory brainstem response waveforms (Porter et al., 2022), tongue pressure measurements (Szynkiewicz et al., 2023), otoacoustic emissions (Pacheco et al., 2022), and acoustic measures of voice (Dahl & Stepp, 2023), or measuring both behaviors (speech recognition, effort ratings) and physical properties (pupillometry) to assess listening effort (Lau et al., 2019).

Researchers conducting nonempirical investigations make use of existing information instead of gathering new data. Nonempirical research ranges from loosely structured term papers and literature reviews to carefully constructed theoretical analyses or systematic reviews of a body of research. Another way to characterize different forms of research is the distinction between *qualitative* and *quantitative* research. Qualitative research and quantitative research differ with regard to the way questions or problems are formulated and investigated. A commonly identified difference, however, is in the type of information or data a researcher gathers. Qualitative research data often include verbal information. This might take the form of highly detailed descriptions of a person's behavior or perhaps direct quotes of a person's statements. Quantitative research, as you might expect, relates to numerical information such as frequency counts and measures of size or other physical properties. Sometimes researchers gather both types of data and report both numerical and verbal information.

Within the category of quantitative research, we often make a distinction between studies that are experimental and those that are nonexperimental. In experimental research, researchers identify one or more factors that they will manipulate or control during the experiment. For example, a researcher might compare different approaches for improving a person's communication abilities and could manipulate how much or what type of approach participants experience. The researcher manipulates or controls the conditions so that some participants have a different experience during the experiment than others. According to Newhart and Patten (2023), a true experiment meets two criteria. The first is the researcher's creation of different conditions or experiences by manipulating one or more factors during the experiment, and the second is that the conditions participants experience are determined randomly. A true experiment has random assignment of the participants to different experimental groups. Experimental research that lacks random assignment to groups is sometimes referred to as quasi-experimental research. Generally speaking, a study that meets both standards, experimental manipulation and random assignment, provides stronger evidence than a quasi-experimental study.

One of the most common kinds of experiments is one in which a researcher compares the performance of two groups, each experiencing a different experimental manipulation or treatment. In audiology and speech-language pathology, such comparisons might involve traditional treatment as compared to some new treatment approach. As noted, when the participants are divided at random into groups, the study is considered a true experiment. Sometimes researchers find it impractical or impossible to assign their participants randomly, however. Perhaps the researchers want to compare two different classroom-based interventions. Children in school settings are seldom assigned to their classrooms in a random manner. Therefore, if researchers decide to conduct the experiment with two existing classrooms, they are conducting quasi-experimental research rather than a true experiment.

As you read research articles in the field of communication sciences and disorder, you also are likely to find articles that are identified as representing a *Phase I* to *IV* clinical trial. Such terminology refers to experimental research that focuses on treatment for a condition or disorder. A *Phase I trial* is an early, exploratory study of a treatment usually with a small number of participants (National Institutes of Health [NIH], 2022). A *Phase II trial* is a true experimental study with a large number of participants and a strong research design. A *Phase III trial* is confirmatory research, often with multiple sites and research groups, and many participants. Finally, *Phase IV* research includes studies of application of the treatment in clinical practice in real-world settings (NIH, 2022). Phase IV research is sometimes called *translational research* or implementation science (Campbell & Douglas, 2016; Douglas et al., 2022).

In contrast with experimental research, nonexperimental research includes a wide variety of studies in which the researcher investigates existing conditions. Some forms of nonexperimental research are descriptive in nature. Studies that provide information about the typical communication behaviors of persons of various ages fall into this category. Such studies might include measures based on speech and language samples, measures of physical properties of speech such as fundamental frequency or intensity, and psychoacoustic responses to speech. Other examples of nonexperimental research include case studies, surveys, studies of relationships or correlations between measures, and comparison or case-control studies (Newhart & Patten, 2023). In comparison or case-control studies, researchers include groups of persons with preexisting differences, rather than create differences via an experimental manipulation. Some examples include comparisons of 3-year-olds and 5-year-olds, persons with a particular type of hearing loss and persons with normal hearing, adults with functional voice disorders and those with normal voices, or children with specific language impairment and those with typical language.

Another important distinction for research in communication sciences and disorders is the difference between *group* and *single*-subject research. This difference is not associated with the number of research participants in a literal way. That is, one might encounter a small group study with just five participants in each group or single-subject research with several participants. Nor is single-subject research the equivalent of a nonexperimental case study. Nonexperimental case studies involve descriptive research, whereas single-subject research is experimental in nature. The most important differences between group and single-subject research concern how participants are treated during the study and how their data are reported. In single-subject research, a participant experiences both the experimental and control conditions, and results for each participant are reported separately. When experimental and control conditions are compared in group research, usually the participants in one group experience the experimental condition and the participants in another group experience the control condition. The results from group research are aggregated and reported for each of the comparison groups and not for individual participants.

Variables

Two additional terms are useful for understanding how researchers talk about their studies. Usually researchers have identified some characteristic or manipulation they want to investigate. The characteristic or manipulation the researcher wants to study is called the *independent variable*. In experimental research, the independent variable might be an experience such as receiving a treatment or a way of presenting information that the researcher manipulates. In nonexperimental research, the independent variable might be an existing characteristic such as the presence or absence of a communication disorder or the age of the participants. Often the independent variable has two or more categories or levels that the researcher wants to compare in some way (Newhart & Patten, 2023). Keep in mind that experimental and nonexperimental studies may have more than one independent variable, and sometimes researchers study the effects of both an experimental manipulation and an existing characteristic in the same investigation. An example of this would be a researcher who studies the effects of a treatment manipulation, such as giving feedback in two different ways, for children in two different age groups. The researcher could determine in a random way which participants receive a particular type of feedback during their treatment, but the age of the children is an existing characteristic that cannot be manipulated.

When researchers want to compare the performance of their participants, they need to identify ways of measuring that performance. The measures that researchers use to determine the outcomes of their experimental or nonexperimental research are called dependent variables. In a sense, you might think of independent variables as the inputs and dependent variables as the outputs of the research. If the experimental manipulation or existing characteristics make a difference, researchers will see these differences in the values of their dependent variables or outcome measures.

Getting Started With Research

One of the best ways to become familiar with the various types of research is to read the research reports published in our professional journals. Sometimes students express frustration with the notion of reading professional research. They find the articles highly detailed and confusing. When reading a research report, keep in mind that the key information in nearly any such report is a question or problem the researcher investigated and the answer(s) provided by the researcher's observations or data. Thus, the most important goal in reading a research report is to find out the research question(s) and to learn what the author(s) wrote in answering those questions.

Silverman (1998) suggested a five-part strategy for reading and taking notes on a research article. He suggested you needed to obtain complete reference information, the research question(s), a brief description of the procedures, a brief description of the outcome measures or observations, and the answer to the research question. Some examples of this question-and-answer format are included on pages 7 to 9 in Silverman's book.

One approach you might consider is to read the article in a nonlinear way. Most research reports follow a very similar structure. The articles include an abstract, introduction and review of literature, methods, results, and discussion sections.

Most journals require an abstract, and this is a logical place to begin reading the article. The abstract provides a brief overview of the article's contents, but because the information is a summary, you will not be able to judge the quality of the research or fully understand the theoretical basis, results, and implications without reading the full article. Some journals now use a format called a structured abstract. If you read an article in a recent volume of the *Journal of Speech-Language-Hearing Research*, for example, you will see abstracts with headings such as Purpose, Method, Results, and Conclusion. The inclusion of headings of this type allows the reader to quickly identify the question(s) addressed in the study, typically in the purpose section, and the tentative answers, typically in the results and conclusion sections.

In the main body of the article, the first section is the *introduction and review of literature*. In some journals, this section may not have a heading but will be the initial information presented. This section will introduce the topics relevant to the research and what is currently known and unknown about these topics. The authors discuss the significance of the topics and build a logical argument for why their research question is important. Some articles have a separate heading identifying the research question(s). However, many articles embed the research question at the end of the introductory section, as this represents the culmination of all the background information.

The next main section of the article is the *methods*. This is where authors provide significant detail on how the research was conducted in order that other researchers can replicate the study and readers can critically appraise and appropriately apply the research findings. The methods section is typically divided up into subsections including participants (who participated in the research), materials or equipment (describing what was used to complete the research), and procedures (describing how, when, and where the research was conducted).

Following the methods is the *results* section. This includes the findings of the qualitative and/or quantitative analyses (often the dependent variables observed or measured by the researchers). In quantitative research, this section includes descriptive and/or inferential statistics.

The *discussion* section usually begins with statements summarizing the results. The authors address how the current study supports, conflicts with, or adds to the body of literature on the topic. This section often includes the authors' reflection on limitations to the study and ideas for future research.

Once you have a broad understanding of the content of an article from reading the abstract, you have some idea whether the article is relevant to the topic you are researching. When you read the full article, we suggest you begin by identifying the research question or the problem being studied by the author(s). In almost every research article you read, the research question(s) will appear in the paragraph or two immediately preceding the methods section. Sometimes, you will see a series of actual questions listed in these paragraphs, although at other times, you might read a statement of purpose. We will learn more about the various forms a research question or problem might take in Chapter 3. Once we know the question(s), we typically want to know the tentative answers next. Usually, in a well-written article, the authors will provide their interpretation of results and the possible answers to their research questions in the discussion section of the article. You might even find that the various questions or purposes of the research are clearly identified with subheadings in the discussion section. Once you have a general understanding of the research questions and possible answers, you are better prepared to read the full article. You will begin with the introduction and review of literature, and because you know the questions addressed in the study, you will have a good understanding why the author included certain topics in this review. As you read the methods section, you should be considering whether the way in which the researchers designed the study and collected their data gives you confidence in the results of the study. A course in research methods should provide you with the knowledge you need to critically evaluate the articles you read. Finally, as you read the results section, you will be able to judge how the numerical (quantitative) or verbal (qualitative) information reported there relates to the interpretation and conclusions the authors presented in their discussion section.

As you read an article, you should take notes on the most important information. From the introductory section, you might note any controversies, key findings from previous research, and, most importantly, the research question or statement of purpose that generally appears at the end of the introductory section. From the methods, your notes should include a brief description of the participants, information on the design of the study, and a summary of the most important procedures. Notes from the discussion section should cover answers to the research question or interpretations related to the purpose of the study, as well as possible limitations of the study. When taking notes, you should try to paraphrase from memory, rather than rewriting the exact words from the research paper (Stolley et al., 2014). You might initially use sentence fragments that capture the main points and develop these more fully later in the writing process. When you write about another person's work, you need to avoid, even inadvertently, using their words as your own; otherwise, you risk plagiarism. If you find it difficult to paraphrase or summarize a particular statement, you might copy a direct quote, but make sure you identify this material with quotation marks in your notes, along with the source's page number. In writing about others' research, most of your text should be your own summaries and paraphrases with only sparing use of direct quotes from the authors.

Summary

As noted previously, research is an essential component of the professional practice of audiologists and speech-language pathologists. In your clinical practice, you will utilize research on a regular basis because our professional research is the basis of our clinical practice from decisions about diagnosis and etiology to the approaches we use in treatment. Furthermore, speech-language pathologists and audiologists might need to consult existing research directly on behalf of specific clients. This might occur when these professionals are required, perhaps by a funding agency, to document the effectiveness of a proposed treatment, or perhaps when the audiologist or speech-language pathologist needs additional information to decide on the best course of treatment.

Professionals who investigate the existing research literature on behalf of their clients or for their own professional development are acting in the role of a consumer of research. Audiologists and speech-language pathologists working in clinical settings have many good reasons, however, to participate in designing and conducting original research as well. Some of the skills associated with the diagnosis and treatment of communication disorders could transfer to the research setting. Professionals already engage in a scientific approach to problem solving and regularly participate in observation and measurement of communication behaviors to document the effectiveness of their services (ASHA, 2023). Using these skills to generate new information for the professions could be a natural extension for some audiologists and speech-language pathologists. The motivation for such work might come from unanswered questions encountered in the clinical setting, as well as the need for research generated in an ecologically valid setting: the work settings of audiologists and speech-language pathologists. For some types of research, particularly assessment or treatment research, audiologists or speech-language pathologists working regularly in the field might obtain higher-quality data because of their clinical skills and experience.

Review Questions

1. What is the first step in the scientific method?

2. What phrase refers to the use of scientific evidence to guide clinical decisions?
    a. Systematic inquiry
    b. Hypothesis testing
    c. Evidence-based practice
    d. Single-subject research

3. Define cost-effectiveness research.

4. Which of the following statements is true?
    a. Empirical research involves the collection of new information through observation and measurement.
    b. Empirical research involves a systematic review of existing information identified through a literature search.

5. In _____ research, data often include verbal information such as a detailed description of behavior or a direct quote.

6. What are the two characteristics of a *true* experiment?

7. Match the following terms.

    Independent variable
    Dependent variable
    True experiment

    a. Outcome measure
    b. Random assignment
    c. Experimental manipulation

8. What kind of research includes case studies, surveys, studies of correlations between measures, or studies of preexisting differences?

9. Which of the following statements is true?

a. Single-subject research is descriptive research in which a researcher provides a detailed report on the characteristics of an individual participant.
b. Single-subject research is experimental research in which a participant experiences both the experimental and control conditions.

10. When reading a research report, where are you most likely to find the research questions or statement of purpose?

11. List the typical parts of a research report. When you start reading a research report, which part would you read first? Which part would you read next?

12. Which of the following statements is true?
a. Some of the skills associated with the diagnosis and treatment of communication disorders are similar to the skills required to conduct scientific research.
b. The skills required to conduct scientific research are entirely different from the skills associated with the diagnosis and treatment of communication disorders.

References

American Speech-Language-Hearing Association. (2004). *Evidence-based practice in communication disorders: An introduction* [Technical report]. https://www.asha.org/policy/TR2004-00001/

American Speech-Language-Hearing Association. (2005). *Evidence-based practice in communication disorders* [Position statement]. https://www.asha.org/policy/PS2005-00221/

American Speech-Language-Hearing Association. (2023). *Code of ethics* [Ethics]. http://www.asha.org/policy

American Speech-Language-Hearing Association. (2024). *Evidence maps.* http://www.asha.org/Evidence-Maps/

Barnett, W. S. (2000). Economics of early childhood intervention. In J. P. Shonkoff & S. J. Meisels (Eds.), *Handbook of early childhood intervention* (2nd ed., pp. 589–610). Cambridge University Press.

Campbell, W., & Douglas, N. (2016, November). Research with an impact: Launching an academic career in knowledge translation and implementation science. *Clinical Practice Research, CREd Library.* https://doi.org/10.1044/CRED-PVD-C16007

Chute, P. M. (2013, August). Clinician-researcher collaborations: Strengthening clinical outcomes through science. *Academics & Research in Context.* https://academy.pubs.asha.org/2013/08/clinician-researcher-collaborations-strengthening-clinical-outcomes-through-science/

Cortez-Aoyagi, M., Gufstason, E., Murphy, A., & van Mersbergen, M. (2023). A measure of swallow effort using the Borg Category Ratio 10 Perceived Exertion Scale. *American Journal of Speech-Language Pathology, 32*(6), 2846–2857. https://doi.org/10.1044/2023_AJSLP-23-00090

Dahl, K. L., & Stepp, C. E. (2023). Effects of cognitive stress on voice acoustics in individuals with hyperfunctional voice disorders. *American Journal of Speech-Language Pathology, 32*(1), 264–274. https://doi.org/10.1044/2022_AJSLP-22-00204

Dollaghan, C. A. (2007). *The handbook for evidence-based practice in communication disorders.* Brookes Publishing.

Douglas, N. F., Feuerstein, J. L., Oshita, J. Y., Schliep, M. E., & Danowski, M. L. (2022). Implementation science research in communication sciences and disorders: A scoping review. *American Journal of Speech-Language Pathology, 31*(3), 1054–1083. https://doi.org/10.1044/2021_AJSLP-21-00126

Ebert, K. D., & Williams, L. (2023). Perceptions of racism among graduate students of color in audiology and speech-language pathology. *American Journal of Speech-Language Pathology, 32*(6), 2982–2998. https://doi.org/10.1044/2023_AJSLP-23-00163

Fissel Brannick, S., Wolford, G. W., Wolford, L. L., Effron, K., & Buckler, J. (2022). What is clinical evidence in speech-language pathology? A scoping review. *American Journal of Speech-Language Pathology, 31*(6), 2943–2958. https://doi.org/10.1044/2022_AJSLP-22-00203.

Gallagher, T. M. (2002). Evidence-based practice: Applications to speech-language pathology. *Perspectives on Language Learning and Education, 9*(1), 2–5.

Lau, M. K., Hicks, C., Kroll, T., & Zupancic, S. (2019). Effect of auditory task type on physiological and subjective measures of listening effort in individuals with normal hearing. *Journal of Speech, Language, and Hearing Research, 62*, 1549–1560. https://doi.org/10.1044/2018_JSLHR-H-17-0473

Liberati, A., Altman, D. G., Tetzlaff, J., Mulrow, C., Gøtzsche, P. C., Ioannidis, J. P. A., Clarke, M., Devereaux, P. J., Kleijen, J., & Moher, D. (2009). The PRISMA statement for reporting systematic reviews and meta-analyses of studies that evaluate health care interventions: Explanation and elaboration. *BMJ, 339*, 2700. https://doi.org/10.1136/bmj.b2700

Moher, D., Liberati, A., Tetzlaff, J., Altman, D. G., & the PRISMA Group. (2009). Preferred reporting items for systematic reviews and meta-analyses: The PRISMA statement. *Annals of Internal Medicine, 151*(4), 264–269. https://doi.org/10.7326/0003-4819-151-4-200908180-00135

Mues, M., Zuk, J., Norton, E. S., Gabrieli, J. D. E., Hogan, T. P., & Gaab, N. (2023). Preliteracy skills mediate the relation between early speech sound production and subsequent reading outcomes. *Journal of Speech, Language, and Hearing Research, 66*(8), 2766–2782. https://doi.org/10.1044/2023_JSLHR-22-00142

National Institutes of Health. (2022, October 3). The basics. *NIH clinical research trials and you.* https://www.nih.gov/health-information/nih-clinical-research-trials-you/basics.

Newhart, M., & Patten, M. L. (2023). *Understanding research methods: An overview of the essentials* (11th ed.). Routledge Taylor & Francis Group.

Oliva, A., West, J. S., Smith, S. L., Huang, R. J., & Riska, K. M. (2023). Association between hearing handicap and life-space mobility in a patient population. *American Journal of Audiology, 32*(2), 360–368. https://doi.org/10.1044/2023_AJA-22-00052

Pacheco, D., Rajagopal, N., Prieve, B. A., & Nangia, S. (2022). Joint profile characteristics of long-latency transient evoked and distortion otoacoustic emissions. *American Journal of Audiology, 31*(3), 684–697. https://doi.org/10.1044/2022_AJA-21-00182

Pindzola, R. H., Plexico, L. W., & Haynes, W. O. (2016). *Diagnosis and evaluation in speech pathology* (9th ed.). Pearson.

Porter, H. L., Dubas, C., Vicente, M., Buss, E., & Kaminski, J. (2022). Auditory brainstem responses at 6 and 8 kHz in infants with normal hearing. *American Journal of Audiology, 31*(4), 1279–1292. https://doi.org/10.1044/2022_AJA-22-00100

Roberts, M. Y., & Kaiser, A. P. (2011). The effectiveness of parent-implemented language interventions: A meta-analysis. *American Journal of Speech-Language Pathology, 20*, 180–199. https://doi.org/10.1044/1058-0360(2011/10-0055)

Schmitt, M. B., Justice, L. M., & Fey, M. E. (2021). Evidence-based decision making in communication assessment and intervention. In R. Paul & E. S. Simmons (Eds.), *Introduction to clinical methods in communication disorders* (4th ed., pp. 65–82). Paul H. Brookes Publishing.

Schwob, S., Eddé, L., Jacquin, L., Leboulanger, M., Picard, M., Oliveiran, P. R., & Skoruppa, K. (2021). Using nonword repetition to identify developmental language disorder in monolingual and bilingual children: A systematic review and meta-analysis. *Journal of Speech, Language, and Hearing Research*, *64*(9), 3578–3593. https://doi.org/10.1044/2021_JSLHR-20-00552

Silverman, F. H. (1998). *Research design and evaluation in speech-language pathology and audiology: Asking and answering questions* (4th ed.). Prentice-Hall.

Spencer, T. D., Tolentino, T. J., & Foster, M. E. (2023). Impact of discourse type and elicitation task on language sampling outcomes. *American Journal of Speech-Language Pathology*, *32*(6), 2827–2845. https://doi.org/10.1044/2023_AJSLP-22-00365

Stolley, K., Brizee, A., & Paiz, J. M. (2014). *Avoiding plagiarism*. The Purdue Online Writing Lab. https://owl.english.purdue.edu/owl/resource/589/01/

Szynkiewicz, S. H., Drulia, T., Griffin, L., Mulheren, R., Murray, K. L., Lee, T., & Kamarunas, E. (2023). Flexibility for intensity dosing in lingual resistance exercises: A large randomized clinical trial in typically aging adults as proof of principle. *American Journal of Speech-Language Pathology*, *32*(6), 3021–3035. https://doi.org/10.1044/2023_AJSLP-23-00113

Trochim, W. M. K., Donnelly, J. P., & Arora, K. (2016). *Research methods: The essential knowledge base* (2nd ed.). Cengage Learning.

Waechter, S., & Jönsson, A. (2022). Hearing aids mitigate tinnitus, but does it matter if the patient receives amplification in accordance with their hearing impairment or not? A meta-analysis. *American Journal of Audiology*, *31*(3), 789–818. https://doi.org/10.1044/2022_AJA-22-00004

Wisenburn, B., & Mahoney, K. (2009). A meta-analysis of word-finding treatments for aphasia. *Aphasiology*, *23*, 1338–1352. https://doi.org/10.1080/02687030902732745

APPENDIX 1–1

Tips for Reading a Research Article

1. Read the abstract for an overview of the article.
2. Identify the research question, typically located at the end of literature review just prior to the Methods section (this may be a question, purpose statement, hypothesis, or if-then statement; see Chapter 3).
3. Identify the type of research (see Chapter 1), purpose of research (e.g., describe, relate, compare; see Chapter 3), and any dependent and/or independent variables (see Chapters 1 and 3).
4. Find the answer to the research question, typically located in the first paragraph(s) of the Discussion section and/or the Conclusions/Summary section.
5. Read the article, taking notes in your own words.
6. Critically evaluate the article and identify limitations, for example:
   a. Were ethical principles upheld? (see Chapter 2)
   b. Were the measures used in the study valid and reliable? (see Chapter 7)
   c. What did the study add to previous literature/knowledge? (see Chapters 4 and 5)
   d. Were the methods appropriate for the research question and conclusions? (see Chapters 6, 7, 8, and 9)
   e. Was the data analysis appropriate for the study design and purpose? (see Chapters 10 and 11)

2

Ethical Considerations

Main Points

- You have multiple roles and each role has its own ethical considerations and guidelines. These include academic, professional, and research ethics.
- A common ethical consideration across these roles is the accurate attribution of ideas (e.g., citing your sources). This includes honest submission of your own original work and always acknowledging when content is not your own original work and directing readers to the source of the information.
- The Belmont Report is a foundational document for ethics in research. It established three main principles when involving humans in research. An institution (e.g., a university, a health care entity) has a review board (i.e., institutional review board) that oversees that all research conducted at that institution conforms to these ethical principles.
    - Respect for persons
    - Beneficence
    - Justice
- The American Speech-Language-Hearing Association Code of Ethics (2023) is an example of professional ethical guidelines. It contains four main principles.
    - Welfare of persons
    - Professional competence and performance
    - Responsibility to the public
    - Uphold dignity and autonomy of the professions

Regardless of their work setting, audiologists and speech-language pathologists who consider carrying out an original research project have many questions and concerns. They might wonder if they have sufficient time to conduct the research, the skills to perform certain procedures, or the equipment and other resources needed for the project. One hopes that one of their foremost concerns will be their ability to conduct the research in an ethical manner. When you behave in an ethical way, you act according to a set of moral standards that characterize appropriate conduct. Professionals in fields such as audiology and speech-language pathology have formal codes established by national and state organizations (e.g., American Speech-Language-Hearing Association, American

Academy of Audiologists, the various state speech-language-hearing associations). Certainly, there are ethical standards that guide us through all phases of a research project from identifying a problem and formulating research questions, to conducting the research and data gathering, to the eventual dissemination and possibly publication of your findings.

Protection of Human Participants

One of the primary considerations in the ethical conduct of research is protecting the well-being of the persons who participate in that research. Policies and regulations that guide us in protecting participants in research have been established by federal agencies and professional associations, as well as at the local level. Agencies that receive federal funds for research, such as universities, major medical centers, and school districts, need to have guidelines in place for the ethical conduct of research. Specific protections for human participants are specified in the "Federal Policy for the Protection of Human Subjects," often referred to as the "Common Rule" (U.S. Department of Health & Human Services [HHS], n.d., 2009). Some of the essential protections for human participants include the requirement that participation be voluntary and not coerced, that researchers safeguard participants from any psychological or physical harm, that participants have an appropriate amount of information about the nature and purpose of the research before they are asked to take part (i.e., the notion of informed consent), that researchers take steps to maintain confidentiality and protect their participants' privacy, and finally, that participants understand they have a right to discontinue participation in the research study, even if they previously gave their consent. Even if researchers work in settings that are not covered by federal regulations, protections for human participants are embedded in the code of ethics for our professional organizations (American Academy of Audiology [AAA], 2023; American Speech-Language-Hearing Association [ASHA], 2023).

These protections for research participants have their roots in a pioneering federal document, the Belmont Report, from the U.S. Department of Health and Human Services (National Commission, 1979). The authors of the Belmont Report identified three basic principles of culturally acceptable behavior that were also very important in the conduct of research. These included "respect of persons, beneficence and justice" (National Commission, 1979, Part B: Basic Ethical Principles, paragraph 1). *Respect of persons* involves recognizing persons' ability to make their own choices and decisions. Potential participants in research are able to make informed decisions when researchers provide them with sufficient information about the study and when their decision to participate is completely voluntary. For such a decision to be truly voluntary, potential participants should not be coerced or enticed with rewards they could only earn by participating in the research. For example, university professors sometimes encourage their students to participate in research by providing extra credit toward a better course grade. This might be an inappropriate enticement unless the professor also provides alternate ways, unrelated to research participation, for students to earn the extra credit. Similarly, provision of audiology and speech-language pathology services to individuals with speech, language, or hearing disorders should never be contingent on the person's agreeing to participate in research. Some persons, such as children or persons with cognitive disabilities, might have difficulty making an informed decision about their participation. Researchers need to provide special protections to such persons. This does not mean that children or persons with disabilities cannot participate in research, but it does mean that researchers need to consider consent more broadly and obtain permission from parents, guardians, or significant others.

The principle of *beneficence* relates to researchers' obligation to protect the well-being of the persons who participate in a study. In proposing a study, researchers consider whether they are providing a direct benefit to the participants or at least are obtaining information that contributes to the good of society. The former might occur when a researcher finds that a new treatment is more effective than the traditional, accepted practice. The latter might occur in a study that uncovers information about the nature of a disorder or principles of behavior change that will contribute to more effective treatment in the future. An essential requirement of beneficence in research is to protect participants from harm. You might recognize the dictum "Above all, do no harm" as a statement from the oath that guides physicians and other medical professionals.[1] Researchers too must plan their studies in such a way that they expect to "do no harm" to their participants (National Commission, 1979). The nature of research is to investigate the unknown or the untried, however, and researchers might not be able to anticipate the potential harm a new experimental procedure could do. Thus, a second guideline for researchers is to "maximize possible benefits and minimize possible harms" (National Commission, 1979, Part B: Basic Ethical Principles, paragraph 7).

Let's consider some examples of the ways that researchers might conduct a study to minimize possible harms, even unanticipated ones. You might be familiar with the studies that major pharmaceutical companies conduct to test the effectiveness of new drugs. The various news reporting agencies and news websites often include information about these drug trials. When researchers undertake such a study, they might not be able to anticipate the negative side effects of a new drug. To minimize the risk for participants, however, they would carefully monitor each individual's health through periodic medical examinations. They also would monitor the rate of occurrence of any adverse side effects in the group receiving the new drug and in a comparison or control group. Researchers have an obligation to reevaluate the advisability of continuing such a study if they observe an abnormally high rate of adverse side effects in their treatment group.

Audiologists and speech-language pathologists sometimes need to compare different treatment approaches as well. In speech-language pathology, these types of studies often involve comparing a new treatment approach that the researcher expects to be more effective and a traditional approach with a long history. The researcher most likely has concluded, based on indirect evidence such as theoretical principles or evidence of effectiveness in other fields, that the new treatment approach should be more effective than the traditional approaches. Treatment comparisons are important for audiologists to assess best practices in a changing landscape with

---

[1] The statement "Above all, do no harm" is often attributed to the Hippocratic Oath. Although Hippocrates wrote about similar concepts, this statement is not actually found in the Hippocratic Oath (C. M. Smith, 2005).

over-the-counter amplification devices and service delivery models compared with traditional hearing aids with audiologist/clinical service delivery (see, for example, Brody et al., 2018; Humes et al., 2017, 2019) or to compare different hearing aid processing strategies (see, for example, Kirby et al., 2017; Salorio-Corbetto et al., 2019). In audiology and speech-language pathology, the adverse side effects for participants are unlikely to be physical symptoms or life threatening. However, persons in the experimental group might receive a treatment that turns out to be less beneficial. For example, persons receiving an experimental, behavioral treatment for acquired motor speech disorders might have less improvement in accuracy of sound production or speech intelligibility than those receiving traditional treatment. Maybe persons with hearing loss who were fitted with an experimental hearing aid technology received lower scores on tests of speech discrimination and rated their user satisfaction lower than persons who were fitted with a different hearing aid technology. These would be unintended yet adverse effects of participating in the research. Audiologists and speech-language pathologists need to be aware of adverse effects such as these and carefully monitor the progress of the persons who participate in their research, as well as their reactions during any testing or measurement procedures.

Given concerns about protecting the well-being of persons who participate in research, you might wonder why governmental agencies, professional organizations, and universities, among others, encourage research endeavors. The reason is that the benefits of research usually outweigh the potential risks. In a sense, a researcher weighs the potential risks and benefits when deciding to conduct a study. When researchers have reasons to expect substantial benefits either for the individual participants or a societal group (e.g., persons with speech disorders, persons with hearing loss), then they have justification for conducting a study. The beneficial outcomes are obvious when the research results in a treatment for a previously untreatable illness or condition or greater improvement or more rapid improvement in speech, language, or hearing outcomes.

The concept of *justice* relates to the need to make equitable decisions regarding who is invited to participate in research. Sometimes individuals want to participate in research because a study might provide a personal benefit. This might be the case when a person has a disorder with no known treatment, and an experimental approach is the only option. Researchers' decisions to include or exclude particular groups should have a sound, scientific basis. The Code of Ethics of the American Speech-Language-Hearing Association (ASHA) specifically addresses this issue in the following statement: "Individuals shall not discriminate in the delivery of professional services or in the conduct of research and scholarly activities" (ASHA, 2023, Principles of Ethics I, C). The ASHA Code of Ethics specifically prohibits discrimination related to variables such as "the basis of age; citizenship; disability; ethnicity; gender; gender expression; gender identity; genetic information; national origin, including culture, language, dialect, and accent; race; religion; sex; sexual orientation; or veteran status" (ASHA, 2023, Principles of Ethics I, C).

On the other hand, research participants might experience some adverse effects during a study making involvement in the study less desirable. In the case of possible adverse effects, the burden of participating in the research should be shared equally. Ideally, the persons who are invited to participate would come from the group of persons most likely to benefit from the research. If the benefits of the research will be widespread, then the participants should be drawn from a widely representative group.

Special Protections

Certain groups might be particularly vulnerable to exploitation in research and have been identified as needing special protections under federal law. These persons include prisoners, children, pregnant women and their fetuses, and persons with impaired consent capacity (Centers for Disease Control and Prevention [CDC], 2010; Secretary's Advisory Committee on Human Research Protections, 2008/2009; U.S. HHS, 2009). The need for special protections sometimes stems from concerns about persons' ability to make a free choice without undue influence. The case of persons in prison exemplifies why special protections might be needed. Persons in a prison are confined against their will and are living in circumstances where voluntary consent has little meaning. A prison environment usually provides limited opportunities to enrich one's life with respect to choices of entertainment, food, living space, and so forth. A person in prison might be overly influenced by the offer of a reward for participation in research and thus more likely than persons outside prison to volunteer to take part in a somewhat risky study.

The special protections afforded persons in prison or other institutional settings, children, pregnant women and their fetuses, and persons with impairments that would affect their ability to make decisions encompass all three principles of human participant protection: respect of persons, beneficence, and justice. Respect of persons relates to providing individuals with appropriate information so they can make voluntary decisions about participation in research. Special protections related to informed decision-making could include writing the consent document in language appropriate for the person's reading level or providing appropriate, not excessive, rewards or incentives, because excessive rewards for participating might overly influence a person's judgment about the level of risk associated with a study. Other examples of special protections include limiting research with protected populations to studies that have minimal risk and a direct benefit. Who benefits from the research is an important consideration; for special populations, the expectation is that the research should directly benefit the individual or benefit a group of persons in similar circumstances.

Although we usually think of special protections in the context of shielding vulnerable populations from unwarranted risks, systematically excluding protected populations from research participation also could be detrimental to the individuals' well-being. Let's consider the situation of persons who have a medical condition that has no known treatment. An individual with an untreatable illness, whether relatively young, in prison, or cognitively impaired, might desire an opportunity to receive even an experimental treatment. Similarly, persons receiving audiology and speech-language pathology services might want to participate in a study that could lead to improved outcomes for themselves or others with similar communication disorders. Thus, the principle of justice means protecting persons from unfair burden in assuming the risks of research, while at the same time providing equitable opportunities to participate in beneficial research (Kiskaddon, 2005).

Historical Perspective

Recognition of the need to protect research participants emerged largely in response to reported instances of mistreatment or exploitation of persons in the conduct of scientific research. Sometimes the reports became public many years after the end of the studies, although in some instances, the reports coincided with the need to stop research with unacceptable, negative consequences. Considering why some studies prompted strong public and professional reaction is worthwhile for persons who might be conducting their own original research in the future. Three studies that are noteworthy, either because the study influenced current policies on protection of research participants or because the study triggered extensive discussion of research ethics, are the Tuskegee Syphilis Study (King, 1998), the hepatitis study at Willowbrook State School (Moreno, 1998; Nelson, 1998), and the Tudor study at the University of Iowa (Goldfarb, 2006; Tudor, 1939). In discussing each of these studies, our focus is on learning the lessons each teaches regarding protection of research participants and specifically regarding respect of persons, beneficence, and justice. A thorough examination of the ethical issues associated with each study is beyond the scope of this chapter and has been addressed in other sources (Fairchild & Bayer, 1999; Goldfarb, 2006; Kahn et al., 1998).

The Tuskegee Syphilis Study is one of the most notorious research projects ever conducted in the United States. The study began in 1932 and continued for 40 years, ending in 1972 after the particulars of the study first became widely known and published in sources available to the general public (CDC, n.d.; King, 1998). The study was conducted by the U.S. Public Health Service, and its purpose was to study the effects of untreated syphilis. The participants in the study were 399 African American men with syphilis and 201 African American men without syphilis who served as controls (CDC, n.d.; King, 1998). What are the characteristics of the Tuskegee study that made it notorious for violating the basic ethical principles of respect of persons, beneficence, and justice?

- With regard to respect of persons, the participants were never told the true nature of their disease (Fairchild & Bayer, 1999); the researchers offered an enticement of free medical checkups, which might be regarded as a coercive inducement for participation given the participants had almost no access to health care and lived in poverty.
- With regard to beneficence, the men never were told about or offered a treatment that was available in 1930,[2] nor did the researchers inform the participants of an effective treatment, penicillin, which became available in the mid-1940s, an even more disconcerting fact (King, 1998).
- Finally, with regard to justice, the way the researchers conducted the study, particularly the disregard for the health and well-being of participants over a long period of time, suggested

---

[2]According to a document available on the CDC (n.d.) website, a treatment with mercury and bismuth was available by 1932. This treatment had a low cure rate and major toxic side effects; however, participants should have received information about this treatment option and been able to make a decision about seeking this option on their own.

exploitation of a vulnerable, less privileged population. The participants were vulnerable because their poverty prevented them from seeking adequate health care. The participants may have had less privilege because of their race. The way African American men were treated in the Tuskegee study reflected the racial discrimination that was prevalent in society when the study began (King, 1998).

The Tuskegee Syphilis Study is often cited in discussions of research ethics (Kahn et al., 1998). According to Fairchild and Bayer (1999), the study "has come to symbolize the most egregious abuse on the part of medical researchers" (p. 1). The study participants and their families were eventually awarded $10 million in an out-of-court settlement that followed their 1973 class-action lawsuit, and reaction to the study helped shape current national policies regarding the protection of research participants (National Commission, 1979).

Another example often cited in discussions of protection of research participants is a series of studies of hepatitis infection that took place at the Willowbrook State School in New York (Nelson, 1998). The study took place from 1955 through the early 1970s. The Willowbrook studies had several elements that were at odds with ethical and responsible conduct of research.

- Regarding respect of persons and informed consent, the researchers did obtain permission from the children's parents before enrolling them in the study, but in a manner that critics regarded as misleading and coercive. The consent process involved a meeting with a social worker as well as a group meeting where parents learned about the research (Diekma, 2006), but the information was incomplete and possibly misleading (Freedman, 2001) and possibly led parents to think their children would receive a vaccination for the virus, although the actual intent of the study was to infect children with a strain of the hepatitis virus under controlled conditions (Rothman, 1982).
- Regarding coercive influence, some parents received a letter regarding the study shortly after learning that the institution had no openings currently and their child would be placed on a waiting list; they were offered an earlier placement in the institution that was contingent on their child's participation in the research (Ramsey, 2002).
- Regarding beneficence, the Willowbrook study involved deliberately infecting children with a strain of the hepatitis virus that posed more than minimal risk; the researchers argued that the risks were not more than that of any child living at Willowbrook and perhaps less due to the controlled circumstances of the infection and the better medical care afterwards (Krugman, 1971). Critics of the study disagreed with this contention and suggested that the researchers could have made a positive difference for the children at Willowbrook if improving the children's living conditions had that been their focus (Rothman, 1982).
- Finally, regarding justice, the participants in the Willowbrook

studies were perhaps among the most vulnerable in our society because they were children with disabilities who lived in an institutional environment. Any involvement of children in nontherapeutic research is controversial (Bartholome, 1978; Jonsen, 2006; Ramsey, 1978, 2002) and even more controversial for children with additional vulnerability due to their disability or living conditions. Diekma (2006) summarized thinking on children's participation in research as follows:

> Because children represent a vulnerable subject population, their involvement in research can be justified only if the level of risk entailed in the research is very low, or if there is the potential for direct benefit to the child by participating in the research project. (p. S7)

The Willowbrook studies were conducted with the full knowledge of several medical boards and committees that reviewed the studies ahead of time and provided oversight for the research (Nelson, 1998). Thus, both the researchers who conducted the study as well as those responsible for administration of the school and oversight of the research could be the focus of criticism. Eventually, the Willowbrook State School was involved in legal action that sought to improve conditions at the school and to move residents out of this large institutional environment (Grossman, 1987).

The final research example we consider is a study conducted in 1939 at the University of Iowa by a graduate student, Mary Tudor, under the direction of Dr. Wendell Johnson (Goldfarb, 2006; Tudor, 1939). In comparison to the Tuskegee and Willowbrook studies, Tudor's study was relatively unknown and had little impact on current national policy regarding the protection of participants in research. The study had few participants, 22 children in total, only 6 of whom prompted concerns about the conduct of the study. The study is interesting in communication sciences and disorders because Wendell Johnson was one of the pioneers in the field of speech-language pathology (Goldfarb, 2006), as well as because the study has lessons to teach regarding our current thinking about treatment of child participants in research. The way the study was first reported in the popular press also teaches lessons regarding accurate, careful dissemination of information (Yairi, 2006).

The purpose of Tudor's research was to study how verbal labeling affected children's speech fluency (Tudor, 1939; Yairi, 2006). The participants in the study were 22 children who were residents at the Iowa Soldiers and Sailors Orphans' Home. Ten of the children were considered stutterers before the study, and 12 were children who were considered normal speakers.[3] To test the effects of verbal labeling, Tudor met with the children several times over a 5-month period. During these meetings, she spoke to the children in different ways. Half of the children who stuttered received positive comments suggesting that their speech was fine, and half of the children with normal speech received highly negative comments

---

[3]Yairi (2006) discussed the Tudor study in detail. He noted that the fluency levels among the children regarded as stutterers and those regarded as normal speakers were not clearly distinct and the two groups overlapped to a considerable degree.

suggesting they were having trouble speaking, that they had the signs of stuttering, and that they should try not to stutter (Silverman, 1988[4]; Yairi, 2006). Tudor also gave the staff at the children's home information about the children's "diagnoses." With respect to the original research questions, Tudor's results were unremarkable. The procedures produced no consistent changes in the fluency levels of the participants. Tudor's research notes suggested, however, that some of the children in the normal speaking group who were subjected to negative comments changed in other ways. For example, they showed signs of being reluctant or self-conscious about speaking, and some commented on having difficulty with speaking (Reynolds, 2006; Tudor, 1939).

The six children whom Tudor subjected to negative comments were at the center of a controversy that emerged more than 60 years later, after the publication of an article about the study in the *San Jose Mercury News* (Goldfarb, 2006). The sensationalized way the study was reported is one reason it became briefly infamous when it surfaced in 2001. The newspaper article suggested the researchers set out to turn children into stutterers, and Wendell Johnson, in an effort to avoid criticism, concealed the results of the study and never published it. Furthermore, the study had a colorful nickname, the "monster" study,[5] a label taken from a 1988 *Journal of Fluency Disorders* article (Silverman, 1988). The information in the popular press misrepresented the actual research questions Tudor and Johnson investigated, as well as the nature of their findings.[6]

For professionals in the field of communication sciences and disorders who inevitably viewed the Tudor study through the lens of contemporary thinking about protection of research participants and professional ethics, learning about the Tudor study was disturbing. Clearly, this study would not be conducted as originally designed under current research guidelines and policies (Schwartz, 2006; Yairi, 2006). Considering why professional and public reaction to the study was so strong could help us better understand current thinking about children's participation in research.

Because of their vulnerability, children are regarded as needing special protections in research. Generally, researchers accept that the types of studies children participate in should be limited to those with minimal risks or those that might provide a direct, personal benefit. In the Tudor study, only the children who already stuttered who received positive verbal comments stood to benefit from the research. Because the concept of risk encompasses psychological as well as physical risks, the children with normal speech who received negative verbal comments were exposed to some degree of risk. Some authors have argued that, when research involves more than minimal risks, parents or guardians should not be able to give consent for their children to participate (Ramsey, 1978, 2002).

The Tudor study also had features that illustrate the need to consider beneficence

---

[4]For readers who are interested in the exact nature of Tudor's comments, Silverman (1988) provides a few lengthy excerpts from the thesis manuscript.

[5]In a 1988 article, Silverman stated that Tudor's study "was labeled the 'monster' study by some of the persons who were associated with the Stuttering Research Program at the University of Iowa during the 1940s and 1950s and who knew of its existence" (p. 225). However, Silverman never elaborated on the exact reasons these individuals had for using this label.

[6]Ambrose and Yairi (2002) and Yairi (2006) provided a scholarly critique of Tudor's study, and Yairi (2006) also discussed how the study was reported in the popular press.

and justice in the design of research. With regard to beneficence, the possibility that either Tudor or Johnson intended to cause any harm to the children seems remote (Yairi, 2006). Tudor's research notes, as well as statements from the participants more than 60 years later, however, suggested some unintentional harm did occur (Reynolds, 2006). Tudor intended to study changes in the children's fluency, but what she observed were general communication changes associated with being reluctant or self-conscious about speaking. One lesson that researchers can learn from this is to be observant of unintended changes in participant behavior, as Tudor was, but also to be willing to modify or even stop research that is causing these changes. Rothman (1982) noted that sometimes researchers become overly focused on completing their studies. In such instances, researchers might overlook the possible negative effects the research procedures are having on their participants.

With regard to justice, the fact that the children were residents of an institution for orphaned or abandoned children was noteworthy. Historically, persons who resided in institutions of various types were exploited in research, leading to guidelines identifying prisoners and persons in other institutions as uniquely vulnerable populations in need of special protections (Moreno, 1998; National Commission, 1979). Ideally, the benefits and risks of research should be shared in an equitable way. The questions addressed in Tudor's study regarding the effects of verbal labeling on dysfluency were questions that were important to children and parents in general, not just to children living in a home for orphans. Reportedly, Tudor and Johnson conducted their study at the orphanage because the University of Iowa had a prior research relationship with the institution (Reynolds, 2006). As a sample of "convenience," the six children in Tudor's research took on more than their fair share of risk when they participated in the study. Current research guidelines, such as those for persons in prison (U.S. HHS, 2009), suggest that permissible research would address questions unique to the institutional environment, including the conditions that led to imprisonment, or providing a personal benefit to the participants, such as an opportunity to receive new, more effective treatment for an illness.

Although the Tudor study reflected the research ethics of its time, it raised questions of respect of persons, beneficence, and justice when it became widely known over 60 years later. In 2002, a lawsuit was brought against the State of Iowa on behalf of the three surviving participants and the estates of three other participants ("Iowa to Pay," 2007). These were the individuals who, as 6- to 15-year-old children, were the targets of Tudor's attempts to increase dysfluency. In August 2007, the State of Iowa agreed to settle this lawsuit for $925,000 ("Iowa to Pay," 2007).

Institutional Review Boards

One way that protections for research participants have been enhanced is through the process of institutional review (Balon et al., 2019). Organizations such as universities, medical research facilities, and other research institutions that conduct research under federal regulations are required to provide institutional oversight through the process of an *institutional review board* (IRB). The role of an IRB is to evaluate proposed studies before the researchers begin collecting data. Researchers provide the

IRB with a description of their proposed study, including information about the research design, participants, procedures, participant recruitment, and informed consent. The IRB reviews these materials and determines if the study adheres to guidelines associated with respect of persons, beneficence, and justice. A particular role of the IRB is to conduct a risk/benefit analysis of the proposed research to determine if risks to participants are minimal or justifiable based on potential benefits to the participants themselves or to society (Balon et al., 2019). Although individual researchers still should endeavor to design projects that adhere to federal guidelines as well as the ethical standards of their professional associations, the IRB provides an opportunity for researchers to receive guidance from a qualified panel and an additional layer of protection for potential research participants.

Current Perspective

Given the protections for human participants codified in federal law and the enhanced processes for institutional oversight, we might anticipate that violations of human participant protections would be minor and rare instances. Unfortunately, violations of research ethics have occurred despite current participant protections. The U.S. Department of Health & Human Services Office of Research Integrity lists case summaries of recent research ethics violations on a website (https://ori.hhs.gov/content/case_summary). The website lists 8 case summaries for 2022 and 10 for 2023. The list includes the names of researchers with current sanctions of some type. The cases primarily involved some form of data falsification or misrepresentation in grant applications, publications, or presentations. This form of misconduct might not result in direct harm to a human participant, but it does general harm by misleading other researchers and the public.

Other fairly recent examples of ethics violations either did harm or had the potential to harm actual research participants. One of these incidents occurred in 1999 during an early phase, exploratory study of a new gene therapy (White, 2020). One of the participants, 18-year-old Jesse Gelsinger, died a short time after receiving the trial therapy. In a subsequent inquiry, investigators found issues related to respect of persons/informed consent and beneficence.

- Regarding beneficence, Jesse should not have been a participant in the study because he had a mild form of the disorder; Jesse's current management with a special diet and medication was effective; and because of the mild form of the disorder and effective management, Jesse did not meet the inclusion/exclusion criteria for the study and took on unwarranted risk when he received the experimental gene therapy (Sibbald, 2001; White, 2020).
- Regarding respect of persons and informed consent, investigators questioned whether Jesse had been fully informed about the possible risks of the trial. According to Sibbald (2001), several previous study participants had experienced significant side effects. Additionally, in an earlier trial with monkeys, three of the animals died from adverse reactions to the gene therapy injection.

Following the investigation, the U.S. Food and Drug Administration suspended the study and took steps to enhance participant protections in clinical trials with gene therapy. The researcher, a medical geneticist who led the clinical trial, eventually returned to medial research and now advocates for far more caution and care in studying new treatments (Wenner, 2009; Wilson, 2009).

Another recent violation of research ethics came to light in 2017 in a warning letter from the U.S. Food and Drug Administration, Center for Drug Evaluation and Research (USDA, 2017). The violation involved a prominent medical researcher in the field of ophthalmology (Racino & Castellano, 2019a). The findings in this case included violations of the principle of beneficence and respect of persons as well as other research misconduct.

- Regarding beneficence, the research team did not conduct the study according to the written clinical investigation plan; the team enrolled five participants who were ineligible for the study because their vision tested better than the level in the eligibility criteria and the team failed to pretest another participant before administering treatment (USDA, 2017); the USDA report indicated that ineligible participants had unwarranted risk compared to individuals with lower vision levels who might have benefited from the treatment; and at the time of the investigation, which occurred relatively early in the clinical trial, ineligible individuals represented a significant proportion of study participants (Racino & Castellano, 2019a).
- Regarding respect of persons and informed consent, the research team conducted HIV testing on participants without their prior consent (USDA, 2017).
- Regarding other forms of misconduct, several units of a drug used in the study went missing, the research team did not keep adequate records or appropriately document patient follow-up, and the medical geneticist who was the lead investigator had not completed the ethics training required for conducting a stem cell study (Racino & Castellano, 2019a; USDA, 2017).

Research laboratories often function with a team of individuals. The lead investigator has the responsibility for providing appropriate oversight, ensuring strict adherence to study protocols, and protecting the well-being of all study participants. The medical researcher who was the lead investigator on the vision clinical trial was suspended and ultimately resigned his university position (Racino & Castellano, 2019b; Sawant, 2019).

Although protection of human participants in research is one of the researcher's primary ethical responsibilities, it is not the only one. The topic of research integrity encompasses other issues as well, such as data management practices, mentorship, authorship and assigning credit for intellectual effort, accurate attribution of ideas and citing sources, accuracy and honesty in reporting information, and potential conflicts of interest (American Psychological Association [APA], 2016; ASHA, 2009; D. Smith, 2003; Steneck, 2007). The final sections of this chapter address each of these topics in turn.

Research Integrity

The general topic of research integrity relates to attitudes, behaviors, and values associated with the responsible conduct of research. Besides protection of human participants, the Office of Research Integrity has identified protection of nonhuman animals, conflicts of interest, care in data acquisition and handling, relationships with mentors/mentees and collaborators, accuracy and honesty in publishing research findings, peer review, and avoiding research misconduct as topics critical to the responsible conduct of research (Horner & Minifie, 2011a, 2011b, 2011c; Jones & Mock, 2007; Steneck, 2007). Audiologists and speech-language pathologists who participate in research—whether as students, clinician-investigators, or full-time researchers—need to make a commitment to act with high integrity and ethical standards, and to seek appropriate training through research coursework, online resources (Office of Research Integrity, 2015), and personal reading.

Avoiding Conflicts of Interest

Individuals face the possibility of a conflict of interest when they perform more than one role. Sometimes the obligations of one role are at odds with the responsibilities of other roles. Researchers who perform clinical research, such as audiologists and speech-language pathologists who study the nature, assessment, and treatment of speech-language-hearing disorders, might experience such conflicts. For example, researchers might want to investigate the effectiveness of a new treatment program that, in theory, should be stronger than treatment approaches currently used in the field. However, the researchers cannot be certain the new approach is better until they gather some evidence. Professionals in this situation must balance their desire to investigate the new treatment with their desire to provide known, effective treatment to their clients with communication disorders. If they lean too heavily toward their research role, they might try experimental treatments with clients that have little chance of success. If they lean too heavily toward their clinician role, however, they might miss opportunities to advance the professions through research that leads to more effective clinical procedures.

Another possible conflict of interest is when speech-language pathologists and audiologists in the dual roles of researchers and clinicians recruit participants for their studies. If researchers recruit participants from among persons they serve clinically, they must be equally supportive of their clients' decisions, whether the clients agree to participate or decline to participate in any studies. The fact that a client was or was not a research participant should have no impact on the quality of speech-language or audiology services they receive. Keeping the clinician-client and researcher-participant roles separated is particularly challenging because clients might assume their clinical services might be negatively affected. That is, the client's consent to participate might be coerced through fear of losing access to treatment, even if that never was the researcher's intention. Perhaps the best way to manage this conflict between clinician and researcher roles is to ask a third party to manage the process of participant informed consent. That way the clinician-researchers avoid talking directly to any of their clients about participating in their research.

Another example of a conflict of interest is a conflict between the roles of researcher and product developer. Perhaps a speech-language pathologist or audiologist developed a product they think will improve assessment or treatment of communication disorders. One factor potential purchasers of this product might consider is whether or not the new product is superior to the assessment and treatment tools they already use. If the product developers design and conduct research to demonstrate its superiority, this might constitute a conflict of interest. What would happen if the researcher-developers found evidence that existing assessment or treatment products were more effective? They might be tempted to conceal that evidence or to redesign their study in hopes of obtaining more favorable results. In this case, the desire of the developers to market their product might be at odds with conducting and accurately reporting the results of their research. Ideally, product developers should recruit independent researchers to evaluate the superiority of new products or conduct research on new assessment and treatment instruments before making plans to market those instruments.

D. Smith (2003) identified another possible conflict of interest, a conflict between the roles of instructor and researcher. One example of this is common in psychology when course instructors recruit their students to participate in research projects (D. Smith, 2003). In some courses, participating in research is a course requirement; in other courses, students receive extra credit for participating in research. Instructors should be careful to provide students who choose not to participate in research with alternative ways to earn course or extra credit. Otherwise, instructors could be perceived as coercing their students into taking part in research. The principles of informed consent include the requirement that participants make their decision to participate free of coercion. Instructor-researchers might face another conflict of interest when the students in their courses also work as their research assistants. In this case, researchers need to be careful about how much work they ask their assistants to do or how they set up their schedules. Students who are research assistants might agree to a work overload or a burdensome work schedule because they think refusing could have a negative impact on their course grade (D. Smith, 2003). Instructor-researchers should be aware of this potential conflict, carefully monitor the hours their research assistants work, and encourage their assistants to communicate with them about workload issues.

Credit for Intellectual Effort

In a way, receiving credit for intellectual effort relates to researchers' sense of ownership and desire to earn rewards for their ideas. This issue links to several aspects of research integrity, including mentorship, collaboration, and publication practices (Horner & Minifie, 2011b, 2011c). When a researcher works alone on a project, identifying who "owns" and receives credit for a study is fairly straightforward. However, researchers often work together in teams or are students working under the direction of a faculty adviser (D. Smith, 2003). Ideally, in such instances, the individuals involved should discuss their perceptions of their roles and contributions early in the planning process. That way, the research team can avoid any misunderstanding before they reach a critical point in the project. One of the major rewards for conducting research is having an opportunity to present or publish the results of the study. D.

Smith (2003) noted that this particular form of reward has taken on special importance in some research settings, such as universities, where decisions about retention and promotion are partially based on how much a person has published. Smith characterizes this as a "competitive 'publish or perish' mindset" (p. 56). Conversely some researchers, particularly those in senior positions who have a long record of publication, might be tempted to be very generous in sharing credit for research. In sharing the rewards of their work, however, researchers need to be careful to give credit only to those who have made an actual contribution, as well as to consider the significance of that contribution (APA, 2020; ASHA, 2009). Sometimes, the appropriate form of credit might be an acknowledgment rather than authorship; however, if the individual made an important contribution, they should be included as one of the authors. According to D. Smith (2003), when researchers "contribute substantively to the conceptualization, design, execution, analysis or interpretation of the research reported, they should be listed as authors" (p. 56).

Attribution of Ideas

Another way the researchers receive credit for their work is when others cite it in their own writing. Researchers publish the results of their studies because they hope to influence the work of other researchers and to inspire new projects. As writers, we need to acknowledge the original author whenever we include an idea in our work that comes from another source. The ASHA Code of Ethics includes the following statement on the use of others' work: "Individuals shall reference the source when using other persons' ideas, research, presentations, results, or products in written, oral, or any other media presentation or summary" (ASHA, 2023, Principles of Ethics IV, L). When writers use information from another source, they often paraphrase it in their own words. Even when paraphrasing information, you still should give credit to the original source. Beginning professional writers sometimes ask, "How do I know when to attribute information to a particular source?" One possible answer is to consider if the information is common knowledge in the profession or unique to a particular source. It is essential to cite the source when the information you use reflects the special expertise of another author. Sometimes the same information might be found in several sources but still reflects the special expertise of those authors. For example, several authors who are experts on the topic of spoken language disorders might define this term in similar ways, or authors who are experts on the topic of central auditory processing disorders might provide similar guidance regarding appropriate testing. In instances of this type, you should cite all of the sources for the information. Certainly, deciding whether information is common knowledge or reflects some special expertise is a subjective judgment. However, if you have any doubt, you should include your sources. Providing a few citations unnecessarily is better than mistakenly taking credit for another person's ideas.

Another issue for beginning writers is distinguishing between an accurate paraphrase of another author's work and plagiarism. Students sometimes ask, "How much do I need to change the original author's work to avoid plagiarism?" The key to avoiding plagiarism and generating your own paraphrase is not to start with statements written by another author. Small modifications such as changing a few words in a sentence by using synonyms, putting the key phrases in a different order, changing from present to past tense, and so forth are all writing strategies to avoid. A better strategy is to begin by trying to understand a passage when you read it (Purdue Online Writing Lab [OWL], n.d.-a; UW Madison Writing Center, 2020). Once you are comfortable with your understanding, write down some notes using short phrases or words that are your own. Later you can use these notes to generate a summary or paraphrase of the information.[7] The following are steps to generate an accurate paraphrase in your own words (Purdue OWL, n.d.-a). The suggestions include reading for comprehension even if you have to read a passage more than once, writing your notes or paraphrase from memory, rereading the original text and comparing it with your paraphrase to check your accuracy, identifying any unique terms or phrases that you took directly from the source by using quotation marks, and including the information you will need for an accurate citation with your notes.

A final point to address in your writing is when and how often to use direct quotes. A direct quote from the original author could be the best approach when you find yourself struggling to restate or paraphrase a point. A direct quote is preferable to making small changes in the original and risking plagiarism. Similarly, a direct quote is preferable when the original sentence or passage is particularly clear and any paraphrase, even a well-written one, weakens the line of reasoning. Writers use direct quotes for other reasons as well. For example, a writer might choose a direct quote from a recognized expert in a field to add credibility to an argument, or a writer might use a direct quote when presenting an opinion that is contrary to the writer's own point of view (Purdue OWL, n.d.-b). A key point when using a direct quote is to identify it with quotation marks for a shorter quote or use an indented block style for longer quotes (APA, 2020). Usually, you also should include the page number where you found the quoted statement.

Accuracy in Reporting Information

Another aspect of research ethics is the accurate representation of findings in your reports and presentations. Authors sometimes inadvertently report inaccurate findings due to mistakes in collecting, entering, or analyzing their results. This is not the kind of misrepresentation that raises ethical concerns. Usually when authors discover they made an inadvertent error, they make sure that their publisher or an appropriate organization issues a correction. The kind of misrepresentation that raises ethical concerns is the deliberate misrepresentation of results (Gross, 2016). Changing a number or two to increase the significance of your findings, reporting findings that you fabricated, or representing another person's findings as your own are all examples of deliberate misrepresentation of information. Any form of deliberate misrepresentation is considered *scientific misconduct* and, depending on the nature of the deception, could lead to serious penalties (Gross, 2016; Horner & Minifie, 2011c; Jones & Mock, 2007; Kin-

---

[7]Any readers who are uncomfortable with their ability to write in their own words could benefit from a simple Internet search using terms such as *paraphrase* or *avoiding plagiarism*. You will find resources at several university websites such as the Purdue OWL and the Writing Center at the University of Wisconsin–Madison. These resources include examples as well as practice items.

tisch, 2005). Certainly, deliberate misrepresentation is a violation of the codes that define scientific and professional ethics (AAA, 2023; APA, 2016; ASHA, 2023).

Given the possibility of facing serious penalties as well as professional embarrassment, you might wonder why any researcher would risk falsifying information in their presentations and publications. One reason might be to increase the likelihood of receiving research funding (Kintisch, 2005). The competition for research grants is highly intense, and receiving this type of funding is very important in some fields of study and work settings. Another reason researchers might be tempted to falsify data is to increase the possibility of getting a study published. If you perused the research publications in any field, including audiology and speech-language pathology, you would learn that most published research involves significant findings. In many universities and other research settings, professional prestige is based to a large degree on having a strong track record of publication. For at least a few researchers, the desire for grant funding and professional recognition overpowers their sense of professional ethics (Brainard, 2000). Furthermore, identifying instances of misrepresentation of findings is very difficult in the typical review process for research publications and presentations (Kintisch, 2005). Rather, scientific misconduct usually is uncovered when it is reported by those who observed it, frequently research colleagues or even students (Couzin, 2006; Gross, 2016).

Data Management

Data management encompasses topics such as data quality, data ownership and sharing, and data storage and security. Ideally, the product of any study will be a set of data that is accurate and appropriate for answering the research question. To ensure that their data are trustworthy, researchers need to take steps such as establishing a detailed research protocol prior to starting the study, employing reliable and valid methods of measurement, monitoring the implementation of the protocol throughout the study, and keeping accurate data records. The term *treatment fidelity* refers to the strategies researchers employ to make sure their study is executed in an accurate and consistent manner (S. W. Smith et al., 2007). In addition to steps to ensure treatment fidelity, researchers also should consider the issue of data ownership and sharing prior to the study. Horner and Minifie (2011b) identified several issues that make data ownership a complicated matter.

> Data ownership is a complex matter that is determined by who created the data (e.g., an individual, an employee, a university, or a commercial entity); who subsidized the collection of data (e.g., the federal government, a state institution, or a private-commercial entity); where the data are stored (e.g., a private database or a public repository); and, most critically, what the contracts, regulations, licenses, or other legal arrangements are that govern the data. (pp. S339–S340)

Steneck (2007) noted that providing access to your data after publication is a general expectation in the research community and allows scientists outside the original research group to verify the data analysis (Horner & Minifie, 2011b) and perhaps apply new analyses. Additionally, if a group of researchers played a role in gathering the data, the research group should consider an a priori agreement about who will be responsible to secure storage of the data and who will have ready access to the data in the future. Conflicts sometimes arise between students who work as laboratory assistants and their research mentors. Students who participate in data collection and analysis as part of their graduate studies often feel they should have access to their data for possible future projects. This is an issue that students should discuss with their mentors before beginning a study, rather than make an assumption that might lead to later conflicts.

Confidentiality and Privacy

A final issue related to data management is the need for researchers to maintain the confidentiality and privacy of information they obtain from research participants (AAA, 2023; ASHA, 2023). Some basic procedures to ensure confidentiality include using identification codes rather than participants' names on all research documents, avoiding any mention of participants' names in any publications or presentations, and maintaining all documents, particularly consent forms that include identifying information, in a secure location. D. Smith (2003) identified several other concerns associated with confidentiality and privacy. For example, researchers need to consider the extent to which they might want to share their data before they obtain informed consent from their participants. Unless participants know that other researchers might examine and use their responses when they sign the consent form, only the original research team should typically have access to the data. Smith also noted that researchers need to make sure others cannot overhear them when discussing participants and to be aware of computer security issues, particularly those associated with networked computers.

Data collection approaches that use video or audiotapes of participants present special concerns for maintaining confidentiality. Participants usually can be identified from a visual image and sometimes even from an audio recording. Sometimes participants make statements during recording that could identify them or comment in ways that could be embarrassing to them or their families. Thus, researchers need to be particularly careful about handling and storing participant recordings. Some precautions could include storing recordings in a secure laboratory or office, making sure research team members review recordings only in designated locations, and having a plan for how long to keep recordings and how to dispose of them at the end of the study.

Health Insurance Portability and Accountability Act

Some research might involve medical records covered under the Health Insurance Portability and Accountability Act (HIPAA; U.S. HHS, 2003a). The "Privacy Rule" is an important aspect of HIPAA that provides regulations to protect the privacy of an individual's "protected health information" (Horner & Wheeler, 2005; U.S. HHS, 2003a). Although HIPAA rules and regulations cover health information and not research specifically, clinician-investigators must comply with the Privacy Rule when they are affiliated with a covered organization and/or they are conducting research using protected health information obtained from a covered organization. Covered organizations subject to HIPAA regulations generally include "a health plan, a health care clearinghouse, or a health care provider who transmits health information in electronic forms" (U.S. HHS, 2003a, p. 24). Clinician-investigators might be health care providers themselves, might work for a covered organization, or might be students within a covered organization. Thus, in some circumstances, researchers need to comply with both the rules for protecting human research participants and the rules for protecting privacy of health information (Horner & Wheeler, 2005). Not all researchers who gather health information from participants are included under HIPAA regulations. If researchers obtain health information in the course of their data gathering but do not work for a covered organization, they still must protect the confidentiality and privacy of their participants' information as specified in the Common Rule for protecting human research participants; they are not, however, subject to the additional regulations under the Privacy Rule (U.S. HHS, 2003a). On the other hand, researchers are subject to HIPAA privacy regulations, even if they are not affiliated with a covered health care agency, if they want to use protected health care records from a covered agency in their studies (Institutional Integrity and Risk Management Privacy Office, 2024; U.S. HHS, 2003a). U.S. HHS (2003a) listed several types of medical records that would be covered under the Privacy Rules: "from medical records and epidemiological databases to disease registries, hospital discharge records, and government compilations of vital health statistics" (p. 1).

Recognizing that access to health information is essential for some forms of research, the HIPAA rules and regulations provide some options for covered health care agencies to allow access to protected health information (Institutional Integrity and Risk Management Privacy Office, 2024; U.S. HHS, 2003a). These options include:

- Access to "deidentified" health information with identifying information removed. The rules specify 18 categories of information to remove, including name and address, e-mail, images of a person's face, specific dates such as a date of birth, date of hospital entry or discharge, any numerical identifiers such as Social Security and account numbers, and so forth.
- Access to health information after it has been de-identified through some generally accepted statistical method.
- Access to a limited data set with 16 categories of identifying information removed. A limited data set contains some information about geographic location, such as the city and state where an individual resides. If the researchers are not affiliated with the covered health care agency providing the data, they need to develop a data use agreement that states what and how the protected health care information will be used.
- Access to health information after obtaining written authorizations from the individuals covered in the data set. Just as with informed consent forms, a written authorization must cover certain topics. See "HIPAA Authorization for Research" for sample language (U.S. HHS, 2003b).
- Access to health information after obtaining a waiver of authorization from an institutional review board or privacy board. A waiver of authorization might cover all of a study or only one part. For example, researchers might obtain

a waiver of authorization just to access records for the purpose of recruiting participants.

If you need more specific information about the Privacy Rule and are affiliated with a covered health care agency, your institution might have a designated individual who serves as a privacy officer. Additionally, you might review educational materials provided by the Department of Health and Human Services, such as the booklet, "Protecting Personal Health Information in Research: Understanding the HIPAA Privacy Rule" (U.S. HHS, 2003a).

Summary

In this chapter, we reviewed a number of ethical considerations that guide all phases of research from initial planning to the final analysis and publication of our findings. Among the primary considerations is the need to protect the well-being of human participants. Both governmental regulations and professional ethics provide researchers with guidance on aspects of human subject participation such as informed consent, protecting the well-being of participants, maintaining confidentiality of participants' information, and ensuring equitable distribution of the risks and rewards of research. Ethical conduct in research also encompasses other areas such as credit for intellectual effort in publishing research findings, maintaining high standards of accuracy and honesty in reporting findings when citing the work of others, and recognizing potential conflicts of interest between the role of researcher and other professional roles. Under some circumstances, researchers also may need to comply with the privacy rules governing access to individual health care records.

Review Questions

1. What are the three basic principles of protection of human research participants identified in the Belmont Report?

2. Which of the three basic principles of protection of human participants means persons make their own, informed decisions about participating in research?

3. Given concerns about protecting the well-being of persons who participate in research, why do governmental agencies, professional organizations, and universities, among others, encourage research endeavors?

4. Which principle of protection of human participants means researchers need to make equitable decisions regarding who is invited to participate in research?

5. Identify two groups of research participants who receive special protections under federal law. What are the reasons for these special protections?

6. Provide an example of coercive or undue influence in recruiting participants for a research study.

7. Provide an example of a violation of the principle of beneficence in the conduct of a research study.

8. What is the role of an institutional review board?

9. Provide a brief explanation for each of the following terms.

a. Attribution of ideas
   b. Credit for intellectual effort
   c. Conflict of interest

10. Is it ever appropriate to use another author's words in your writing? Explain your answer.

11. What kind of information is covered under the HIPAA "Privacy Rule"?

12. Do researchers have to follow the HIPAA "Privacy Rule" when managing data for a research project? Explain your answer.

Learning Activities

1. The following websites have information on ethical conduct in research and protection of human participants. Visit one of these websites and explore some of the educational materials provided.
   a. American Speech-Language-Hearing Association: Ethics Resources at https://www.asha.org/Practice/ethics/
   b. American Psychological Association–APA Office of Research Ethics at https://www.apa.org/science/programs/research
   c. American Psychological Association–APA Publishing Policies at https://www.apa.org/pubs/journals/resources/publishing-policies
   d. United States Department of Health and Human Services–Office for Human Research Protections at https://www.hhs.gov/ohrp/

2. Alternatively, conduct a web search on a topic such as "protection of human participants" or "ethical conduct of research" and explore some of the information you retrieve.

3. Visit one or more of the following Internet sites and participate in the training activities provided.
   a. Collaborative Institutional Training Initiative (CITI) at the following web address: https://about.citiprogram.org/en/homepage/
   The CITI site provides training on many topics, including modules on protection of human research participants and the responsible conduct of research. Different modules are provided for biomedical research and social and behavioral research, with additional modules on specific topics such as HIPAA and conflicts of interest.
   b. The Office of Research Integrity online simulations "The Lab" at https://ori.hhs.gov/content/thelab and "The Research Clinic" at https://ori.hhs.gov/research-clinic
   The Office of Research provides online, interactive simulations addressing issues relating to the responsible conduct of research and protecting human participants. Participants in the simulation choose to play different roles, such as a principal investigator, graduate student, postdoctoral research fellow, research assistant, and IRB chair.
   c. The Office of Research Integrity "RCR Casebook: Stories About Researchers Worth Discussing" at https://ori.hhs.gov/rcr-casebook-stories-about-researchers-worth-discussing
   The RCR Casebook has many brief case studies on research

ethics topics, such as authorship, research misconduct, conflicts of interest, and mentor/mentee relationships.

4. Read the case study "Responsible Conduct of Research Scenario" provided in Appendix 2–1. Consider how you would answer each of the discussion questions and compare your answers with those of your peers.

References

Ambrose, N., & Yairi, E. (2002). The Tudor study: Data and ethics. *American Journal of Speech-Language Pathology, 11*(2), 190–203. https://doi.org/10.1044/1058-0360(2002/018)

American Academy of Audiology. (2023, April). *Code of ethics.* https://www.audiology.org/sites/default/files/about/membership/documents/Code%20of%20Ethics%20with%20procedures-REV%202018_0216.pdf

American Psychological Association. (2016). *Ethical principles of psychologists and code of conduct: Including 2010 and 2016 amendments.* https://www.apa.org/ethics/code/

American Psychological Association. (2020). *Publication manual of the American Psychological Association* (7th ed.). https://www.apa.org/pubs/books

American Speech-Language-Hearing Association. (2009). *Guidelines for the responsible conduct of research: Ethics and the publication process* [Guidelines]. https://www.asha.org/policy/GL2009-00308/

American Speech-Language-Hearing Association. (2023). *Code of ethics* [Ethics]. http://www.asha.org/policy

Balon, R., Guerrero, A. P. S., Coverdale, J. H., Brenner, A. M., Louie, A. L., Beresin, E. V., & Roberts, L. W. (2019). Institutional review board approval as an educational tool. *Academic Psychiatry, 43,* 285–289. https://doi.org/10.1007/s40596-019-01027-9

Bartholome, W. G. (1978). Central themes in the debate over the involvement of infants and children in biomedical research: A critical examination. In J. van Eys (Ed.), *Research on children: Medical imperatives, ethical quandaries, and legal constraints* (pp. 69–76). University Park Press.

Brainard, J. (2000). As U.S. releases new rules on scientific fraud, scholars debate how much and why it occurs. *Chronicle of Higher Education, 47*(15), A26.

Brody, L., Yu-Hsiang, W., & Stangl, E. (2018). A comparison of personal sound amplification products and hearing aids in ecologically relevant test environments. *American Journal of Audiology, 27,* 581–593. https://doi.org/10.1044/2018_AJA-18-0027

Centers for Disease Control and Prevention. (n.d.). *U.S. Public Health Service syphilis study at Tuskegee: The Tuskegee timeline.* https://www.cdc.gov/tuskegee/timeline.htm

Centers for Disease Control and Prevention. (2010). *CDC policy on human research protections.* https://www.cdc.gov/os/integrity/docs/cdc-policy-human-research-protections.pdf

Couzin, J. (2006, September). Scientific misconduct: Truth and consequences. *Science, 313*(5791), 1222–1226. https://doi.org/10.1126/science.313.5791.1222

Diekma, D. S. (2006). Conducting ethical research in pediatrics: A brief historical overview and review of pediatric regulations. *Journal of Pediatrics, 149,* S3–S11. https://doi.org/10.1016/j.jpeds.2006.04.043

Fairchild, A. L., & Bayer, R. (1999, May 7). Uses and abuses of Tuskegee. *Science, 284*(5416), 919–921. https://doi.org/10.1126/science.284.5416.919

Freedman, R. I. (2001). Ethical challenges in the conduct of research involving persons with mental retardation. *Mental Retardation, 39*(2), 130–141. https://doi.org/10.1352/0047-6765(2001)039<0130:ECITCO>2.0.CO;2

Goldfarb, R. (Ed.). (2006). *Ethics: A case study from fluency.* Plural Publishing.

Gross, C. (2016). Scientific misconduct. *Annual Review of Psychology, 67,* 693–711. https://doi.org/10.1146/annurev-psych-122414-033437

Grossman, J. B. (1987, Winter). Review: Beyond the Willowbrook Wars: The courts and institutional reform. *American Bar Foundation Research Journal, 12*(1), 249–259.

Horner, J., & Minifie, F. (2011a). Research ethics I: Responsible conduct of research (RCR)—historical and contemporary issues pertaining to human and animal experimentation. *Journal of Speech-Language-Hearing Research, 54,* S303–S329. https://doi.org/10.1044/10924388(2010/09-0265)

Horner, J., & Minifie, F. (2011b). Research ethics II: Mentoring, collaboration, peer review, and data management and ownership. *Journal of Speech-Language-Hearing Research, 54,* S330–S345. https://doi.org/10.1044/10924388(2010/09-0264)

Horner, J., & Minifie, F. (2011c). Research ethics III: Publication practices and authorship, conflicts of interest, and research misconduct. *Journal of Speech-Language-Hearing Research, 54,* S346–S345. https://doi.org/10.1044/10924388(2010/09-0263)

Horner, J., & Wheeler, M. (2005, November). HIPAA: Impact on research practices. *ASHA Leader, 10,* 8–27. https://doi.org/10.1044/leader.FTR2.10152005.8

Humes, L. E., Kinney, D. L., Main, A. K., & Rogers, S. E. (2019). A follow-up clinical trial evaluating the consumer-decides service delivery model. *American Journal of Audiology, 28,* 69–84. https://doi.org/10.1044/2018_AJA-18-0082

Humes, L. E., Rogers, S. E., Quigley, T. M., Main, A. K., Kinney, D. L., & Herring, C. (2017). The effects of service-delivery model and purchase price on hearing-aid outcomes in older adults: A randomized double-blind placebo-controlled clinical trial. *American Journal of Audiology, 26,* 53–79. https://doi.org/10.1044/2017_AJA-16-0111

Institutional Integrity and Risk Management Privacy Office. (2024). *HIPAA.* University of North Carolina at Chapel Hill. https://privacy.unc.edu/protect-unc-information/hipaa/

Iowa to pay subjects $925K for stuttering study. (2007, August 17). NBC News. https://www.nbcnews.com/health/health-news/iowa-pay-subjects-925k-stuttering-study-flna1c9469063

Jones, S. M., & Mock, B. E. (2007). Responsible conduct of research in audiology. *Seminars in Hearing, 28*(3), 206–215. https://doi.org/10.1055/s-2007-982902

Jonsen, A. R. (2006). Nontherapeutic research with children: The Ramsey versus McCormick debate. *Journal of Pediatrics, 149,* S12–S14. https://doi.org/https://doi.org/10.1016/j.jpeds.2006.04.044

Kahn, J. P., Mastroianni, A. C., & Sugarman, J. (Eds.). (1998). *Beyond consent: Seeking justice in research.* Oxford University Press.

King, P. A. (1998). Race, justice, and research. In J. P. Kahn, A. C. Mastroianni, & J. Sugarman (Eds.), *Beyond consent: Seeking justice in research* (pp. 88–110). Oxford University Press.

Kintisch, E. (2005, March). Scientific misconduct: Researcher faces prison for fraud in NIH grant applications and papers. *Science, 307*(5717), 1851. https://doi.org/10.1126/science.307.5717.1851a

Kirby, B. J., Kopun, J. G., Spratford, M., Mollak, C. M., Brennan, M. A., & McCreery, R. W. (2017). Listener performance with a novel hearing aid frequency lowering technique. *Journal of the American Academy of Audiology, 28*(9), 810–822. https://doi.org/10.3766/jaaa.16157

Kiskaddon, S. H. (2005). Balancing access to participation in research and protection from risks. *The Journal of Nutrition, 135*(4), 929–932. https://doi.org/10.1093/jn/135.4.929

Krugman, S. (1971, May 8). Experiments at the Willowbrook State School [Letter to the editor]. *Lancet, 1*(7706), 966–967. https://doi.org/10.1016/S0140-6736(71)91462-0

Moreno, J. D. (1998). Convenient and captive populations. In J. P. Kahn, A. C. Mastroianni, & J. Sugarman (Eds.), *Beyond consent: Seeking justice in research* (pp. 111–130). Oxford University Press.

National Commission for the Protection of Human Subjects of Biomedical and Behavioral Research. (1979). *The Belmont Report:*

Ethical principles and guidelines for the protection of human subjects of research. U.S. Department of Health and Human Services. https://www.hhs.gov/ohrp/regulations-and-policy/belmont-report/index.html

Nelson, R. M. (1998). Children as research subjects. In J. P. Kahn, A. C. Mastroianni, & J. Sugarman (Eds.), *Beyond consent: Seeking justice in research* (pp. 47–66). Oxford University Press.

Office of Research Integrity. (2015). *General resources.* https://ori.hhs.gov/general-resources

Purdue Online Writing Lab. (n.d.-a). *Paraphrase: Write it in your own words.* https://owl.purdue.edu/owl/research_and_citation/using_research/paraphrase_exercises/index.html

Purdue Online Writing Lab. (n.d.-b). *Quoting, paraphrasing, and summarizing.* https://owl.purdue.edu/owl/research_and_citation/using_research/quoting_paraphrasing_and_summarizing/index.html

Racino, B., & Castellano, J. (2019a, April 18). UCSD eye doctor broke human research rules, putting patients at risk. *inewsource.* https://inewsource.org/2019/04/18/kang-zhang-ucsd-human-research-violations/

Racino, B., & Castellano, J. (2019b, July 6). UCSD doctor resigns amid questions about undisclosed Chinese businesses. *inewsource.* https://inewsource.org/2019/07/06/thousand-talents-program-china-fbi-kang-zhang-ucsd/

Ramsey, P. (1978). Ethical dimensions of experimental research on children. In J. van Eys (Ed.), *Research on children: Medical imperatives, ethical quandaries, and legal constraints* (pp. 57–68). University Park Press.

Ramsey, P. (2002). *The patient as person: Explorations in medical ethics* (2nd ed.). Yale University Press.

Reynolds, G. (2006). The stuttering doctor's "monster study." In R. Goldfarb (Ed.), *Ethics: A case study from fluency* (pp. 1–12). Plural Publishing.

Rothman, D. J. (1982). Were Tuskegee and Willowbrook "studies in nature"? *Hastings Center Report, 12*(2), 5–7.

Salorio-Corbetto, M., Baer, T., & Moore, B. C. J. (2019). Comparison of frequency transposition and frequency compression for people with extensive dead regions in the cochlea. *Trends in Hearing, 23*, 1–23. https://doi.org/10.1177/2331216518822206

Sawant, T. (2019, May 6). UCSD eye doctor suspended for objectionable study conditions. *The Guardian.* https://ucsdguardian.org/2019/05/06/ucsd-eye-doctor-suspended-objectionable-study-conditions/

Schwartz, R. G. (2006). Would today's IRB approve Tudor's study? Ethical considerations in conducting research involving children with communication disorders. In R. Goldfarb (Ed.), *Ethics: A case study from fluency* (pp. 83–96). Plural Publishing.

Secretary's Advisory Committee on Human Research Protections. (2008/2009). *Attachment: Recommendations regarding research involving individuals with impaired decision-making (SIIIDR).* https://www.hhs.gov/ohrp/sachrp-committee/recommendations/2009-july-15-letter-attachment/index.html

Sibbald, B. (2001). Death but one unintended consequence of gene-therapy trial. *Canadian Medical Association Journal, 164*(11), 1612. https://www.cmaj.ca/

Silverman, F. H. (1988). The "monster" study. *Journal of Fluency Disorders, 13*, 225–231. https://doi.org/10.1016/0094-730X(88)90049-6

Smith, C. M. (2005). Origin and uses of primum non nocere—above all, do no harm! *Journal of Clinical Pharmacology, 45*(4), 371–377. https://doi.org/10.1177/0091270004273680

Smith, D. (2003). Five principles for research ethics. *Monitor on Psychology, 34*(1), 56. https://www.apa.org/monitor/jan03/principles

Smith, S. W., Daunic, A. P., & Taylor, G. G. (2007, November 1). Treatment fidelity in applied educational research: Expanding the adoption and application of measures to ensure evidence-based practice. *Education and Treatment of Young Children, 30*(4), 121–134. https://doi.org/10.1353/etc.2007.0033

Steneck, N.H. (2007). *ORI: Introduction to responsible conduct of research* (D. Zinn, Illus.). https://ori.hhs.gov/ori-introduction-responsible-conduct-research

Tudor, M. (1939). *An experimental study of the effect of evaluative labeling on speech fluency*

(Unpublished master's thesis). University of Iowa, Iowa City.

U.S. Department of Health & Human Services. (n.d.). *Federal policy for the protection of human subjects ("Common Rule")*. https://www.hhs.gov/ohrp/regulations-and-policy/regulations/common-rule/index.html

U.S. Department of Health and Human Services. (2003a, April). *Protecting personal health information in research: Understanding the HIPAA privacy rule*. https://privacyruleandresearch.nih.gov/pdf/hipaa_privacy_rule_booklet.pdf

U.S. Department of Health and Human Services. (2003b, May). *HIPAA authorization for research*. https://privacyruleandresearch.nih.gov/authorization.asp

U.S. Department of Health & Human Services. (2009, January 15). Protection of human subjects, 45C.F.R. § 46. https://www.hhs.gov/ohrp/regulations-and-policy/regulations/45-cfr-46/index.html

U.S. Food and Drug Administration, Center for Drug Evaluation and Research. (2017, January 31). *Warning letter*. https://www.fda.gov/inspections-compliance-enforcement-and-criminal-investigations/warning-letters/kang-zhang-md-phd-511374-01052017

UW-Madison Writing Center. (2020). *Writer's handbook*. https://writing.wisc.edu/handbook/

Wenner, M. (2009, September 1). Gene therapy: An interview with an unfortunate pioneer (previously published with the title "Tribulations of a trial"). *Scientific American, 301*(3), 14. https://doi.org/10.1038/scientificamerican0909-14

White, J. M. (2020). Why human subjects research protection is important. *The Ochsner Journal, 20*(1), 16–33. https://doi.org/10.31486/toj.20.5012

Wilson, J. M. (2009). Lessons learned from the gene therapy trial for ornithine transcarbamylase deficiency. *Molecular Genetics and Metabolism, 96*(4), 151–157. https://doi.org/10.1016/j.ymgme.2008.12.016

Yairi, E. (2006). The Tudor study and Wendell Johnson. In R. Goldfarb (Ed.), *Ethics: A case study from fluency* (pp. 35–62). Plural Publishing.

APPENDIX 2–1

Research Scenario

Responsible Conduct of Research Scenario

Please note that the following case description is a work of fiction. It is not intended to represent any actual individuals or events.

Dr. P. T. Smith has worked as an audiologist in an outpatient clinic at a small hospital since graduating with an AuD degree approximately 4 years ago. As a graduate student, PT embraced the concept of clinician-investigator and completed an empirical research project under the direction of audiology faculty member, Dr. R. Star. PT particularly enjoyed Dr. Star's mentorship and individual attention as they worked together on the research project. Knowing PT's interest in completing a research project, Dr. Star had recruited PT to work on an idea that was already partially developed. Dr. Star had the notion of developing a follow-up program for new hearing aid users based on adult learning theory. PT liked the idea right away and could appreciate its clinical relevance. Dr. Star's idea was relatively undefined, however, and PT had put in considerable time studying the literature on adult learning: developing a script for the follow-up training, planning a set of short activities to orient new patients to the features of their devices, and developing some listening activities that simulated the experience of listening in different conditions. PT and Dr. Star obtained permission to run their study from their university's institutional review board. The design of the study involved randomly assigning persons who were new hearing aid users to either PT's new follow-up training or the traditional follow-up that had been used in the campus clinic for many years. The participants completed a user satisfaction questionnaire 1 month after receiving their hearing aids and 6 months later. Ultimately, because of the time spent in developing the training protocol, PT only had time to run 10 individuals through the study, 5 who completed PT's training protocol and 5 in the control group. PT's only disappointment with the research was that they did not find any significant differences in user satisfaction. Even though the mean scores for PT's experimental follow-up procedures were higher than for the control group, these differences were not very strong. Dr. Star still praised PT's work and stated that the study would be a very good pilot study for future work on the topic.

About a year after PT graduated, R. Star took a job at a larger university known for its strong research programs. PT kept track of R. Star's work through the audiology literature. One day when perusing one of the audiology journals, PT was surprised to see an article by R. Star and a new doctoral student. The article was on the same topic as PT's graduate research project. In reading the article, PT noted one sentence acknowledging "preliminary work on this topic in an unpublished research paper" (Smith, 2018). When PT read the full article, however, it seemed as though the methods in this new paper were identical to the ones PT had developed for the smaller study 4 years previously. PT was disappointed that Dr. Star had not acknowledged this contribution in the Methods section. PT would have enjoyed publication credit and wondered if the pilot study and work on the methods warranted inclusion as an author. In a sense, PT felt betrayed. Shouldn't Dr. Star have at least acknowledged PT's role in developing the experimental training protocol? Rightly or wrongly, PT felt some sense of ownership over the experimental protocol.

Discussion Questions

1. What are the issues in this case that relate to research ethics?

2. In your opinion, how should Dr. Star have acknowledged PT's work on the experimental training protocol? Was the brief mention about preliminary work sufficient? Be prepared to explain your answer.

3. Would your answer to Question 2 change if Dr. Star used the data from PT's study and simply collected data from more participants for the published work?

4. How could researchers such as PT and Dr. Star avoid this type of conflict in the future?

3

Identifying and Formulating Research Questions

Main Points

- When developing a research question, consider your interest in the topic, the practicality of the question, and the importance of finding an answer to the question.
- Three generalized goals of research studies are to describe, relate, or compare.
- Research questions can be formatted in different ways.
  - Hypothesis
  - Question
  - Purpose statement
  - If-then
  - Evidence-based practice (EBP)
- Well-written research questions utilize operational definitions and are constructed to yield valid and reliable conclusions.

The starting point for most research projects is a problem that requires a solution or a question that needs an answer. Most of us have encountered problems or questions in our daily lives and engaged in some kind of investigation to find a solution to the problem or an answer to the question. Perhaps our automobile needed service and we had to find a reliable repair shop that would provide the service in a timely way and at a reasonable cost. Maybe we decided to upgrade to a new laptop computer and wondered which seller would provide good service as well as a reasonable cost. Once we formulated our problem or question, we started to make some telephone calls, to talk with friends or family, to complete an Internet search, and perhaps to visit some retailers and consult some consumer publications. We began to gather information after identifying the problem or question. Similarly, researchers begin their process of inquiry by identifying some unknown information, which they express as a problem to resolve or as a question to answer. How researchers and consumers differ is in the precise way researchers state their questions and in the process of preliminary investigation that researchers use to revise and refine their questions. Another type of question that audiologists and speech-language pathologists sometimes need to investigate is an evidence-based practice question. With these types of questions, audiologists and speech-language pathologists investigate existing research to identify information that applies to persons they serve clinically. Although evidence-based practice questions might not lead to original research, generating a well-formed question is still an important consideration.

Identifying Important Questions

Sometimes students at the beginning of their professional training have asked how to find a viable research topic. Often, these questions arise when students consider the requirements of their graduate programs, many of which require some type of research paper or offer the option of a research paper or thesis. When these questions are addressed to us, our advice always is to consider your professional interests. Although all audiologists and speech-language pathologists complete a broad program of study that encompasses all areas of the profession, most find certain areas of study more inherently interesting than others. Some examples to consider are the work setting you find most attractive (e.g., medical, school, private practice), any special interests you have in certain communication disorders (acquired cognitive or language disorders, phonological disorders in children, central auditory processing disorders), or an area of clinical practice you particularly enjoy (such as evaluation and diagnosis, counseling clients and their families, providing direct treatment, hearing aid fitting). Once you have identified a general focus for your research, a good strategy is to follow up by reading extensively in your particular areas of interest.[1]

Occasionally, speech-language pathologists and audiologists discover interesting questions even though they were not planning to conduct research. Rosenthal and Rosnow (2008) identified two forms of inspiration that could apply in clinical settings. The first example is finding inspiration for research from a case study. Perhaps a clinician encountered a particularly interesting case that inspired interest in research. Sometimes audiologists or speech-language pathologists encounter individuals in their clinical practice with unique needs that are not covered in the existing research. This might inspire a research interest to better understand these unique individuals and to provide them with more effective treatment. The second example is finding inspiration in contradictory or paradoxical situations or behaviors (Rosenthal & Rosnow, 2008). An example of this form of inspiration might involve encountering a client whose evaluation results are contradictory or who responds to treatment in a contrary manner. Perhaps an audiologist has encountered several clients whose problems on certain perceptual tasks are much worse than would be predicted from other audiological test results, or a speech-language pathologist has identified several clients whose speech production errors in conversational speech are very different from those exhibited in single-word productions. Contradictions of this type might inspire clinicians to further explore the reasons why these clients behaved in unpredicted ways and eventually to even formulate research questions to investigate.

Researchers also should consider several practical issues when they choose a question to investigate. Finding a question

---

[1] Another way to follow up on your professional interests is to find a mentor who conducts research in a similar area. In many scientific fields, graduate students work for several years in their mentors' laboratories before developing an independent line of research.

that is both interesting and practical is particularly important for students in graduate programs that might last only 2 to 4 years, depending on whether they are pursuing a master's degree, clinical doctorate, or research doctorate. Some of the practical considerations include how much time you have, whether you have the required skills, whether or not you have access to an appropriate group of participants, what equipment and facilities you have available, and what persons you need for support in conducting the research (Cohen et al., 2018). Another consideration, particularly for students who are developing as investigators, is whether or not a mentor who is knowledgeable in your interest area is available to guide the research.

A few examples might clarify the challenge of finding a research question that is both motivating and practical. Some questions require that you gather information over a long period of time. One of the most impressive studies we have read was a study of the impact of participating in a preschool program on children's subsequent achievement in school and in life (Barnett, 2000). The researchers who conducted this study followed their participants from the time they were preschool children into adulthood. The study yielded important information about the lasting effects of the preschool program but required the researchers to follow their participants for more than 15 years. Studies of this type are important for any field but are not practical to undertake in the typical time frame of a graduate program.

Some research questions might be practical only in research facilities associated with major medical centers. Perhaps the questions you find most interesting center on the development of speech perception in young children following a cochlear implant, neuroimaging studies of listeners' reactions to certain speech stimuli, or the genetic bases of speech, language, and hearing disorders. These are just a few examples of very interesting avenues of research that might be practical in only a few facilities where the researchers have access to experts from other professions as well as expensive, highly specialized equipment.

A final factor to consider when choosing research questions is the importance to your field of study. Researchers in communication sciences and disorders might ask, "Would answering this question make a significant contribution to audiology, speech-language pathology, or speech and hearing science?" Judging the value of a research question is a subjective process, but you might find evidence in your reading to support your judgments. For example, an author who is highly respected in your field of study might have identified certain questions as worthwhile. When reading in your areas of interest, you might look for suggested research questions in review articles or in the discussion sections of research reports. Often authors of research articles include suggestions for future research toward the end of their discussion sections. After discussing the results of existing research, authors will extend their discussion to address areas for further studies. Another way to identify significant questions is to consider questions that were posed and investigated but not answered in a definitive manner (Silverman, 1998). The original study might have weaknesses that you or other authors identified, such as a small sample size, inadequate outcome measures, or uncontrolled, extraneous variables that might have influenced the results. Perhaps the original study was well designed but left a number of related, unanswered questions. You might see ways to extend the original research in new directions. Consider some of the following possibilities:

1. Extend the study to a new research population such as a new age group, a different diagnostic group, or persons from a different linguistic or cultural background.
2. Apply different outcome measures such as using measures from spontaneous speech if the original study used formal tests and/or measures from elicited speech samples, or perhaps use a newly developed measure, such as a new approach for assessing speech perception.
3. Address questions of social validity by determining the functional impact of observed changes for the participants or their families (Foster & Mash, 1999; Strain et al., 2012).
4. Change the stimuli used to elicit responses or the procedures for presenting stimuli to test whether findings are specific to certain stimuli or conditions.
5. Change the setting in which an evaluation or treatment occurs to provide either a more naturalistic setting or a setting that more closely matches real clinical situations.
6. Use up-to-date instrumentation in testing and analyzing participants' responses for approaches that might be outmoded.

These are just a few suggestions for how one might modify an existing research approach to provide more complete and accurate answers to a question. The idea is to read existing research reports in an analytical way, considering how ideas presented in an article or perhaps approaches to measurement and analysis might differ from what you have learned.

Perhaps the research question that was most interesting is an original idea that emerged from your reading or professional experiences. An original research question might emerge as an inspiration as we discussed previously. Another way that original questions emerge is through researchers' familiarity with work in other fields of study. Researchers in communication sciences and disorders have found relevant ideas in many related disciplines, such as linguistics, psycholinguistics, developmental psychology, information processing, neuropsychology, and physiology, to name just a few. When supporting the importance of a question that emerged from work in other disciplines, researchers might include an explanation of the findings, procedures, theory, or principles and an explanation of their potential application in communication sciences and disorders. Explaining the importance of finding answers to particular questions generally involves making explicit the thought process that led you to formulate those questions, whether they emerged from a critical review of previous research, from reading research reports from other disciplines, or from your own professional experiences.

Readers might ask why it is important to investigate a worthwhile and relevant question, and why simply having a strong, personal interest in the question is not sufficient justification. A casual answer to such a question is that in some cases, a strong personal interest in a question would be sufficient justification. Investigating relevant questions of broad interest in communication sciences and disorders is most important when researchers might want to publish their findings in the future, receive recognition for their efforts from peers or administrators, or possibly compete for financial support to conduct their research (Silverman, 1998). However, in most professional settings, a researcher must justify the importance of a proposed study to a review board before ever gathering data. Therefore, even if researchers were willing to forgo future publication opportunities or other recognition, they still need a well-thought-out rationale for any questions they want to investigate.

Formulating Research Questions

Once researchers decide what questions they want to investigate, their next task is to frame the questions in an unambiguous way. When you read a well-written research question, you learn something about the design of the study as well as the kind of data the researchers obtained from their participants. A well-written question has enough detail to make clear what measurements or observations the researchers might obtain to formulate an answer. One of the first things to consider when writing a research question is how to specify what you are going to investigate. Usually, interesting subjects to investigate are things that change or vary as the situation or circumstances change. Researchers use the term *variables* to refer to the phenomena they plan to observe. When studying a variable, researchers might study naturally occurring differences or manipulate the circumstances to create changes in a variable. The research is *nonexperimental* when the study centers on naturally occurring changes or differences and *experimental* when the study centers on the researchers' manipulations to create changes.

Depending on the kind of the research, the question might specify both independent and dependent variables. *Independent variables* are the conditions or manipulations the researcher is interested in studying. In nonexperimental research the independent variables could include existing differences such as age groups, diagnostic categories, language backgrounds, and so forth. A common nonexperimental approach to research in communication sciences and disorders is to compare persons with communication disorders and those without communication disorders. For example, persons with moderate-to-severe hearing loss might be compared with persons with normal hearing, or children with language impairments might be compared with children matched for chronological age and/or language age. In experimental research, the independent variables could include differences the researcher created by manipulating some circumstance. For example, the researcher might create two different versions of a task to determine how that manipulation affected the performance of the research participants, or the researcher might compare two different treatment programs to determine if either one is more effective.

The *dependent variables* in a study are the observations or measures a researcher obtains. For example, participants with communication disorders and those with normal communication might both complete a set of tests selected by the researchers. This type of study would be a nonexperimental comparison and the participants' scores on the tests would be dependent variables. A similar example for an experimental study would involve administering the test before and after treatment. If researchers administered the test to two different treatment groups, they could compare the groups' scores. In this example, the test scores would be the dependent variable and the different treatment groups would be the independent variable. In experimental research, the dependent variables are the researchers' outcome measures.

Another consideration in formulating a research question is the intent of the research. The way a research question is framed will depend on whether the researchers' aim is to describe persons or circumstances, to discover relationships between or among variables, or to identify differences between groups (Rosenthal & Rosnow, 2008). Consider the example of researchers who were interested in studying speech and language development in preschool children. The researchers decided to study several measures of speech development or speech perception. Through their reading prior to designing a study, the researchers discovered several measures they thought were worthy of further investigation. Examples of such measures were the consonant-vowel (CV) ratio and a new test of speech perception in noise. The researchers considered a series of studies beginning with a descriptive approach, then a relational approach, and finally a study of differences. For these studies, they framed questions such as those posed in Table 3–1.

The sample questions in Table 3–1 illustrate how researchers might represent different types of studies, including descriptive, relational, and difference approaches. However, a researcher would need to refine these example questions before using them to guide the design of an investigation. We cover some of the criteria for developing well-formed research questions in a follow-

Table 3–1. Research Questions That Illustrate Differences Among Descriptive, Relational, and Difference Studies

Descriptive Study	1. What is the CV ratio for preschool children at ages 18 months, 24 months, 30 months, and 36 months?
Relational Study	2. What is the relationship between CV ratio and mean length of utterance in preschool children from ages 18 months to 36 months?
	3. What is the relationship between scores on a new measure to assess recognition of speech in noise and performance on the Quick Speech-in-Noise (QuickSIN) test?
Difference Study— Nonexperimental	4. What is the difference in CV ratio between children with normal hearing and those with moderate-to-severe hearing loss at 24 months?
Difference Study— Experimental	5. What is the difference in CV ratio for 24-month-old children with expressive language delay who participated in an 8-week intervention program compared to 24-month-old children with expressive language delay who received no intervention?
	6. How do adults with hearing loss perform on a test of speech recognition when fitted with hearing aids that employ two different noise reduction algorithms?

ing section, but before dealing with that issue, we consider various ways researchers might state the problem(s) they intend to investigate.

Ways to Formulate a Research Problem

One of the first steps in conducting a study is to clearly define the problem that the researchers intend to investigate. Although researchers frequently choose to state the problem or focus of their study in a research question or series of questions, research questions are not the only option. Some other approaches include formal hypotheses, a statement of purpose, or even conditional if-then statements.

Whether researchers use formal hypotheses, research questions, or a statement of purpose depends in part on the type of study they are conducting. For example, a researcher who is conducting a descriptive study is more likely to use research questions or a statement of purpose than formal hypotheses; a researcher who is conducting a relational or difference study, particularly one that involves statistical analyses, could use any approach, including formal hypotheses, a statement of purpose, or research questions. For many studies, the approaches to formulating a research problem are essentially interchangeable, and the one you use is a matter of personal preference.

Traditionally, researchers conducting quantitative studies developed formal hypotheses when defining the problem that they intended to investigate. A *hypothesis* is a formal statement of the predicted outcome of a study (Trochim et al., 2016). Actually, in stating the predicted outcome of a study, researchers often formulate two versions of their hypothesis. The first is called a *null hypothesis* and is sometimes abbreviated as H_0. The alternative hypothesis is sometimes called a *research hypothesis* and is abbreviated as H_1 (Newhart & Patten, 2023).

A null hypothesis is stated in the negative and is based on the assumption that the results of a study will yield no significant differences between groups and/or no significant relationships among variables. In Table 3–2, some of the example questions presented in Table 3–1 are restated as null hypotheses and research hypotheses.

The idea of a null hypothesis stems from quantitative studies in which researchers employ statistical procedures to evaluate their findings. The point of many statistical procedures is to test the viability of a null hypothesis. Based on their statistical findings, researchers will either *reject* the null hypothesis, meaning that the null hypothesis is not viable, or *fail to reject* the null hypothesis, meaning that the null hypothesis is viable. In a sense, the null hypothesis is a strategy for maintaining researchers' objectivity. A researcher states there is no relationship or no difference until or unless the data indicate otherwise. Researchers also have to be careful not to say that they have proven a null hypothesis is true. Failing to reject a null hypothesis is not the same thing as concluding or proving that two variables are not related or that two groups are not different.

As previously noted, researchers often formulate a second, alternative version of their hypothesis called the research hypothesis (Newhart & Patten, 2023). The alternative or research hypothesis is usually stated in a positive form. The research hypothesis is a statement of what the researchers expected to find when they conducted their study. For example, theoretical models

Table 3–2. Examples of Null Hypotheses (H_0) and Research Hypotheses (H_1) for Relational and Difference Studies

Relational Study	H_0: There is *no* relationship between CV ratio and mean length of utterance in preschool children from ages 18 months to 36 months.
	H_1: There is a significant relationship between CV ratio and mean length of utterance in preschool children from ages 18 months to 36 months.
	H_0: There is *no* relationship between scores on a new measure to assess recognition of speech in noise and performance on the Quick Speech-in-Noise (QuickSIN) test.
	H_1: There is a significant relationship between scores on a new measure to assess recognition of speech in noise and performance on the Quick Speech-in-Noise (QuickSIN) test.
Difference Study—Nonexperimental	H_0: CV ratio will *not* be different in 24-month-old children with normal hearing compared to 24-month-old children with moderate-to-severe hearing loss.
	H_1: CV ratio will be different in 24-month-old children with normal hearing compared to 24-month-old children with moderate-to-severe hearing loss.
Difference Study—Experimental	H_0: CV ratios for 24-month-old children with expressive language delay who participated in an 8-week intervention program will *not* be different from the CV ratios of 24-month-old children with expressive language delay who received no intervention.
	H_1: CV ratios for 24-month-old children with expressive language delay who participated in an 8-week intervention program will be different from the CV ratios of 24-month-old children with expressive language delay who received no intervention.
	H_0: For adults with hearing loss, scores on a test of speech recognition in noise will *not* be different when fitted with hearing aids that employ two different noise reduction algorithms.
	H_1: For adults with hearing loss, scores on a test of speech recognition in noise will be different when fitted with hearing aids that employ two different noise reduction algorithms.

and previous research with other populations might all support the prediction that two variables are closely related. When researchers study these two variables in a new population, they expect the variables to be closely related when measured in the new population as well. This expectation is reflected in their statement of a research hypothesis. Table 3–2 includes examples of the alternative or research hypothesis that corresponds to each of the null hypotheses.

The research hypothesis might be stated as a *directional* hypothesis or as a *nondirectional* hypothesis (Cohen et al., 2018). Each of the example research hypotheses in Table 3–2 was a nondirectional hypothesis.

Although the researchers stated that they expected to find significant relationships between two variables or a significant difference between two groups, they did not indicate whether the relationship would be positive or negative, or which group would achieve higher scores. If researchers had reason to expect a particular outcome, such as a positive relationship between two variables or significantly higher scores for children in a treatment group, the researchers could formulate directional research hypotheses. In the examples in Table 3–3, each of the nondirectional research hypotheses from Table 3–2 is restated as its corresponding directional version.

Although the research and null hypotheses are a traditional way of defining the problem in quantitative studies, most authors of recent research articles choose other ways to state their problem. A perusal of articles published in the field of communication sciences and disorders in the past 5 years revealed that most articles include either research questions or a statement of purpose. The differences among research hypotheses, research questions, and statements of purpose, however, are more differences in the form of the statement than differences in the content. Often a research question or statement of purpose includes the same information one would find in a research hypothesis.

Let's consider the following hypothetical study. A group of researchers developed a measure for assessing the intelligibility of conversational speech. They felt their new approach would be less time-consuming and just as accurate as several existing measures of speech intelligibility. However, they needed to conduct a study to determine if these assumptions about their new measure were true. We call the new measure the *conversational speech intelligibility*

Table 3–3. Examples of Directional Research Hypotheses (H_1) for Relational and Difference Studies

Relational Study	*Directional H_1:* There is a significant *positive* relationship between CV ratio and mean length of utterance in preschool children from ages 18 months to 36 months.
	Directional H_1: There is a significant *inverse* relationship between scores on a new measure to assess recognition of speech in noise and performance on the Quick Speech-in-Noise (QuickSIN) test.
Difference Study— Nonexperimental	*Directional H_1:* CV ratio will be *higher* in 24-month-old children with normal hearing compared to 24-month-old children with moderate-to-severe hearing loss.
Difference Study— Experimental	*Directional H_1:* CV ratios for 24-month-old children with expressive language delay who participated in an 8-week intervention program will be *higher than* the CV ratios of 24-month-old children with expressive language delay who received no intervention.
	Directional H_1: For adults with hearing loss, scores on a test of speech recognition in noise will be significantly higher when fitted with hearing aids that employ noise reduction Algorithm A, as compared to noise reduction Algorithm B.

index or CSII. The researchers decided to conduct a study to compare scores on their CSII to scores on an existing speech intelligibility test. They expected to find a strong relationship between CSII performance and performance on the speech intelligibility test. Thus, they formulated the following research hypothesis:

H_1: There is a significant relationship between scores on the conversational speech intelligibility index and scores on an existing speech intelligibility test in children between the ages of 3 and 5 who have been diagnosed with a phonological disorder.

Meanwhile, the researchers could just as easily have stated the same information in the form of a research question. With some minor rewording, you could develop a question like the following:

1. Is there a significant relationship between scores on the conversational speech intelligibility index and scores on an existing speech intelligibility test in children between the ages of 3 and 5 who have been diagnosed with a phonological disorder?

Many research reports include yes/no questions like the above example. For some topics, researchers are less interested in discrete yes/no answers and more on the amount or degree of difference (Newhart & Patten, 2023). For those researchers, formulating "what" or "how" questions is preferable. Changing a yes/no question to generate a question starting with what, how, and so forth is relatively easy. For example, the question above could be restated as a what question:

2. For children between the ages of 3 and 5 who have been diagnosed with a phonological disorder, what is the relationship between scores on the conversational speech intelligibility index and scores on an existing speech intelligibility test?

Stating a research question as a what or a how question allows a researcher to give an answer that is less discrete and more elaborate. For example, in answering the what version of our example research question, a researcher could discuss the existence of a relationship between the measures, the direction of any relationship (e.g., positive or negative), and the strength of the relationship. Given a lack of consistent guidance regarding how to formulate research questions, deciding whether to use a yes/no version or a what/how version is largely a matter of personal preference.

Researchers also have the option of presenting the problem they intend to investigate in a *statement of purpose*. Like research questions, a statement of purpose usually includes the same kinds of information one would find in a formal hypothesis. A statement of purpose is a highly flexible form, however, not tied closely to quantitative research and statistical analysis. A statement of purpose would be an appropriate way to explain the focus of nearly any type of research, including descriptive, relational, and difference studies. Using our previous example, we could generate a very similar statement of purpose for our hypothetical study. Such a statement might read as follows:

The purpose of this study was to investigate the relationship between a new measure of speech intelligibility, the conversational speech intelligibility index, and an existing speech intelligibility test when used with children between the ages of 3 and 5 who have been diagnosed with a phonological disorder.

When you begin reading research reports on a regular basis, you will occasionally encounter an additional approach to the problem statement, a *conditional* or *if-then* statement. When a study has theoretical implications, researchers sometimes prefer to state the problem in a conditional format. The general basis of conditional statements is that if the findings turn out one way, the study supports a certain conclusion, but if the findings turn out another way, the study supports a different conclusion. In a recent study, Coady et al. (2007) used conditional statements to express possible outcomes for their study of speech perception in children with specific language impairment (SLI). The following examples of if-then statements are from Coady et al. (2007):

> If children with SLI [specific language impairment] are sensitive to speech quality, then they should perceive synthetic speech series less categorically than naturally spoken series. If they are sensitive to the lexical status of test items, then they should perceive nonsense-syllable test series less categorically than real-word test series. If their performance suffers from both of these manipulations, then only their perception of naturally spoken real words should match that of age-matched control children. (p. 43)

As noted in Chapter 1, authors usually explain the focus of their study in a paragraph that immediately precedes the methods section of a research report. Thus, when you read an article, look for the research hypotheses, questions, or statement of purpose right before the methods section. When you read these questions or statements, you might find it helpful to look for information about how the outcomes were measured, that is, the dependent variables and, if appropriate, what variables the authors compared or manipulated (the independent variables).

Evidence-Based Practice Questions

In the previous section, we covered the kinds of research questions and statements that guide empirical research. Empirical research involves gathering new information to answer questions that are important in the field of communication sciences and disorders. Another kind of research question, an *evidence-based practice question*, however, is of critical importance to audiologists and speech-language pathologists who are providing clinical services. When clinicians ask an evidence-based practice (EBP) question, they generally expect to find an answer to their question in the existing, published research literature. Sometimes clinicians have questions about the evidence associated with a particular etiology (e.g., Casby, 2001; Chau et al., 2010) or the reliability and validity of an assessment procedure, but most often clinicians have questions about the effectiveness of treatment for a particular disorder (e.g., Law et al., 2011; Waechter & Jönsson, 2022; Wisenburn & Mahoney, 2009).

Sometimes audiologists and speech-language pathologists have EBP questions that are general in nature. For example, they might need to document the effectiveness of a particular intervention approach to meet a requirement of their work setting or of a funding or regulatory agency, or they might need information about a particular etiology to answer questions from a client or a client's family. These broad questions might take a form like the following:

1. What evidence is available to document the effectiveness of language intervention for children in elementary school?
2. What evidence is available to document the effectiveness of behavioral treatment for adults who stutter?
3. What evidence is available to document the effectiveness of remote microphone hearing assistance technologies (HAT)?

Most often, EBP questions take the form of a Patient/Population, Intervention, Comparison, and Outcome (PICO) question (American Speech-Language-Hearing Association, n.d.; Baker & McLeod, 2011). In your reading, you may see variations or additions to the PICO strategy, such as addressing the study design (PICOS) or the length of time (PICOT). When creating a PICO question, clinical researchers try to be fairly specific about each of the components. The population description minimally includes the disorder, such as fluency disorder, speech sound disorder, sudden-onset hearing loss, or aphasia following stroke, but usually includes additional information such as an age range, severity, and length of time since onset. The intervention of interest is stated in a specific way as well, such as naturalistic language intervention, fluency shaping, bilateral cochlear implants, or auditory osseointegrated devices. The comparison would encompass alternate possible interventions for the population in question or no intervention. Finally, the desired outcome varies depending on the population and the clinician's focus. Some example outcomes include increased expressive vocabulary, reduction in number of dysfluencies in conversational speech, improved scores on a speech recognition test, and improved speech intelligibility. Some EBP questions may focus on broader goals, such as increased ability to participate in activities of daily living or higher scores on a quality-of-life questionnaire. Robey (1998) noted that clinicians also might be interested in more specific questions addressing how treatment effectiveness is influenced by factors such as the amount of treatment, the severity of the person's disorder, or the kind of disorder. For additional information on constructing a PICO question and subsequent steps in the EBP process, you might consult web-based tutorials, for example from the American Speech-Language-Hearing Association (n.d.), or University of Washington, Health Sciences Library (2020). Although intervention questions are the most common EBP questions, the PICO approach can be adapted to other EBP topics, including diagnosis, etiology, and prognosis. The following list illustrates the variety of EBP questions.

- Etiology: Research that focuses on the underlying causes of disorders, possibly by comparing individuals with a disorder and those who are disorder free, or by following individuals with a disorder longitudinally to determine the disorder's impact.
- Diagnosis/screening: Research that focuses on the ability of diagnostic or screening tools to accurately identify persons with and without a particular disorder.
- Treatment: Research that focuses on comparisons of a treatment approach compared to a no-treatment control or alternate treatments.
- Prognosis: Research that focuses on predictions of future outcomes

for individuals with a disorder and the extent to which treatment improves those outcomes.
- Cost-benefit: Research that focuses on the cost of delivering treatment compared to the benefits to the persons with a disorders and society, including future financial savings due to a reduced need for special services.
- Quality of life: Research that focuses on the impact of a disorder on the everyday living experiences of individuals and the extent to which treatment reduces or eliminates those impacts.
- Client perspectives: Research that focuses on the experiences, opinions, and preferences of clients on issues such as access to speech, language, and hearing services; perceptions of quality of services; and experiences of barriers and supports.

Figure 3–1 illustrates the application of the PICO format to several types of EBP questions, including etiology, diagnosis, treatment, prognosis, and client perspectives.

Articles addressing EBP questions have started to appear fairly frequently in journals in the field of communication sciences and disorders. Some of the topics addressed in the published EBP reviews include early communication interventions (Pak et al., 2023), treatment for persons who stutter (Bothe et al., 2006), acute cognitive improvement with amplification for adults (Kalluri et al., 2019), comparing traditional hearing aids and personal sound amplification products (PSAPs) (Maidment et al., 2018), effects of electrical stimulation on

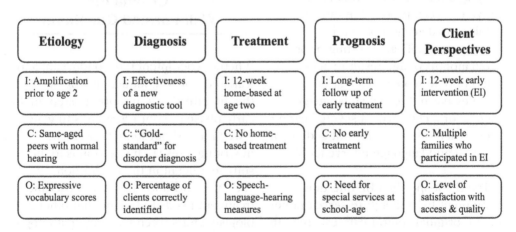

Figure 3–1. Examples of population, intervention, comparison, outcome (PICO) for different evidence-based practice topics.

swallowing (Clark et al., 2009), patient perspectives on treatment outcomes (Cohen & Hula, 2020), and word-finding treatments for persons with aphasia (Wisenburn & Mahoney, 2009).

Another way that audiologists and speech-language pathologists might approach EBP is to ask client-specific questions (Gallagher, 2002). When looking for evidence on behalf of an individual client, the clinician formulates a question that includes information about the client's disorder, their age, and the severity of the disorder (Gallagher, 2002). If clinicians have a question about intervention, they might include information about the specific form of treatment, the amount and/or frequency of treatment, and perhaps the expected amount of improvement (Gallagher, 2002). Each of the following example questions illustrates the features of a client-specific treatment question.

1. Will minimal pair phonological treatment, provided for two 30-minute individual treatment sessions per week for 16 weeks, produce a 20% gain in percentage of consonants correct in spontaneous speech for a 5-year-old child with a moderately severe speech production disorder?
2. Will early detection of hearing loss and amplification fitting prior to 6 months of age result in age-appropriate scores on a test of expressive and receptive language at age 2 for a child with a severe hearing loss when provided without additional speech and language intervention?

The client-specific EBP question is the starting point for a literature search rather than for original, empirical research. In searching the literature, the clinician will focus on those studies that more closely match the client and treatment characteristics specified in the question. For Question 1 above, the clinician would look for studies that addressed minimal pair phonological treatment, included participants who were approximately 5 years of age, and ideally had moderate-to-severe speech production disorders. For Question 2, the clinician would look for studies of early detection and treatment of children with severe hearing loss that included long-term follow-up and assessment of the children's speech and language development at approximately age 2. When audiologists and speech-language pathologists search for research evidence on behalf of an individual client, they need to keep in mind that they might not find studies that perfectly fit the criteria of their question. In such instances, clinicians need to decide if studies that meet only some of their criteria are useful. For example, they need to consider whether or not research conducted with participants who were a different age, had less severe disorders, or had different language backgrounds is useful for guiding their clinical decisions.

Criteria for Well-Formed Questions

Whether your intent is to conduct an empirical study or to conduct an EBP search of the literature, an important step in the early phase of your research is to generate a well-formed question. One consideration in writing a research question is to include sufficient detail in the descriptions of your variables. Additionally, the experimental treatment needs to be one that other audiologists and speech-language pathologists could carry out in a similar way (i.e., reliable procedure). The term *operationalize* refers to a process in which researchers provide a precise, specific description of the independent and dependent variables in their study. An independent variable could be described in terms of the procedures associated with an experimental treatment, whereas a dependent variable could be defined in terms of a specific measure or test. Although a well-written research question should include specific information, a researcher might only partially define the variables in the questions or statement of purpose and provide a full description in the methods section of a research report. Table 3–4 includes a set of statements illustrating the difference between general and specific descriptions of both independent and dependent variables.

Another characteristic of a well-written research question is that the variables are defined in a way that leads to valid and reliable conclusions.[2] When choosing ways to measure outcomes, researchers should consider the validity and reliability of the measures. The *validity* of a measurement refers to how accurately a test or measure represents the knowledge, skill, or trait you set out to assess. Furthermore, an instrument has an intended purpose and conclusions about validity are based on the extent to which it accomplishes that purpose (Newhart & Patten, 2023).

Table 3–4. Statements Illustrating the Difference Between General and Specific Descriptions of Research Variables

General Statement	*Specific Statement*
1. Children with language disorders	1. Children who scored more than 1.5 standard deviations below the mean on the Test of Language Development–Primary, 5th Edition
2. Adults with aphasia	2. Adults who received a score of 90 or less on the Aphasia Quotient of the Western Aphasia Battery
3. Children with bilateral hearing loss	3. Children with 3 frequency pure-tone averages of 50 dB HL or poorer, bilaterally
4. Phonological treatment	4. Hodson's cycles phonological treatment approach
5. Treatment for voice disorders	5. Sixteen 30-minute sessions of resonance voice therapy over 8 weeks
6. Improved speech production	6. Higher percentage of intelligible words in a 200-word conversational speech sample
7. Improved speech perception	7. Higher scores on the AzBio Sentence test

---

[2]Usually, we apply the concepts of validity and reliability to dependent variables or outcome measurements. Trochim et al. (2016) noted that independent variables also should be implemented in a way that supports the validity and reliability of conclusions regarding experimental manipulations. For example, a researcher testing a new treatment approach needs to plan a treatment that others in the field would recognize as a valuable one (i.e., valid treatment).

The *reliability* of a measure refers to the extent to which the measure yields consistent or repeatable results (Rosenthal & Rosnow, 2008). When judging reliability, one might consider consistency of measurement from one time to another, from one person to another, from one form of a test to another, or from one subset of test items to another. A statement frequently associated with the concepts of reliability and validity is that a measure can be reliable even if it is not valid, but a measure cannot be valid if it is not reliable.[3] The most preferred measures are those that have both high a high degree of validity and high reliability (Rosenthal & Rosnow, 2008). We cover topics related to validity and reliability in greater detail in Chapter 7 of this text.

Summary

The starting point for most research is a question or problem a researcher or clinician wants to explore. Usually, these unanswered questions emerge from our reading of professional literature or from the problems clients present when we provide audiology and speech-language pathology services. A well-written research question provides guidance for designing original research or conducting a literature search. Regardless of the nature of the research —whether it is a descriptive, relational, or difference study, or whether it is an evidence-based practice search—researchers will be more successful if they develop a well-formed research question. In writing their questions, researchers consider ways to describe their manipulations or independent variables and outcome or dependent variables in a precise and specific way. The term *operationalize* refers to this process of defining the variables in a study. Researchers also need to establish that the information they obtain is both valid and reliable. Validity refers to how accurately a measure or procedure represents an actual behavioral construct. Reliability refers to the extent to which a measure or procedure yields consistent or repeatable results. The best measures and procedures for answering researchers' questions are those that have both high validity and reliability. Chapter 7 has more detailed information about validity and reliability.

Review Questions

H_0: Children who participate in the dynamic intervention approach will have intelligibility scores and accuracy of sound production in conversational speech after 12 weeks of treatment that are not different from children who participate in the traditional articulation approach.

H_1: Children who participate in the dynamic intervention approach will have intelligibility scores and accuracy of sound production in conversational speech after 12 weeks of treatment that are higher than those of children who participate in the traditional articulation approach.

1. The statement labeled H_0 above is called a _____, and the statement labeled H_1 is called a _____.

2. In either H_0 or H_1 above, what is the independent variable? The dependent variable?

---

[3]Although generally accepted as true, this statement may have some exceptions. Rosenthal and Rosnow (2008) described a rare situation in which a measure could be valid even though it was not reliable.

3. Is H_1 in the example directional or nondirectional? If it is directional, rewrite it to be nondirectional. If it is nondirectional, rewrite it to be directional.

4. Another approach to defining the focus of a study is to write a research question. Rewrite H_1 above as a research question.

5. How might an author of a research paper include the information in these examples in a statement of purpose? Write an example.

6. Consider the dependent variable(s) in H_0 or H_1. How might you *operationalize* the dependent variable(s) to make them more measurable?

7. Provide an example for each of the following components of an evidence-based practice question:
   a. Population
   b. Intervention
   c. Comparison
   d. Outcome

8. What would the outcome(s) be for an evidence-based practice question on each of the following topics?
   a. Etiology
   b. Diagnosis/screening
   c. Treatment
   d. Prognosis
   e. Client perspectives

Learning Activities

1. Read the introductory section of one or more of the following research articles. These articles illustrate different ways of defining the focus of a study such as using hypotheses, research questions, or a statement of purpose.

Hypotheses

Cook, S., Donlan, C., & Howell, P. (2013). Stuttering severity, psychosocial impact and lexical diversity as predictors of outcome for treatment of stuttering. *Journal of Fluency Disorders, 38*(2), 124–133. https://doi.org/10.1016/j.jfludis.2012.08.001

Lane, H., Denny, M., Guenther, F. H., Hanson, H. M., Marrone, N., Mathies, M. L., Perkell, J., Stockman, E., Tiede, M., Vick, J., & Zandipour, M. (2007). On the structure of phoneme categories in listeners with cochlear implants. *Journal of Speech-Language-Hearing Research, 50*, 2–14. https://doi.org/10.1044/10924388(2007/001)

Yes/No Questions

Girolametto, L., Weitzman, E., & Greenberg, J. (2012). Facilitating emergent literacy: Efficacy of a model that partners speech-language pathologists and educators. *American Journal of Speech-Language Pathology, 21*, 47–63. https://doi.org/10.1044/10580360(2011/11-0002)

Lundberg, M., Andersson, G., & Lunner, T. (2011). A randomized, controlled trial of the short-term effects of complementing an educational program for hearing aid users with telephone consultations. *Journal of the American Academy of Audiology, 22*(10), 654–662. https://doi.org/10.3766/jaaa.22.10.4

Pfyler, P. N., Lowery, K. J., Hamby, H. M., & Trine, T. D. (2007). The objective and subjective evaluation of multichannel expansion in wide dynamic range compression hearing instruments. *Journal of Speech-Language-Hearing Research, 50*, 15–24. https://doi.org/10.1044/1092-4388(2007/002)

If-Then Statements

Coady, J. A., Evans, J. L., Mainela-Arnold, E., & Kluender, K. R. (2007). Children with specific language impairments perceive speech most categorically when tokens are natural and meaningful. *Journal of Speech-Language-Hearing Research, 50*, 41–57. https://doi.org/10.1044/1092-4388(2007/004)

Statements of Purpose

Jean, Y. Q., Mazlan, R., Ahmad, M., & Maamor, N. (2018). Parenting stress and maternal coherence: Mothers with deaf or hard-of-hearing children. *American Journal of Audiology, 27*, 260–271. https://doi.org/10.1044/2018_AJA-17-0093

Stierwalt, J. A. G., & Youmans, S. R. (2007). Tongue measures in individuals with normal and impaired swallowing. *American Journal of Speech-Language Pathology, 16*, 148–156. https://doi.org/10.1044/1058-0360(2007/019)

Thibodeau, L. (2010). Benefits of adaptive FM systems on speech recognition in noise for listeners who use hearing aids. *American Journal of Audiology, 19*, 36–45. https://doi.org/10.1044/10590889(2010/09-0014)

Zekveld, A. A., Deijen, J. B., Goverts, S. T., & Kramer, S. E. (2007). The relationship between nonverbal cognitive functions and hearing loss. *Journal of Speech-Language-Hearing Research, 50*, 74–82. https://doi.org/10.1044/1092-4388(2007/006)

2. Find a research article on a topic of strong personal interest. Find the research questions or statement of purpose for the study, usually located right before the methods section. How did the authors measure the outcomes of their study? Next, find the section in the methods where the authors discuss outcome measurement. What information could you find about the reliability or validity of the measures?

References

American Speech-Language-Hearing Association. (n.d.). *Evidence-based practice (EBP)*. https://www.asha.org/Research/EBP/

Baker, E., & McLeod, S. (2011). Evidence-based practice for children with speech sound disorders: Part 2 application to clinical practice. *Language, Speech, and Hearing Services in Schools, 42*, 140–151. https://doi.org/10.1044/01611461(2010/10-0023)

Barnett, W. S. (2000). Economics of early childhood intervention. In J. P. Shonkoff & S. J. Meisels (Eds.), *Handbook of early childhood intervention* (2nd ed., pp. 589–610). Cambridge University Press.

Bothe, A. K., Davidow, J. H., Bramlett, R. E., & Ingham, R. J. (2006). Stuttering treatment research 1970–2005: I. Systematic review incorporating trial quality assessment of behavioral, cognitive, and related approaches. *American Journal of Speech-Language Pathology, 15*, 321–341. https://doi.org/10.1044/1058-0360 (2006/031)

Casby, M. W. (2001). Otitis media and language development: A meta-analysis. *American Journal of Speech-Language Pathology, 10*, 65–80. https://doi.org/10.1044/1058-0360(2001/009)

Chau, J. K. Lin, J. R. J., Atashband, S., Irvine, R. A., & Westerberg, B. D. (2010). Systematic review of the evidence for the etiology of adult sudden sensorineural hearing loss. *Laryngoscope, 120*(5), 1011–1021. https://doi.org/10.1002/lary.20873

Clark, H., Lazarus, C., Arvedson, J., Schooling, T., & Frymark, T. (2009). Evidence-based systematic review: Effects of neuromuscular electrical stimulation on swallowing and neural activation. *American Journal of Speech-Language Pathology, 18*, 361–375. https://doi.org/10.1044/10580360(2009/08-0088)

Coady, J. A., Evans, J. L., Mainela-Arnold, E., & Kluender, K. R. (2007). Children with specific language impairments perceive speech most categorically when tokens are natural and meaningful. *Journal of Speech-Language Hearing Research*, *50*, 41–57. https://doi.org/10.1044/1092-4388(2007/004)

Cohen, L., Manion, L., & Morrison, K. (2018). *Research methods in education* (8th ed.). Routledge.

Cohen, M. L., & Hula, W. D. (2020). Patient-reported outcomes and evidence-based practice in speech-language pathology. *American Journal of Speech-Language Pathology*, *29*(1), 357–370. https://doi.org/10.1044/2019_AJSLP-19-00076

Foster, S. L., & Mash, E. J. (1999). Assessing social validity in clinical treatment research: Issues and procedures. *Journal of Consulting and Clinical Psychology*, *67*(3), 308–319. http://www.apa.org/pubs/journals/ccp/index.aspx

Gallagher, T. M. (2002). Evidence-based practice: Applications to speech-language pathology. *Perspectives on Language Learning and Education*, *9*(1), 2–5. https://doi.org/10.1044/lle9.1.2

Kalluri, S., Ahmann, B., & Munro, K. J. (2019). A systematic narrative synthesis of acute amplification-induced improvements in cognitive ability in hearing-impaired adults. *International Journal of Audiology*, *58*(8), 455–463. https://doi.org/10.1080/14992027.2019.1594414

Law, J., Plunkett, C. C., & Stringer, H. (2011). Communication interventions and their impact on behaviour in the young child: A systematic review. *Child Language Teaching and Therapy*, *28*(1), 7–23. https://doi.org/10.1177/0265659011414214

Maidment, D. W., Barker, A. B., Xia, J., & Ferguson, M. A. (2018). A systematic review and meta-analysis assessing the effectiveness of alternative listening devices to conventional hearing aids in adults with hearing loss. *International Journal of Audiology*, *57*(10), 721–729. https://doi.org/10.1080/14992027.2018.1493546

Newhart, M., & Patten, M. L. (2023). *Understanding research methods: An overview of the essentials* (11th ed.). Routledge Taylor & Francis Group.

Pak, N. S., Chow, J. C., Dillehay, K. M., & Kaiser, A. P. (2023). Long-term effects of early communication interventions: A *systematic review and meta-analysis. Journal of Speech, Language, and Hearing Research*, *66*(8), 2884–2899. https://doi.org/10.1044/2023_JSLHR-22-00711

Robey, R. R. (1998). A meta-analysis of clinical outcomes in the treatment of aphasia. *Journal of Speech-Language Hearing Research*, *41*, 172–187. https://doi.org/10.1044/jslhr.4101.172

Rosenthal, R., & Rosnow, R. L. (2008). *Essentials of behavioral research: Methods and data analysis* (3rd ed.). McGraw-Hill.

Silverman, F. H. (1998). *Research design and evaluation in speech-language pathology and audiology: Asking and answering questions* (4th ed.). Prentice-Hall.

Strain, P. D., Barton, E. E., & Dunlap, G. (2012). Lessons learned about the utility of social validity. *Education and Treatment of Children*, *35*, 183–200. https://doi.org/10.1353/etc.2012.0007

Trochim, W. M. K., Donnelly, J. P., & Arora, K. (2016). *Research methods: The essential knowledge base* (2nd ed.). Cengage Learning.

University of Washington, Health Sciences Library. (2020). *Evidence-based practice*. https://guides.lib.uw.edu/hsl/ebp

Waechter, S., & Jönsson, A. (2022). Hearing aids mitigate tinnitus, but does it matter if the patient receives amplification in accordance with their hearing impairment or not? A meta-analysis. *American Journal of Audiology*, *31*(3), 789–818. https://doi.org/10.1044/2022_AJA-22-00004

Wisenburn, B., & Mahoney, K. (2009). A meta-analysis of word-finding treatments for aphasia. *Aphasiology*, *23*, 1338–1352. https://doi.org/10.1080/02687030902732745

Completing a Literature Search

Main Points

- A literature search is how you find sources to gain knowledge about a topic. You might conduct a literature search to find out if a question has already been answered, what research has been done in the same or related fields, or what methods, procedures, or outcome measures have been used to investigate a topic.
- There are many tools available to help you conduct a literature search. These include web-based search engines and databases, professional organizations, and cited reference searches.
- You will want to access databases and search engines that are geared toward professional, scientific literature. Some are free, and some may be available through an institutional subscription or license.
- Utilize key words, synonyms, logical/Boolean operators, truncation operator, and limits to either narrow or broaden your literature search.

Audiologists and speech-language pathologists working in clinical settings, as well as researchers planning an original study, need to be skilled at finding, evaluating, and summarizing information. *Information literacy* is a term often used to refer to the skills associated with finding, evaluating, summarizing, and using information (American Library Association, 2024). For audiologists and speech-language pathologists, the emerging emphasis on evidence-based practice (EBP) has made information literacy skills even more important. For researchers, information literacy skills have always been an essential part of finding problems to study and of defining and researching those problems in ways that yield valid and reliable answers.

When professionals, such as those in communication sciences and disorders, medicine, or psychology, look for information, we usually conduct a *literature search*. The intent of a literature search is to find information within a body of written work that pertains to our topic. Audiologists and speech-language pathologists might search within the body of written work for communication sciences and disorders, or within the body of written work for related fields like education, medicine, neuroscience, or psychology. A successful literature search depends on information literacy skills such as knowing how to search, where to look, and how to define your topic. In the following sections of this chapter, we cover the reasons for conducting a literature search, some general information about planning and conducting searches, and some beginning skills for reading, evaluating, and documenting information. In Appendix 4–1, we practice some sample searches to learn more about planning and conducting searches, and how to use some of the more readily available search tools. Some of you might skip this last section if you already feel comfortable with your ability to plan a search and find appropriate information on a topic.

Purposes of a Literature Search

Audiologists and speech-language pathologists have many reasons to conduct a literature search. Sometimes the goal of the search is to *find an answer* to your question in the existing literature. This would be the case when conducting a search for evidence to answer clinical questions pertaining to the etiology, assessment, prognosis, or treatment of communication disorders. In EBP research, the aim is to find information that already exists in the body of written work in a particular field (Duke University and University of North Carolina at Chapel Hill, 2019). Furthermore, some of the published work in the field of communication sciences and disorders is nonempirical in nature. In empirical research, the goal is to generate original evidence; however, in nonempirical research, the goal is to identify all of the existing evidence on a particular topic. The author of a nonempirical work, such as a theoretical discussion or a systematic review, needs to conduct a thorough literature search in order to find all of the published work relevant to the topic. Even researchers who are planning an empirical study need to conduct a literature search to find out if their question has already been answered in an earlier study.

For those who are planning to conduct original, empirical research, finding that someone else has conducted a study similar to the one you were planning does not necessarily mean you should abandon your idea. A field with a strong body of empirical research should have some studies that replicate the findings of earlier work. Sometimes the research in a field becomes outdated for reasons such as changes in population characteristics or the emergence of new tests or instruments to measure outcomes. Even for relatively recent studies, researchers could plan a study that replicates the results with slightly different procedures or participants.

Another reason for conducting a literature search is to find the *previous research on a topic*, even if that research does not answer your question directly. The previous research might be relevant even if it addressed a different population from the one you intended to study, looked at a different set of outcome measures, or even examined a different approach to treatment. For example, researchers interested in studying the use of classroom amplification in college and university classrooms might find very little research in the college setting. They could include several studies of use of classroom amplification in elementary school classrooms, however, in their review of literature. Researchers who designed a study of a particular approach to treatment, such as a treatment for persons with functional voice disorders, aphasia, or specific language impairment, usually would include information about other approaches to treatment in their review of prior research. In an EBP search, you might not find a study that exactly matches your client's age and severity of disorder or examined the treatment you wanted to investigate. The related research you do find, however, might provide meaningful guidance for your clinical decisions.

Researchers who want to conduct an original, empirical study might conduct a literature search to *identify a problem* to study. The researchers might know the general topics in communication sciences and disorders they want to investigate but not have an idea for a specific research question. As we discussed in Chapter 3, sometimes the authors of a research report include specific suggestions for future studies in their discussion sections. Sometimes when you read a few articles on the same research topic, you find that the findings of the studies conflict. This is another way to find an interesting research question. You might consider any differences in the conflicting studies. For example, were the participants different in some way? Did one study include participants with more severe disorders or participants from different age groups? Or perhaps the researchers in one study administered their treatment for a longer time or measured their outcomes in different ways. Any differences you find could be good independent variables to investigate in a new study.

Perhaps you have an interest in another field of study in addition to communication sciences and disorders. You could find important questions to research by searching the literature to *identify methods from other fields of study*. If you looked at the reference lists for research articles in communication sciences and disorders, you might find citations from journals covering cognitive psychology, developmental psychology, neuroscience, psycholinguistics, and so forth. For example, a published article on auditory working memory and comprehension in school-age children and the effects of noise included citations from journals such as *Child Development, Journal of the Acoustical Society of America, Journal of Verbal Learning and Verbal Behavior, Memory and Cognition, Noise and Health*, and *The Quarterly Journal of Experimental Psychology: Human Experimental Psychology* (Sullivan et al., 2015). A 2014 study of word learning in adult, monolingual speakers included citations from journals such as *Behavior Research Methods, Cognition, Cognitive Psychology, Journal of Cognitive Neuroscience, Journal of Epidemiology and Community Health, Journal of Memory and Language, Nature Neuroscience, Psychological Review*, and *Psychological Science* (Storkel et al., 2014).

Even when researchers know the research question they want to investigate, they might conduct a literature search to *generate background information* for use when writing their research report (Newhart & Patten, 2023). This background information might include theories or models that pertain to the focus of the study, statistical information on the prevalence of a disorder, or definitions of important concepts. Finally, researchers might need to search the literature to *identify procedures or outcome measures* to use in their research. Possibly a researcher has a need to describe participants or document a treatment outcome in terms of the impact of the person's communication impairment on activity and participation and quality of life (American Speech-Language-Hearing Association [ASHA], 2004, 2006; Baylor et al., 2013; Heuer & Willer, 2020). This researcher could do a literature search to identify ways to document activity, participation, and quality of life. Other researchers might be interested in using a reaction time measurement in their study and might search the literature to determine how other researchers measured reaction times in their experiments.

A search of the existing research literature is an important early step in planning a study. Such a search might aid the researcher to find an interesting problem to study, to find new research approaches, or to find the background information they need to develop a strong justification for their research ideas. In the following section, we cover some of the tools a researcher could use to complete the important step of a literature search.

Planning and Conducting a Search

Search Tools

As you plan a literature search, one of the first considerations is how to find trustworthy, professional information in an efficient way. Generally, the most efficient way to find information is to use a *web-based search engine*. You might already be familiar with very popular search engines such as *Google* (https://www.google.com/), *Bing*™ (https://www.bing.com/), *DuckDuckGo* (https://duckduckgo.com), or *Yahoo! Search* (https://search.yahoo.com). These search engines provide a large amount of information on a topic in a short time. However, none of the general search engines would be an ideal choice when looking for literature in the field of communication sciences and disorders. When conducting an EBP search or planning scientific research, audiologists and speech-language pathologists need to search the evidence published in professional journals or presented at professional conferences. Usually, professional journals have procedures for peer review of submissions designed to ensure that published articles meet the journal's standards, are well written, and report on well-designed research. Although Google, Bing, DuckDuckGo, or Yahoo! searches generally uncover some professional literature, you also retrieve other kinds of information from commercial and even personal websites. Thus, when conducting a search for high-quality information in communication sciences and disorders, you should use a search engine designed to retrieve peer-reviewed journal articles from various scientific disciplines.

Researchers have many search engines to employ when looking for professional literature. Covering all of the possible search engines is beyond the scope of this chapter; however, we will cover some of the most important search tools for audiologists and speech-language pathologists. Listed below are several of many possible search engines. The first six are either free or have free options; the other databases require subscriptions but may be available to individuals with a university affiliation.

1. Education Resources Information Center (ERIC)
2. PubMed
3. Professional association websites
4. Google Scholar and Google Books
5. WorldCat
6. Trip (https://www.tripdatabase.com/)
7. CINAHL
8. ComDisDome via ProQuest
9. Communication and Mass Media Complete
10. Linguistics and Language Behavior Abstracts

11. ProQuest Dissertations & Theses
12. PsychInfo
13. ScienceDirect
14. speechBITE
15. Web of Science

The online search engines listed above are not necessarily ordered according to which would be the best choice for a search. However, some of the search engines are provided without a fee and should be available to you throughout your professional career. Others are premium services that might be available on many college and university campuses via site licenses.

The first two online search tools we cover are databases provided by the U.S. government. The *ERIC database* is a research tool provided by the Institute of Education Sciences (https://eric.ed.gov/) and the U.S. Department of Education. ERIC provides a way to search more than 1,000 journals in the field of education, including articles from journals in communication sciences and disorders (https://eric.ed.gov/). The ERIC database includes other sources as well, such as publications from government agencies, professional associations, and conference papers. Although researchers usually use several online search engines, ERIC could be the primary search tool for research focusing on education, preschool and school-age children, language and literacy, and so forth. An ERIC search yields citation information such as author(s), title, journal, and usually an abstract of the article. Some articles in the ERIC database are available in full text form. The ERIC website provides both basic and advanced search strategies. Appendix 4–1 includes a description of a search using the ERIC advanced search option for those who would like specific information about using this tool.

PubMed is a web-based tool for searching the Medline database, a major database of journal articles in medicine and other life science disciplines (National Center for Biotechnology Information [NCBI], n.d.-a, n.d.-b). PubMed is provided as a service of the National Library of Medicine and the U.S. National Institutes of Health. Like an ERIC search, a literature search with PubMed yields information such as the author(s), title, journal, and usually an abstract of the article. If a journal publisher has a website with full-text versions of articles, a PubMed search also returns a link to that website. PubMed could be your primary search tool when looking for information on a variety of topics: medical audiology or speech-language pathology; speech, language, or hearing disorders with an anatomical or physiological basis; and adult-onset disorders like sensorineural hearing loss, aphasia, and voice disorders. The PubMed search engine provides some helpful search tools, such as the ability to set limits on publication dates, language, age groups, and type of article, and the process of automatic term mapping provides matches on semantically similar terms (e.g., treatment, therapy) and grammatical variations (e.g., stutter, stuttering). You can view the results of the automatic term mapping process in the "Search Details" box on the right side of your browser after you conduct a PubMed search. Appendix 4–1 includes a description of a PubMed search in which some of these tools are illustrated.

Professional associations such as the American Academy of Audiology (AAA), American Speech-Language-Hearing Association (ASHA), and American Psychological Association (APA) publish professional documents and journals as a service to their members. One way to find articles in these journals is to search the association website. Usually, even nonmembers are able to conduct a search of an association website, but they might not be able to view full-text versions of the articles they retrieve. Members of the association often have access to an electronic form of the article as well as the usual citation information such as author, title, and abstract. The strategy for searching these specific websites is similar to a Google search, but the information returned is only from that association website. The advantage is that the search is highly focused, but the disadvantage is that you only retrieve information prepared by that professional association. A search of a specific association website, however, yields documents that you might not be able to retrieve with other search engines, such as information on professional ethics, clinical practice guidelines, and position statements. We list examples of professional societies for communication sciences and disorders below.

1. Academy of Doctors of Audiology
2. American Academy of Audiology
3. American Auditory Society
4. American Speech-Language Hearing Association
5. Association for Research in Otolaryngology
6. Dysphagia Research Society
7. Educational Audiology Association
8. International Association of Logopedics and Phoniatrics
9. International Society for Augmentative and Alternative Communication
10. The Voice Foundation

Google Scholar is another search tool that you can access via the web without a subscription (https://scholar.google.com/). Google Scholar is a specialized search service provided by Google that is designed to search the professional literature from many disciplines. Although a search constructed for Google Scholar looks very similar to one for the general version of Google, the content searched is very different. A general Google search returns a wide variety of content, including information from websites with primarily a commercial purpose. On the other hand, Google Scholar searches within a narrower body of information with an emphasis on articles in peer-reviewed journals, books from academic publishers, and content from the websites of professional associations and universities (About Google Scholar, n.d.). Google Scholar provides some valuable tools that might help you refine or extend your search. To find the most recent publications on a topic, select the option "Any time since [year]" when displaying results or use the "dated between" option on the advanced search page. Researchers also have the option to restrict their searches to a particular journal or a particular subject area (Google Scholar, n.d.). One very helpful tool is the Cited By option. If a Google Scholar search uncovers a particularly appropriate article, you can quickly identify additional articles in which the first article was cited and included in the reference list. Citation searching is an efficient way to find recent information on a specific topic and, therefore, is covered in more detail in a following section. Because Google Scholar is a free search service with several helpful features, an example search using this search engine is included in Appendix 4–1.

The Trip Database (https://www.tripdatabase.com/) has free and premium versions. Trip database searches have a clinical research focus. The search engine offers general search features but also has a unique PICO structured search option. We tried a search using the following search terms.

P: aphasia following a stroke

I: treatment

C: no treatment

O: expressive language, communication

The above search yielded 252 results using the free version, and the search engine offered several filter options such as systematic review, evidence-based synopses, clinical trials, and so forth.

One online database within the ProQuest search engine, the *Communication Sciences and Disorders Dome* or ComDisDome, is specialized for audiologists and speech-language pathologists (ProQuest, n.d.-a). An advantage of using a tool such as the ComDisDome is that your searches should be more efficient because the Dome only scans content in speech, language, and hearing sciences and disorders. Thus, you should retrieve fewer irrelevant articles compared to other search engines such as Google Scholar, even when using the same search terms (ProQuest, n.d.-a). One of the unique features of the Dome is that, once you complete a topic search, you can sort the results to view just scholarly journal articles, dissertations, and other similar sources. Researchers usually search the ProQuest databases such as ComDisDome database via site licenses for libraries affiliated with colleges, universities, and other institutions.

ScienceDirect is another premium service usually licensed by institutions like colleges and universities (https://www.sciencedirect.com/). ScienceDirect includes journals in life and health sciences, as well as physical and social sciences. A search with ScienceDirect includes the Medline database and other health sciences information sources. Because of the large amount of information included in the ScienceDirect database, searches are more efficient if you limit the databases you search; for example, the Medicine and Dentistry, Neuroscience, or Psychology databases may be most relevant for topics in communication sciences and disorders. An advantage of ScienceDirect is that the site includes full-text versions of journal articles. You will only be able to access the journals included in your institution's subscription, however, or those that are from open-access journals.

Often current research is available in a doctoral dissertation before publication in a peer-reviewed journal. The online *ProQuest Dissertations and Theses* database is one way to find a doctoral dissertation on your topic (ProQuest, n.d.-b). Most university libraries provide access to this database.

When you begin a literature search, one or more of these online search services is a good starting point. However, you might miss some references if you rely entirely on an electronic search. For example, a journal might not be included in the database you search or the terms you searched might not retrieve an important article. A simple supplemental strategy is to *browse the key journals* in your field. Many publishers make the tables of contents and abstracts for their journal articles available on their websites, and sometimes researchers enjoy a trip to their library to spend time browsing the current issues of their favorite journals. For example, the PubMed database does not include articles from the *Journal of Medical Speech-Language Pathology*, and although articles from this journal are included in ComDisDome, you may miss some articles when you search. Once, when preparing a presentation on evidence-based practice, one of the authors searched for articles on treatment of childhood apraxia using PubMed, ComDisDome, and other search engines. Although the searches uncovered several articles, an article by Strand and Debertine (2000) on integral stimulation treatment never appeared. She knew about the article, however, because of browsing issues of the *Journal of Medical Speech-Language Pathology* in which this article was published.

Another good supplemental strategy is to *find a bibliography or review article* on your topic or to check the references from a previous research report. The intent of a bibliography is to provide a list of all the important work on a particular topic; sometimes a bibliography includes annotations or brief descriptions of the articles as well. The authors of review articles also cover all the important work on a topic but present an organized narrative and interpretation of the work. By checking the reference lists prepared by other authors, you can be more certain of finding the key work on your topic.

A final strategy for finding information on a topic is to complete a *citation search* for articles that cite a source you already found. Let's consider some graduate students who had an interest in the topic of word production theories. They read a review article on the topic "Models of Word Production," by Levelt (1999), but the article was several years old, and the students wanted to find more recent information. These students could conduct a citation search to identify authors who cited Levelt in their articles. Earlier, we discussed the fact that Google Scholar provides a tool for conducting a citation search. The students decided to search the title of Levelt's review, "Models of Word Production," in Google Scholar.[1] This search revealed that more than 400 articles included Levelt in their reference list and allowed the students to find the most recent work on the topic of word production models.

The *Web of Science* is another online search engine that provides for citation searching (Clarivate, n.d.). You need a subscription to use the Web of Science, but many major university libraries have an institutional subscription. Although the unique uses of Web of Science involve searches for articles that cite other published work, you also can complete general searches, such as those you would conduct on PubMed or ERIC (Clarivate, n.d.). Once you find a key article on your topic, you have the options of viewing subsequent articles with citations either in list format or in a citation map. For example, a search on the topics of "auditory evoked potentials" (e.g., event related) and "traumatic brain injury (TBI)" yielded an article on electrophysiological assessment in TBI patients that was published in 2011. This article subsequently was cited in 50 other articles, one of which was a review article with more than 159 references. Using *Web of Science* as a search tool, a researcher could identify a significant amount of information on a specific topic of interest very quickly.

If the purpose of your search is to find evidence to support treatment decisions in speech-language pathology, the Speech Pathology Database for Best Interventions and Treatment or *speechBITE* is an option to consider (https://speechbite.com/). This database is the work of speech-language pathologists at the University of Sydney. The articles included in the database are prefiltered and include intervention studies the cover all areas of professional practice in speech-language pathology (speechBITE, n.d.). Articles entered into the *speechBITE* database have been rated for quality of evidence, and when you search a topic, the studies that represent the highest quality of evidence appear first in your list.

Finding Information From Books

If you specifically want to find information from a book, a second Google search

---

[1] If you want to search an exact phrase or title in Google or Google Scholar, place the phrase or title in quotations or use the advanced search option "with the exact phrase."

option, Google Books, will be helpful (About Google Books, n.d.). Google Books has some advanced search options that you display by selecting the search tools option. When using Google Books, you generally want to have a fairly specific topic or you will retrieve an extremely large number of sources. Even with a specific topic like "auditory training" and limits on the year of publication (2010 to today), the number of the results from a recent search was fairly large. An advantage of Google Books is that the search usually yields a few preview pages and, in some instances, an entire eBook. Thus, you have an opportunity to review a source to determine how well the information suits your needs.

Another option for searching within books is *WorldCat* (https://www.worldcat .org/). WorldCat has worldwide coverage and provides a way to search for books in more than 10,000 libraries. Although you probably would not be checking out books from most of these libraries, this online search engine provides a means to search within books to identify specific chapters on your topic (Online Computer Library Center, 2001–2020). Sometimes books are collections of chapters by different authors. The individual chapters, although all on related topics, can have very different titles. Thus, to find information on a specific topic within books, you need to be able to search the table of contents. WorldCat is a search engine that lets you accomplish this. As a test, we searched the phrase "motor learning principles" using the basic search option and "Everything." After displaying the results (approximately 2,000), we limited the search to chapters, English, and the last 10 years and found 92 possible chapters. Not all of the chapter titles included our search terms, but some of the terms were within the abstract for the chapter. Notably, the records were organized from the most to least relevant, and chapters with two or three of the terms in their titles were listed first. WorldCat provides other search options, including the option to search both book titles and chapter titles, as well as to limit a search to the most recent years.

Designing a Search Strategy

Although researchers have many online tools to use when looking for previous research on their topics, the quality of the information they retrieve depends on how well they design their search strategy. Researchers want to be both thorough and efficient, so they want to retrieve all of the important information without a lot of irrelevant information. The starting point for most online literature searches is to decide on your *search terms*. Perhaps you are interested in treatment of speech production errors in children with hearing impairments. You might start designing a search strategy by identifying the key words in your topic: *treatment, speech production, children*, and *hearing impairment*. If you only searched with one or two of the terms, you would retrieve too many articles, and much of what you retrieved would be irrelevant. Thus, researchers usually combine several terms when they conduct a literature search. In our example, if you only searched treatment, children, and hearing, you probably would retrieve many irrelevant sources. If you added the term *speech* to your search, you would narrow the topic and retrieve more relevant information. You also need to consider whether or not you need to add some terms to broaden your search. Sometimes, authors use different terms or synonyms to refer to a similar concept. For example, authors might use different terms for treatment like *intervention* or *therapy*. Sometimes, a researcher is primarily interested in retrieving a certain type of article. This might be the case if you were searching for evidence-based practice information. If looking for a specific type of article, include that term in your search, for example, *clinical trial, meta-analysis, or systematic review*. The different search engines provide tools for combining terms to narrow your search as well as ways to include synonyms. In this section, we discuss some general strategies for designing a search, and in Appendix 4–1, we show how these strategies are implemented in several search engines.

Many search tools use the logical operators AND, OR, and NOT from Boolean logic (Eisenberg et al., 2008). Using the AND operator is a way to narrow your search. For example, *language intervention and hearing aids* are very broad topics that would yield an overwhelming number of sources. If you combine these terms with additional terms to narrow your search, terms like *language intervention AND preschool AND children*, or *hearing aids AND preschool AND children*, you reduce the number of sources to a more manageable number. In some online search engines such as Google and Google Scholar, the plus sign (+) and the advanced search option "with all of the words" serve the same purpose as the AND from Boolean logic.

Using the OR operator broadens your search to retrieve sources that use a synonym for one of your terms. As noted previously, the term *intervention* has potential synonyms like *treatment* or *therapy*. Thus, we might want to revise our example search for language intervention approaches as follows: *language AND (intervention OR treatment OR therapy) AND preschool AND children*. The NOT operator is useful when you retrieve many sources that are irrelevant for some reason. For example, a researcher might be looking for information about treatment for fluent aphasia (*treatment AND fluent AND aphasia*) but finds many articles that focus on treatment for nonfluent aphasia. By using the NOT operator, the researcher could eliminate these irrelevant articles (*treatment AND fluent AND aphasia NOT nonfluent*).

Knowing how to use logical operators is helpful for any literature search, but many search engines have advanced search options that help you with this task. For example, the advanced search option for Google Scholar includes the descriptors *with all of the words, with at least one of the words, and without the words* that work like the logical operators AND, OR, and NOT. For some other online search tools, the advanced search option includes dropdown boxes for selecting the logical operators. You need to be careful when using the OR selection this way. Traditionally, terms that were synonyms were placed inside parentheses and then connected with OR [e.g., *speech AND (treatment OR intervention)*]. However, when making selections with the dropdown boxes, sometimes you inadvertently create a search that is very broad (such as speech AND treatment OR intervention). This latter search would retrieve all articles that have both the terms *speech* and *treatment*, as well as any article that has the term *intervention*.

Grammatical variations on terms like *child, children, children's, or stutter, stutterer, stuttering* can cause problems for some search engines. The PubMed search engine handles grammatical variations with its term mapping capability. Using the OR operator is another way to handle grammatical variations (e.g., *child OR children OR children's*). Many search engines allow you to use the *truncation operator* (*) to handle grammatical variations. If a search engine recognizes this operator, typing *child** or *stutter** would retrieve that term and any similar terms with additional letters (children, children's; stutterer, stuttering). You might check the online help option to determine if the search tool you are using recognizes the truncation operator or implements this strategy in a different way.

Finally, many online search tools let you *set limits* on your search to reduce the number of sources you retrieve. Most search engines let you set a publication date when you conduct a search. Setting a minimum date of publication, such as only articles published from 2010 to the present, lets you conduct a slightly broader search while still retrieving a reasonable number of sources. Some other limits are specifying the language (articles written in English), the type of article (clinical trial, review), and the age of participants (adults, school-age children, preschool children).

The options available for the various online search engines are too numerous to cover thoroughly in this chapter. The websites for search engines such as Google Scholar, PubMed, ERIC, and ComDisDome all provide a help option. The help option gives explanations about how to construct a search in that particular search engine and how to use advanced search options to achieve better results.

Organizing and Documenting Your Literature Search

Once you have completed a search, how you use the evidence depends on whether you were conducting a search to find evidence to guide clinical practice, an interesting question to study, or background information and previous research on a research topic. If conducting a search for general clinical evidence, you might identify one or more meta-analyses or systematic reviews and read them to understand how the information relates to your clinical practice. Perhaps you need to include a summary of this evidence in your clinical documentation. If conducting a search for evidence on behalf of an individual client, you might select two or three articles that offer the highest quality evidence and most closely match your client's situation (Gallagher, 2002). After reading and evaluating this information, you might discuss your findings with the client or with family members.

If you conducted a literature search because you plan to write a research paper, you need to begin reading the articles, taking notes on content, and eventually writing content summaries to include in the introductory or review of literature section of your paper. We discuss the process of writing a literature review in Chapter 5.

Summary

In this chapter, we focused on the skills needed to complete a literature search, cite information, and complete a reference list. The term *information literacy* is often used to refer to the skills researchers need to complete a literature search. Audiologists and speech-language pathologists have many reasons to search professional literature in both their clinical and research roles. Clinically, they might need to find answers to clinical or evidence-based practice questions. As a researcher, they might want to find interesting problems to study, previous research on a topic, background information on a topic, relevant information from other studies, or procedures and outcome measures. One of the most efficient ways to conduct a literature search is to use an online search engine. Audiologists and speech-language pathologists can choose from among many web-based search tools, such as ERIC, PubMed, Google Scholar, and speechBITE.

Another aspect of information literacy is knowledge about designing an appropriate search strategy. Audiologists and speech-language pathologists need to know how to identify the key terms for their search, how to determine possible synonyms for these terms, and how to combine these terms to complete a thorough and efficient literature search. The various online search engines provide search aids to help you combine terms, set date limits, and retrieve specific types of articles.

Review Questions

1. What term refers to the skills associated with finding, evaluating, summarizing, and using information?

2. List three reasons why audiologists and speech-language pathologists conduct searches of professional literature.

3. What is the most efficient way to search the professional literature?

4. If your study is focused on children and/or educational topics, which search engine is the best choice for your search?

5. List three search engines that you can use to search the professional literature for free.

6. If your research topic is focused on adults and/or medical issues, which search engine is the best choice for your search?

7. What free search engine provides a way to complete a citation search?

8. What is the role of the AND operator in Boolean logic?

9. Identify the combination of terms that would retrieve fewer sources or would be narrower.
   a. *speech OR language OR hearing*
   b. *speech AND language AND hearing*

10. Identify the combination of terms that would retrieve more sources or would be broader.
    a. *delay OR disorder OR impairment*
    b. *delay AND disorder AND impairment*

Learning Activities

1. Think of a topic for a literature search. Choose two or more of the following databases and conduct a search on that topic. Modify your search by adding an additional term to narrow your search, then broaden your search by choosing one or more synonyms for your search terms.
   a. Education Resources Information Center (ERIC)
   b. PubMed
   c. Google Scholar
   d. Trip database
   e. speechBITE

2. Visit one of the following professional organization websites. What resources are available that relate to research?

a. American Academy of Audiology
b. American Auditory Society
c. American Speech-Language-Hearing Association
d. Dysphagia Research Society
e. Educational Audiology Association
f. International Society for Augmentative and Alternative Communication
g. The Voice Foundation

References

About Google Books. (n.d.). https://www.google.com/intl/en/googlebooks/about/index.html

About Google Scholar. (n.d.). https://scholar.google.com/intl/en/scholar/about.html

American Library Association. (2024). *Information literacy.* https://literacy.ala.org/information-literacy/

American Speech-Language-Hearing Association. (2004). *Preferred practice patterns for the profession of speech-language pathology* [Preferred practice patterns]. http://www.asha.org/policy

American Speech-Language-Hearing Association. (2006). *Preferred practice patterns for the profession of audiology* [Preferred practice patterns]. http://www.asha.org/policy

Baylor, C., Yorkston, K., Eadie, T., Jiseon, K., Chung, H., & Amtmann, D. (2013). The Communicative Participation Item Bank (CPIB): Item bank calibration and development of a disorder-generic short form. *Journal of Speech, Language, and Hearing Research, 56,* 1190–1208. https://doi.org/10.1044/10924388(2012/12-0140)

Clarivate. (n.d.). *Web of Science.* https://clarivate.com/products/scientific-and-academic-research/research-discovery-and-workflow-solutions/webofscience-platform/

Duke University and University of North Carolina at Chapel Hill. (2019). *EBP tutorial: Module 1: Intro to EBP.* https://guides.mclibrary.duke.edu/ebptutorial

Eisenberg, M. B., Lowe, C. A., & Spitzer, K. L. (2008). *Information literacy: Essential skills for the information age* (2nd ed.). Linworth.

Gallagher, T. M. (2002). Evidence-based practice: Applications to speech-language pathology. *Perspectives on Language Learning and Education, 9*(1), 2–5. https://doi.org/10.1044/lle 9.1.2

Google Scholar. (n.d.). *Search help.* https://scholar.google.com/intl/en/scholar/help.html

Heuer, S., & Willer, R. (2020). How is quality of life assessed in people with dementia? A systematic literature review and a primer for speech-language pathologists. *American Journal of Speech-Language Pathology, 29*(30), 1702–1715. https://doi.org/10.1044/2020_AJSLP-19-00169

Levelt, W. J. M. (1999). Models of word production. *Trends in Cognitive Sciences, 3*(6), 223–232.

National Center for Biotechnology Information. (n.d.-a). *Literature.* National Library of Medicine. https://www.ncbi.nlm.nih.gov/guide/literature/

National Center for Biotechnology Information. (n.d.-b). *PubMed overview.* https://pubmed.ncbi.nlm.nih.gov/about/

Newhart, M., & Patten, M. L. (2023). *Understanding research methods: An overview of the essentials* (11th ed.). Routledge Taylor & Francis Group.

Online Computer Library Center. (2001–2020). *What is WorldCat.org?* https://search.worldcat.org/about

ProQuest. (n.d.-a). *ComDisDome.* https://about.proquest.com/en/products-services/cdd-set-c/

ProQuest. (n.d.-b). *Dissertations and theses.* https://www.proquest.com/products-services/dissertations/

speechBITE. (n.d.). *About.* https://speechbite.com/about/

Storkel, H. L., Bontempo, D. E., & Pak, N. S. (2014). Online learning from input versus offline memory evolution in adult word learning: Effects of neighborhood density and phonologically related practice. *Journal of*

Speech, Language, and Hearing Research, *57*, 1708–1721. https://doi.org/10.1044/2014_JSLHR-L-13-0150

Strand, E. A., & Debertine, P. (2000). The efficacy of integral stimulation treatment with developmental apraxia of speech. *Journal of Medical Speech-Language Pathology*, *8*(4), 295–300.

Sullivan, J. R., Osman, H., & Schafer, E. C. (2015). The effect of noise on the relationship between auditory working memory and comprehension in school-age children. *Journal of Speech, Language, and Hearing Research*, *58*, 1043–1051. https://doi.org/10.1044/2015_JSLHR-H-14-0204

APPENDIX 4–1

Electronic Literature Search

The activities in this section provide some practice with web-based search engines for those who have limited experience conducting online searches. For this demonstration, we will conduct an evidence-based practice search for the following sample questions:

1. Will minimal pair phonological treatment, provided for two 30-minute individual treatment sessions per week for 16 weeks, produce a 20% gain in percentage of consonants correct in spontaneous speech for a 5-year-old child with a moderately severe speech production disorder?
2. Will early detection of hearing loss and amplification fitting prior to 6 months of age result in age-appropriate scores on a test of expressive and receptive language at age 2 for a child with a severe hearing loss when provided without additional speech and language intervention?

We will conduct the same search using three different search tools: ERIC, PubMed, and Google Scholar. Our goal will be to retrieve somewhere between 25 and 75 sources. This is a somewhat arbitrary number and we certainly would be comfortable with a few more or less. If you retrieve too few, however, your search might be overly narrow or you might have missed some synonyms. If you retrieve too many, you could go through a large number of sources to find what you want, but that is inefficient. If you have a computer with a relatively current web browser and an Internet connection, you should be able to access ERIC, PubMed, and Google Scholar without any problems. These three search engines are free services. ComDisDome is a commercial product provided for a fee. You might check your institution's library or information services department to determine if you have a site license for this product.

Part 1: Identify Key Terms and Possible Synonyms

1. The first step is to identify key terms from your evidence-based practice or research question. These terms form the basis for your search.
   a. Key terms for Question 1 might include *minimal pair, phonological, treatment, 5-year-old or child*, and *speech production disorder*.
   b. Key terms for Question 2 might include *early detection, hearing loss, amplification, expressive language, receptive language*, and *child*.

2. The next step is to decide which of the key terms to include in your initial search strategy.
   a. For Question 1, you might use *phonological, treatment, child*, and *disorder*. Using a specific treatment approach like *minimal pair* might narrow the search too much, as would including a specific age group. The term *speech production* overlaps with *phonological*, so you could just use the term *disorder*.
   b. For Question 2, you might use *early detection, hearing loss,*

and *language*. The term *child* overlaps with *early detection*, and *amplification* overlaps with *hearing loss*. You could consider adding the term *longitudinal* because you are looking for follow-up studies.

3. The third step is to identify possible synonyms for the terms you picked.
   a. For Question 1, several terms might have synonyms or grammatical variations. Possible synonyms include (I) *treatment, intervention, therapy*; (II) *disorder, delay, impairment*. Terms with possible grammatical variations include *child* and *phonological*. You will need to decide after trying the search whether or not to consider articulation treatment and/or articulation disorders.
   b. For Question 2, some terms might have synonyms such as (I) *early detection, early identification, early intervention*; (II) *hearing loss, hearing impairment*; and (III) *longitudinal, follow-up*. You will need to decide after trying a search if you want to include *speech* as an alternative for *language*.

Part 2: Complete an ERIC Search

Decide whether to search on Question 1 or Question 2. The steps for both questions are the same.

Question 1

1. Begin by going to the ERIC website at https://eric.ed.gov/.
2. For help with your search, look for "Advanced Search Tips" to the right of the search box and click on it.
3. Before you enter search terms, the search box displays the message "Search education resources" in gray text.
4. Begin with a basic search by typing *phonological AND treatment AND children AND disorder* in the search box.
5. Click on the Search button to start your search.
6. This search returned 124 or more results, which is a high number, but still reasonable. We should still consider revising the search by using synonyms and grammatical variations because we might be missing some relevant articles.
7. Use the back arrow on your browser and return to the search box so you can revise the search.
8. This ERIC search engine does not support truncation so we will use synonyms. In the search box, type the following: (phonological OR phonology) AND children AND (treatment OR intervention OR therapy) AND (disorder OR delay OR impairment). Placing the synonyms in parentheses is very important. If you omit the parentheses, your search will be very broad.
9. Click on the search button again. This time you should retrieve more than 558 results. Probably you retrieved too many articles with this search strategy. However, by using synonyms, we are more certain that we did not miss any key articles.
10. Because we retrieved so many articles, let's limit the search by searching for our key terms in the abstract field. This time type the following in the

search box: abstract:(phonological OR phonology) AND abstract:children AND abstract:(treatment OR intervention OR therapy) AND abstract:(disorder OR delay OR impairment). Click on the search button and view the updated results. Searching only the abstract reduced the number of articles to fewer than 304.
11. To further limit the search, select a date option on the far-left side of your browser window, for example, "Since 2020 (last 5 years)." If you click on this option, you will retrieve only the most recent articles. Look over the other options on the far left. You also can limit your results by descriptor, source, education level, and so forth.
12. Scroll down the list to view the articles you retrieved. To see the full abstract of an article, click on the highlighted title of the article. You might experiment with other options in or develop a search strategy for another topic. Then, try this same search in a different web-based search tool.

Question 2

1. Begin by going to the ERIC website at https://eric.ed.gov/.
2. For help with your search, look for "Advanced Search Tips" to the right of the search box and click on it.
3. Before you enter search terms, the search box displays the message "Search education resources" in gray text.
4. Begin with a basic search by typing *early* AND *detection* AND *hearing loss* AND *language* in the search box.
5. Click on the search button to start your search.
6. This search returned only a few results, so we should consider revising it by using synonyms and grammatical variations.
7. Use the back arrow on your browser and return to the search box so you can revise the search.
8. This ERIC search engine does not support truncation, so we will use synonyms. In the search box, type the following: *early* AND (*detection* OR *identification*) AND *hearing* AND (*loss* OR *impairment*) AND *language*. Placing the synonyms in parentheses is very important. If you omit the parentheses, your search will be very broad.
9. Click on the search button again. This time you should retrieve more than 182 results. Probably you retrieved too many articles with this search strategy. However, by using synonyms, we are more certain that we did not miss any key articles.
10. Because we retrieved so many articles, let's limit the search by searching for our key terms in the abstract field. This time type the following in the search box: abstract:early AND abstract:(detection OR identification) AND abstract:hearing AND abstract:(loss OR impairment) AND abstract:language. Click on search button and view the updated results. This time you should retrieve 56 or more results.
11. To further limit the search, select a date option on the far-left side of your browser window, for example, "Since 2015 (last 10 years)." If you click on this option, you will retrieve only the most recent articles. Look over the other options on the far left. You also can limit your results by descriptor, source, education level, and so forth.

12. Scroll down the list to view the articles you retrieved. To see the full abstract of an article, click on the highlighted title of the article. You might experiment with other options in ERIC or develop a search strategy for another topic. Then, try this same search in a different web-based search tool.

Part 3: Complete a PubMed Search

You probably want to search the same question on ERIC and PubMed, so you can compare results. The steps for Question 1 and 2 are the same.

Question 1

1. Begin by going to the PubMed website at https://pubmed.ncbi.nlm.nih.gov/.
2. Look for the word PubMed followed by a long box. For this search, we will use the "Advanced" search option. Select that option underneath the box. On the advanced page, you will see "All Fields" followed by a search box.
3. Click on the box and begin by typing *phonological* AND *treatment* AND *child* AND *disorder* in the box and select "Add." Your search terms will now show up in the "Query" box.
4. Click on the search button to start your search.
5. The search returned quite a few results, more than 930. To view the abstracts for the articles listed, click on the highlighted title of the article.
6. PubMed has a term mapping feature that handles the grammatical variations for most terms fairly well. Thus, you often retrieve more articles using this built-in feature, rather than trying to build the search using truncation. Adding synonyms may be beneficial. Let's try the search again and add some synonyms. After clearing the "Query box," type the following in the search box: phonological AND children AND (treatment OR intervention OR therapy) AND (disorder OR delay OR impairment) and select "Search." This search nearly than doubled the number of results.
7. Because we retrieved too many articles, let's limit the search by searching only for relatively recent publications. On the left side of the page, you can select filters such as "Publication Date." Change this option to *5 years*. Let's set the language to English also. To see the Languages filter, choose the option "Show Additional Filters," select Languages, and click the "Show" button. Then choose Languages on the left side and select English. Your search will update as you apply these filters and display fewer articles, but still more than 350.
8. Looking through over 350 articles would be very time-consuming, so you may want to limit the search field to "Title/Abstract." Selecting "Title/Abstract" will limit your search to just articles that have your terms in their title or abstract. Those articles should be the most relevant.
   To do that, go back to the "Advanced" search option. Keep the filters of 5 years and English. You have two options for entering the search terms and keeping the search to just the article titles and abstracts.

a. Beside the search box, you see "All Fields" with an up and down arrow. Select the arrows and scroll down until you are able to highlight Title/Abstract.
b. Enter the search terms again: phonological AND children AND (treatment OR intervention OR therapy) AND (disorder OR delay OR impairment). Use the search button again.
9. Your revised search should yield approximately 95 articles. You might experiment with other options for filters in PubMed or develop a search strategy for another topic. Afterward, repeat this same search in Google Scholar.

Question 2

1. Begin by going to the PubMed website at https://pubmed.ncbi.nlm.nih.gov/.
2. Look for the word PubMed followed by a long box. For this search, we will use the "Advanced" search option. Select that option underneath the box. On the advanced page, you will see "All Fields" followed by a search box.
3. Click on the box and begin by typing *early* AND *detection* AND *hearing loss* AND *language* in the box and select "Add." Your search terms will now show up in the "Query" box.
4. Click on the search button to start your search.
5. The search returned quite a few results, more than 400. To view the abstracts for the articles listed, click on the highlighted title of the article.
6. PubMed has a term mapping feature that handles the grammatical variations for most terms fairly well. Thus, you often retrieve more articles using this built-in feature, rather than trying to build the search using truncation. However, adding synonyms may be beneficial. Let's try the search again and add some synonyms. After clearing the "Query box," type the following in the search box: *early* AND (*detection* OR *identification*) AND *hearing* AND (*loss* OR *impairment*) AND *language* and select "Search." This search returned over 700 results.
7. Because we retrieved too many articles, let's limit the search by searching only for relatively recent publications. On the left side of the page, you can select filters such as "Publication Date." Change this option to *5 years*. Let's set the language to English also. To see the Languages filter, choose the option "Show Additional Filters," select Languages, and click the "Show" button. Then choose Languages on the left side and select English. Your search will update as you apply these filters and display fewer articles, but still more than 240.
8. Looking through over 240 articles would be very time-consuming, so you may want to limit the search field to "Title/Abstract." Selecting "Title/Abstract" will limit your search to just articles that have your terms in their title or abstract. Those articles should be the most relevant.
9. To do that, go back to the "Advanced" search option. Keep the filters of 5 years and English. You have two options for entering the search terms and keeping the search to just the article titles and abstracts.
a. Beside the search box, you see "All Fields" with an up and down arrow. Select the arrows and scroll down

until you are able to highlight Title/Abstract.
   b. Enter the search terms again: *early* AND (*detection* OR *identification*) AND *hearing* AND (*loss* OR *impairment*) AND *language*. Use the search button again.
10. Your revised search should yield approximately 143 articles. You might experiment with other options for filters in PubMed or develop a search strategy for another topic. Afterward, repeat this same search in either Google Scholar or ComDisDome.

Part 4: Complete a Google Scholar Search

If you want to compare results, you should stay with the same question and terms you searched on ERIC and PubMed.

Question 1

1. Begin by going to the Google Scholar website at https://scholar.google.com/
2. Select the Advanced Search option by clicking on the three horizontal lines (i.e., "hamburger") in the upper left corner of your screen and scroll down until your see Advanced Search.
3. In Advanced Search, you should see the phrase "Find articles" followed by some phrases such as "with all the words, with the exact phrase," and so forth. These are followed by text boxes where you can enter terms.
4. Begin with a basic search by typing *phonological treatment child disorder* in the box following the phrase "with all the words."
5. Click on the Search Scholar button to start your search.
6. You probably retrieved a very large number of sources (more than 75,000).
7. Generally, Google Scholar returns many sources, and you primarily need to narrow your search rather than add synonyms or grammatical variants. Reopen the Advanced Search box where you enter search terms.
8. First, let's try to limit the search to just the titles of articles. Look for the phrase "where my words occur." To the right of this, you should see a highlighted button next to the phrase "anywhere in the article." Click on the button next to the phrase in "the title of the article" to change this option. Click on the search button again. You probably found that this option severely narrowed your search.
9. Let's try some different options for narrowing the search. First, reopen the "Advanced Search" box. Go to where my words occur and reset this to "anywhere in the article."
10. Now limit the search to the most recent articles by entering the year 2020 in the first box following the phrase "Return articles dated between." Finally, I noticed a few of the articles retrieved were about children who stutter and also about children with reading problems. We can eliminate these by typing words such as *stutter stuttering reading* following the phrase "without the words."
11. Let's try the search again by clicking the Search Scholar button. We did retrieve fewer results (over 5,500) this time, but that still would be too many. However, Google Scholar prioritizes the sources and the most relevant

should appear first in your list, so you should not have to view all 5,200 entries. You also could consider a language limiter by adding a term for a language (e.g., *phonological treatment child disorder English*) to your search terms.

12. Finally, let's try the Google Scholar Cited by feature. Perhaps look for an article published between 2020 and 2021. Look for the phrase "Cited by" underneath the entry and find an article cited in several articles. Click on the "Cited by" link to find more recent articles that included this one in their citations and references. You might experiment by trying other options to narrow this search such as using additional terms, entering an exact phrase, or perhaps designing a new search on a topic of your choice.

Question 2

1. Begin by going to the Google Scholar website at https://scholar.google.com/
2. Select the Advanced Search option by clicking on the three horizontal lines (i.e., "hamburger") in the upper left corner of your screen and scroll down until your see "Advanced Search."
3. In Advanced Search, you should see the phrase "Find articles" followed by some phrases such as "with all the words, with the exact phrase," and so forth. These are followed by text boxes where you can enter terms.
4. Begin with a basic search by typing *early detection hearing loss language* in the box following the phrase "with all the words."
5. Click on the Scholar Search button to start your search.
6. You probably retrieved a very large number of sources (more than 800,000).
7. Generally, Google Scholar returns many sources, and you primarily need to narrow your search rather than add synonyms or grammatical variants. Reopen the Advanced Search box where you enter search terms.
8. First, let's try to limit the search to just the titles of articles. Look for the phrase "where my words occur." To the right of this, you should see a highlighted button next to the phrase "anywhere in the article." Click on the button next to the phrase in "the title of the article" to change this option. Click on the search button again. You probably found that this option severely narrowed your search.
9. Let's try some different options for narrowing the search. First, reopen the "Advanced Search" box. Go to where my words occur and reset this to "anywhere in the article."
10. Now limit the search to the most recent articles by entering the year 2020 in the first box following the phrase "Return articles dated between." Finally, I noticed a few of the articles retrieved were about children with otitis media, and others covered a genetic etiology. We can eliminate these by typing words such as *otitis media genetic gene* following the phrase "without the words."
11. Let's try the search again by clicking the Search Scholar button. We did retrieve fewer results (more than 17,000) this time, but that still would be too many. However, Google Scholar prioritizes the sources and the most relevant should appear first in your list, so you should not have to view all 17,000 entries. You also

could consider a language limiter by adding a term for a language (e.g., *early detection hearing loss language English*) to your search terms.
12. Finally, let's try the Google Scholar Cited by feature. Perhaps look for an article published between 2020 and 2021. Look for the phrase "Cited by" underneath the entry and find an article cited by 25 or more authors. Click on the "Cited by" link to find more recent articles that included this one in their citations and references. You might experiment by trying other options to narrow this search such as using additional terms or perhaps designing a new search on a topic of your choice.

5

Writing About Research: Literature Reviews and More

Main Points

- When you start researching a topic, your reading will inform your interest, topic, and your literature search, thus leading to modification and narrowing of your topic to help you come up with a specific research question.
- The literature review is organized into an introduction, a body, and a summary.
- The literature review should reflect your analysis and perspective on what is already known about your research question and make a case for why your research question is important.
- Literature reviews can be narrative, systematic, or scoping reviews.

Most research articles or other scholarly papers include a review of literature, a section that covers the previous work on a topic. The review of literature sometimes constitutes the entire paper and at other times serves as the introduction and background for an original empirical study. The previous work might include original research articles, books, book chapters, and other documents that relate to the topic such as conference presentations, documents from professional associations, nonempirical or theoretical papers, and even unpublished papers. In later sections of this chapter, we will discuss the purposes of a literature review and distinguish different types, such as narrative, scoping, or systematic reviews. Another product that relates to a review of literature is a research proposal. A proposal has additional components that serve to guide the early phases of a research study. Initially, we will consider how a review of literature fits with other phases of research, including identifying a research question and conducting a literature search.

Research Phases

As discussed in Chapters 3 and 4, the early phases of a research project typically involve identifying a research topic or question and conducting a literature search on that topic. Authors frequently discuss the early phases in research as a sequence of steps progressing from the topic or question, to the literature search, to the written literature review (Cronin et al., 2008; Imel, 2011; Jones, 2007; Whittemore & Knafl, 2005). In an actual project, the early phases are mutually influential, as illustrated in Figure 5–1. As researchers complete the initial cycle of identifying articles on a topic and reading those articles, they might discover additional topics to search or ideas for refining their research topic (Pautasso, 2013).

Purposes of a Literature Review

A review of literature has different aims depending on the type of paper you are authoring. Are you writing a paper to fulfill a course requirement, writing the introductory section of an original research report or research proposal, using the literature to answer a focused clinical question, or conducting a systematic review of the literature? If the goal is to introduce a new study, the review of literature typically includes a summary and analysis of the previous work on the topic, an explanation of the need for additional research, and the purpose or research questions (American Psychological Association [APA], 2020; Jones, 2007). Ideally, the analysis and summary of previous work supports the need for additional research.

A stand-alone, *narrative review* of the literature also includes an analysis and summary of previous work on a topic. The authors' aim might be to find answers to a specific clinical question or to uncover common outcomes or possibly conflicting findings within a body of research (Aveyard, 2019; Oliver, 2012). A narrative review most often ends with conclusions that emerged from the authors' reading, analysis, and evaluation of the previous work on the topic (Hart, 1998). The following list gives several possible aims of a review of literature. Please keep in mind that a literature review might cover two or more of these aims, and the list is not exhaustive.

1. Introduce new research
2. Explain the basis for new research
3. Identify a problem or research question
4. Summarize the previous work on a topic
5. Compare and contrast previous research
6. Analyze and synthesize previous work
7. Evaluate previous work
8. Answer a focused clinical question

Organization

A literature review generally starts with an introductory sentence or two in which the authors establish the topic or purpose of the paper. The common elements include (1) an *introduction* or purpose statement(s),

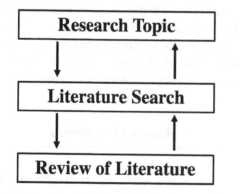

Figure 5–1. Mutually influential early phases of research: identifying the topic, conducting a literature search, and writing the literature review.

(2) a *summary and critique* of prior work, (3) a *conclusion* section, and (4) *references* (Schmidt et al., 2008; Writing Center, 2020). A lengthy review of literature often includes *definitions* of key terminology associated with the topic. A structured review such as a systematic review or meta-analysis also includes a *methods section* with details about the search and article selection criteria (Aveyard, 2019).

For many writers, deciding on a way to introduce their paper creates a period of writer's block. The best solution might be to skip the introduction and begin writing the body of your paper. Completing some of the article summaries and analyzing the findings might provide some new insights that lead to a good approach for introducing the paper. You might discover why a particular topic is critical to audiologists and speech-language pathologists, identify conflicting findings or missing information in the previous research, find an author with a new perspective on the topic, or perhaps discover an emerging consensus regarding best practices in diagnosis and treating a particular communication disorder.

Another way to overcome some initial frustration in starting a paper is to consider the ways other authors started their literature reviews. Some common strategies are to define the primary topic, describe the characteristics of a disorder, state the purpose of the paper, cite information about prevalence, refer to an important issue or challenge, identify an inconsistency, and make a comparison. Table 5–1 provides examples for several of the strategies for introducing a topic. As the examples illustrate, establishing the basis for a new study or stand-alone literature review could take one or more sentences depending on the topic.

The *main section or body* of a literature review consists of a summary and critique of the prior work on the topic. Depending on the type of literature review, the prior work could broadly encompass books, book chapters, review articles, research articles, and presentations on the topic or specifically focus on the prior research. One of the decisions you need to make as an author is how to organize your review of literature. Using a relatively simple strategy such as discussing the prior work in *chronological order* is a temptation, but a chronology is seldom the primary organizing strategy in a well-written review. Often the most appropriate way to organize the prior work emerges after reading and taking notes on many of the articles. As you learn more about the topic through your reading, you might discover a few themes or issues that allow you to group the various articles (Imel, 2011; Jones, 2007). These themes become the primary organizing strategy for your review of literature. Chronological order could be the secondary organizing strategy as you summarize and discuss the articles within a theme.

Authors utilize other approaches to organize the prior work on a topic, such as different methods for studying a problem or trends within a discipline (Oliver, 2012; Writing Center, 2020). If researchers have studied a topic using different methods, organizing articles by those methods could be the best approach (Imel, 2011). You might have broad groupings such as qualitative and quantitative research or nonexperimental and experimental research, or you might have more specific groupings such as nonexperimental case studies, single-subject research, and randomized control trials. In some disciplines, the way researchers approach a topic or views on a topic might undergo a major shift at a particular time. Separating research according to a major shift (i.e., before and after) has a temporal component but is not strictly chronological.

Table 5–1. Examples of Different Strategies for Introducing the Topic of a Literature Review

Type	Example	Source
Assertion	"The ability to initiate new topics of conversation is a basic skill integral to communicative independence and agency . . ."	Leaman and Edmonds (2020, p. 375)
Contrast	"One area related to the distinction between adult and child models involves the use of traditional grid symbol displays versus the use of visual scene displays (VSDs)."	Olin et al., (2019, p. 284)
Definition	"Rehabilitation can be defined as measures required for coping with functional consequences of a disease, defect or trauma."	Kuoppala and Lamminpää (2008, p. 796)
Diagnosis	"Acquired apraxia of speech (AOS) is a neurogenic sensorimotor speech disorder that results in a disruption in spatial and temporal planning or programming in producing speech sounds."	Mauszycki and Wambaugh (2020, p. 511)
Issue	"A proportion of healthy older adults present with differences in voice compared to their younger age equivalents. . . . When assessing individuals for the first time, it can be difficult to separate out what aspects of vocal change are the result of typical aging processes and what changes represent pathology (either vocal or neurological) in older adults."	Rojas et al. (2020, p. 533)
Purpose	"The purpose of this article is to systematically examine the literature on the effectiveness of behavioural interventions for individuals with behaviour problems after traumatic brain injury (TBI) with the goal of deriving possible treatment guidelines."	Ylvisaker et al. (2007, p. 769)
Prevalence	"Hearing loss is the third most common chronic health condition in individuals aged 65 and older, surpassed only by arthritis and hypertension."	Clark et al., 2012 (p. 1936)

When the literature review serves as the introduction to an original empirical study, one of the authors' goals is to justify new research. One way to structure the justification is develop a single topic beginning with works that are broadly related to the topic of the study, then covering the works that are more directly related. You might visualize this as approach as a funnel, with several broadly related articles covered in a brief manner at the top of the funnel and the article most related to the research topic covered in depth at the bottom, narrow end of the funnel. A second possible structure is one that brings two or more separate strands of research that all inform and justify a new study. You might visualize this approach as separate strands of a rope that are twisted together and lead to a single, new research study.

Audiologists and speech-language pathologists are likely to discover other organizing strategies that do not apply to nonclinical fields. For example, an author might determine that various researchers studied a particular assessment or treatment approach with different diagnostic groups and decide to organize a literature review by diagnosis. Another author might have a particular interest in how well a procedure works across different age groups and use age of the participants as an organizing strategy. The strategy you use to organize your paper should be a good fit for the previous work and the focus of your paper.

Note Taking

Having a well-thought-out note-taking strategy and using that strategy consistently as you begin reading articles on your review will save time in the long run. In Chapter 1, we introduced an approach for reading research articles and taking notes. That strategy, outlined below, may work for other types of articles with a few modifications.

1. Reference/source information (e.g., author(s), year, title of article or chapter, journal or book title, volume number for journals, page numbers, DOI number for journal articles, publisher for books)
2. Research purpose or question
3. Methods (e.g., participants and groups, research design, observation or treatment procedures, time frame, measurement plan)
4. Major outcomes or results
5. Conclusions (answers to research questions)
6. Critique of strengths and weaknesses

Cronin et al. (2008) summarized the information you might need from three different types of sources, research articles, systematic reviews and meta-analyses, and other, nonresearch articles. The common elements are the reference or source information, purpose or research questions, conclusions, and critique. Your notes for both research articles and systematic reviews should include the purpose or research questions and methodological information (see Cronin et al., 2008, for detailed guidance). For the most part, the notes on an article should be brief paraphrases *in your own words*. If you copy another author's words verbatim, you need to identify those words as a *direct quote*. If you add a direct quote to your notes, put the sentence(s) in quotation marks and add the page number for the quote. Properly identifying a quote in your notes will help you avoid inadvertently representing another person's work as your own, an ethical violation of plagiarism. Most of what you write, 90% or more, should be in your own words. Taking notes in your own words and **not** copying entire sentences is the first step toward writing a paper that genuinely reflects your own ideas and interpretations.

As you take notes on the content of an article or other source, also record some preliminary thoughts for your critical analysis and evaluation. What are the strengths of this particular article or study and what are its weaknesses? How do the findings and conclusions compare with other articles? Your initial thoughts might include information about the strength of the research design, steps the researcher(s) took to reduce treatment bias in their assessments, and ways to demonstrate that the research procedures and treatments were consistent from one participant to the next. Through your reading and note taking, you also may notice some conflicting findings or perspectives. Adding these ideas to the section of your notes for critical analysis and evaluation supports writing your paper in the future. For more detailed guidance on critical appraisal of articles, you might read a series of articles by Donohue and colleagues that cover systematic and other review articles (Donohue et al., 2021), meta-analyses (Donohue et al., 2022), and randomized control trials (Donohue et al., 2023).

Writing the Paper

Once you have notes from many of the articles selected for your paper, you are ready to begin organizing your notes and writing the paper. How authors organize a writing task depends on their personal work style. Some authors prefer to start with a general outline and add more details. The outline starts with the basic sections of the paper; the authors add details to the outline as ideas and themes emerge in their reading and eventually list specific articles in the different sections. The number of themes, conclusions, and sources will vary depending on your topic and the number of articles your select for each section.

Example of an Outline

1. Introduction
   a. Purpose or Topic
   b. Supporting Details
      i. Source 1
      ii. Source 2
2. Body of the Paper
   a. Theme 1
      i. Source 1
      ii. Source 2
   b. Theme 2
      i. Source 1
      ii. Source 2
3. Summary and Conclusions
   a. Conclusion 1
   b. Conclusion 2
4. References

Some authors prefer a spatial or visual approach. An author might print the notes for each of the articles, review the contents of those notes, and physically arrange them in stacks on their desk or tack them in groups on a bulletin board. Other authors might generate a concept map or graphic organizer—that is, a visual diagram of the key themes and the research that relates to those themes (Aveyard, 2019; Hart, 1998). A visual such as the one in Figure 5–2 could be included in the final paper.

The body of a literature review includes a concise presentation and discussion of each source. An author covers the various articles to a different extent depending on how important the article is for developing a topic. Authors typically write less about articles that provide background or supporting details and more about the key research that contributes to justification for a new study or supports major themes in a standalone literature review. Authors might cite several sources when providing a definition, diagnostic characteristics, or other background information.

A worthwhile literature review comprises more than a description of the prior work on a topic (Oliver, 2012; Pautasso, 2013; Schmidt et al., 2008). According to Jones (2007), writing a paper that is only a series of summaries of the various articles you read is a common mistake. As an author, you should endeavor to analyze and synthesize the prior work by identifying

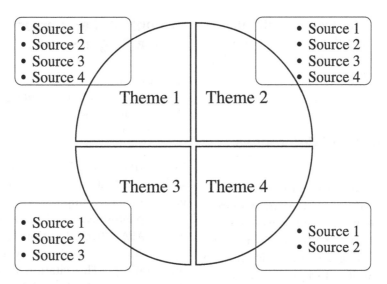

Figure 5–2. Example of a visual diagram illustrating the relationship among themes and sources.

commonalities across multiple studies and contradictions or differences across studies. Authors also use words that reflect the relationships they identified in the prior research. If different research articles support the same conclusion, phrases such as "the findings are similar . . . ," "the results are comparable . . . ," or "like the earlier study. . . " convey that relationship. If some of the studies yielded conflicting results, phrases such as "unlike the earlier study . . . ," "the findings differed . . . ," or "inconsistent with the previous study . . . " alert readers to the differences. In addition to analyzing and synthesizing across studies, authors also critically evaluate the previous work on a topic (Imel, 2011; Pautasso, 2013). The evaluation considers relative strengths and weaknesses within a study in areas such as the research design, number and type of participants, procedural clarity, measurement reliability, and possible sources of researcher bias.

Summary and Conclusions Section

As noted previously, a literature review ends with a summary and conclusions section. This section usually includes a recap of the purpose of the literature review, the organizing scheme, and the most important findings. Authors often include a brief analysis and summary section at the end of each major section within the main part of the literature review. For example, if the review has a thematic organization, the section devoted to each theme ends with a brief summary of the prior work, including a discussion of the similarities and differences and an analysis of the relative strengths and weaknesses of the various sources (Cronin et al., 2008). As Imel (2011) noted, a literature review should be more than just a summary of the existing research. A good goal for authors is to add new perspectives through the ways they organize the literature, the themes they identify, and their critical evaluation of strengths and weaknesses of previous studies (Imel, 2011).

Citations and References

As discussed in the chapter on research ethics, authors need to document their sources carefully when they use the ideas or writing of another person. Usually, this documentation includes citing the source in the text of a paper as well as listing the source in a reference list. A style manual like the *Publication Manual of the American Psychological Association*, seventh edition, provides guidelines for citing sources in an appropriate way and preparing a reference list (APA, 2020). Many journals in communication sciences and disorders follow APA style, so we will review some of the most common citation and reference styles.

Authors should include a citation whenever they use a direct quote from another source or when they paraphrase another author's ideas. In APA style, the text citation includes the author(s) and year and, if a direct quote, also the page number. A quotation is placed in quotation marks if it contains fewer than 40 words and in an indented text block if it contains 40 words or more (APA, 2020). A good writer uses direct quotes from other authors sparingly, so in the examples below, we focus on paraphrases and short quotations.

Example 1: Paraphrase From a Single Source

Fu and Galvin (2006) used simulated speech to investigate cochlear implant users' ability to understand speech over the telephone.

Example 2: Paraphrase From a Single Source

Speaking rate at an early age is one possible predictor of a future reading disability in children with a positive family history (Smith et al., 2006).

In the first example, the source is cited within the text of the sentence, whereas in the second example, the source is cited within parentheses at the end of the sentence (APA, 2020). Citations of the study by Fu and Galvin always would include both authors. The citation of the Smith, Roberts, Smith, Lock, and Bennett (2006) study uses the style for articles with three or more authors. Note how the phrase "et al." replaced all but the first author.

The APA style for including a short quote from another source is similar to the paraphrase except that you need to place the information inside quotation marks and include the page number for the quote.

Example 3: Short Quote Within a Sentence

With regard to children with closed head injury, Hay and Moran (2005, p. 333) noted, "it is important to be able to evaluate how they will cope with the communicative, social, and academic demands that will be placed on them with a return to their normal environment."

Example 4: Short Quote Within Parentheses

With regard to children with closed head injury, "it is important to be able to evaluate how they will cope with the communicative, social, and academic demands that will be placed on them with a return to their normal environment" (Hay & Moran, 2005, p. 333).

Finally, researchers also need to prepare a reference list for their papers. Although you could wait until finishing your paper to complete this list, you might find it helpful to generate the reference list in an ongoing way and to add an entry each time you cite a source. The APA style manual includes specific guidelines for what information to include and how to format your reference list (APA, 2020). A reference list entry generally includes the author(s), date of publication, and title. If the source is a book, the entry also includes publisher information. If the source is a journal article, the entry includes the journal title, as well as volume and page numbers. For information retrieved from a website, the entry includes the website address. Examples of entries for journal articles, a book, a chapter in an edited book, and a website illustrate the different formats for these common types of sources.

Example 1: Entry for a Journal Article From a Print Source

McFadden, T. U. (1998). Sounds and stories: Teaching phonemic awareness in interactions around text. *American Journal of Speech-Language Pathology, 7*(2), 5–13.

If you obtained the article above from an online source, you would modify the listing slightly to include the DOI retrieval informal for the article or, if that is not available, the website for the journal.

Example 2: Entry for a Journal Article With a DOI Number

McFadden, T. U. (1998). Sounds and stories: Teaching phonemic awareness in interactions around text. *American Journal of Speech-Language Pathology, 7*(2), 5–13. https://doi.org/10.1044/1058-0360.0702.05

A DOI number refers to a numerical system of identification, called a Digital Object Identifier (DOI). When an article has a DOI number, you should include this number in your reference list. Whereas the website location for an article might change, DOIs should provide a long-term way to identify and retrieve the article. For articles you retrieve from websites that do not have DOI numbers, you include the journal website, as shown in Example 3.

Example 3: Entry for a Journal Article Without a DOI Number

Malar, G., Sreedevi N., & Suresh, C. (2013). Trends and impact of early intervention for communication disorders at AIISH. *Journal of the All India Institute of Speech & Hearing, 32,* 173–183. https://aiishmysore.in/en/editions-of-jaiish

Example 4: Entry for a Book

Tye-Murray, N. (2024). *Foundations of aural rehabilitation: Children, adults, and their family members* (6th ed.). Plural Publishing.

Example 5: Entry for a Chapter in an Edited Book

Tyler, A. A. (2005). Promoting generalization: Selecting, scheduling, and integrating goals. In A. G. Kamhi & K. E. Pollock (Eds.), *Phonological disorders in children: Clinical decision making in assessment and intervention* (pp. 67–75). Paul H. Brookes.

Example 6: Entry for a Website Document

U.S. Department of Health and Human Services. (2018, March 18). *Special protections for children as research subjects.* https://www.hhs.gov/ohrp/regulations-and-policy/guidance/special-protections-for-children/index.html

Every source you cite, whether a journal article, book, book chapter, or website document, should be in your reference list, called **References**. At the same time, the reference list should include only sources cited in your paper. The correspondence between the citations and reference list is one item to check as you are wrapping up a writing project. The following checklist is one way to double check your work.

Literature Review Checklist

- Well-defined topic or purpose
- Necessary background information
- Definitions of key concepts
- Appropriate number and type of sources
- Current and influential research
- Accurate citations throughout the paper
- Accurate description and summary of prior work
- Thoughtful analysis, evaluation, and synthesis
- Meaningful conclusions by the author(s)
- Accurate reference list; corresponds to citations

Types of Literature Reviews

A literature review involves reading, summarizing, analyzing and evaluating, and writing about the prior works on a topic.

The term *literature review* encompasses more than one type of review. As noted previously, a review of literature might provide background and justification for a new study or as a stand-alone paper. A *narrative review* serves these two purposes, either to cover the prior work needed to justify a new study or to summarize and analyze articles on a well-defined topic (Jones, 2007). A *systematic review or meta-analysis* is a thorough analysis and critical appraisal of the prior research on a focused clinic question (Aveyard, 2019). Systematic reviews have predefined methods for the literature search, selection of articles, and critical appraisal, as well as procedures to ensure inter-reviewer reliability. Systematic reviews often are conducted by a group of researchers. These researchers have exhaustive search strategies for identifying all of the prior research, including unpublished studies. The conclusions in a systematic review come from the combined results of the research that meets the selection criteria. Authors of systematic reviews often employ published methods from the Centre for Evidenced-Based Medicine (https://www.cebm.net/) and the Preferred Reporting Items for Systematic Reviews and Meta-Analyses (PRISMA) website (http://www.prisma-statement.org/).

One additional type of literature review is a *scoping review* (Munn et al., 2018). Similar to a systematic review, scoping reviews are carefully constructed reviews with precise methods for searching, selecting, and evaluating the prior work. The focus of a scoping review is broader than that of a systematic review (Munn et al., 2018). Researchers conducting a scoping review seek to determine how much literature exists and the types of articles available on a topic. The researchers also consider the methods used to study a topic and identify any missing information (Munn et al., 2018).

Writing a Research Proposal

As we noted previously, one of the roles of a review of literature is to serve as the introductory section of a research proposal. Two situations that typically require a research proposal are when presenting an idea for an academic research project such as a thesis or dissertation and when submitting a request for funding to an agency that offers research grants. In some academic settings, the proposal takes the form of a research prospectus. The requirements of a research proposal are variable but often specified by the university or academic department, or the granting agency. In some settings, the proposal is a relatively short document with a concise review of literature (e.g., 10 or so of the most key articles or other sources), whereas in other settings, the proposal would be a lengthier document with a comprehensive review of literature and detailed methods. In proposals to granting agencies, the proposal will also include a budget and timeline for the project.

Most research proposals include a version of the following sections: aim or statement of purpose, review of literature, summary and critique, rationale, project objectives or research questions, methodology, timeline, and budget.

1. Aim or statement of purpose: The aim or purpose of a proposal is a concise, informative statement related to the project objectives or research questions. The aim typically has one to two sentences and is at the beginning of the proposal. It should captivate the readers' interest and motivate them to continue reading. Authors might provide context for the aim by describing the individuals who would benefit from the research or adding a brief rationale.

2. Review of literature: The review of literature covers relevant background information and prior research related to your topic. The content goes beyond a summary of the prior work to include the authors' viewpoint on comparable or conflicting findings within the prior work, strengths and limitations of prior work, and missing perspectives.

3. Summary and critique: A summary and critique includes highlights of the most important findings from prior work as well as the limitations or missing perspectives. The summary and critique serve to connect the aim of the study with rationale, project objectives, and research questions. A lengthy review of literature might have a summary and critique after each major section as well as at the end of the review.

4. Rationale: The rationale is the justification for a project or study; it emerges from the discussion and critique of prior work on the topic. The rationale should clearly state how the research that you propose will address one or more of the limitations of prior studies.

5. Project objectives and/or research questions: Project objectives and research questions connect but are not necessarily the same. A research proposal will have a statement of purpose, hypotheses, or research questions. Often grant proposals have project objectives that relate to the use of research funds, such as purchasing equipment for a laboratory, hiring project personnel, conducting the actual research, and disseminating the findings. The objectives and research questions are measurable outcomes consistent with the nature of the research.

6. Methodology: The methodology section provides information about how you will conduct your study. The typical content includes the study design, population and sample for participants, approach for collecting and analyzing data, and additional information to support the reliability and validity of your data.
7. Timeline: The timeline for your study should cover all phases such as obtaining institutional review board approval, acquiring and setting up any necessary equipment, completing any required training, recruiting and selecting participants, completing procedures with all participants (e.g., pretests if relevant, sessions with participants), organizing and analyzing data, writing, and possibly presenting your final product. The timeline should have specific dates for all planned activities and be realistic.
8. Budget: The budget section is essential for any grant proposal and might be necessary for other research proposals. The budget includes specific categories such as equipment, consumables, personnel, and participant reimbursement. Some grants require matching funds so the source of funding might also be included.
9. References: The references section includes complete source information for any books, chapters, or research papers that you cited.

As we noted above, the requirements for research proposals differ across settings and situations. The differences encompass the requisite sections, the order of sections, and the length of sections and the overall length of the proposal. A budget section is critical for grant proposals but might be optional or excluded from thesis or dissertation proposals. Carefully reading and following any guidelines is crucial for writing a successful proposal. For additional guidance in writing a proposal, you might consult online resources such as Kramer (2023) or Purdue Online Writing Lab (n.d.).

Summary

A review of literature is a paper or section that covers the previous work on a topic. Writing a literature review often follows the early phases of research involving identification of a research topic or question and conducting a literature search on that topic. The common elements of a literature review include (1) an introduction or purpose statement(s), (2) a summary and critique of prior work, (3) a conclusion section, and (4) references. The *main section or body* of a literature review consists of a summary and critique of the prior work on the topic. Depending on the type of literature review, the prior work could broadly encompass books, book chapters, review articles, research articles, and presentations on the topic or specifically focus on the prior research.

The body of a literature review includes a concise presentation and discussion of each source. Besides describing the prior work on a topic, a well-written literature review includes analysis and synthesis of the prior work. Authors appraise the various articles to identify commonalities and contradictions or differences across studies. Authors typically report on the relative strengths and weaknesses within a study in areas such as the research design, number and type of participants, procedural clarity, measurement reliability, and possible sources of research bias.

Additionally, researchers need to know the appropriate way to cite or attribute ideas to their appropriate sources and how to generate a reference list. Usually, a publication like a journal or book uses a particular style for citing sources and formatting a reference list. Journals in the field of communication sciences and disorders commonly use the style described in the *Publication Manual of the American Psychological Association*, seventh edition (APA, 2020).

A review of literature also is an important element in a special form of research writing, the research proposal. The research proposal often is the beginning step in starting a project or in securing grant funding. Although the requirements for proposals vary, common elements include a statement of purpose or the aim of the study, a review and critique of the literature, methods, and a timeline.

Review Questions

1. Identify the true statement.
   a. The early phases of a research project are always a sequence of steps progressing from the topic or question, to the literature search, to the written literature review.
   b. The early phases of a research project are mutually influential, and reading or writing about the literature may lead to refining the topic or a new search.

2. List four of the purposes of a literature review.

3. Complete the following list. Most literature reviews include (1) an introduction or purpose statement, (2) _____, (3) _____, and (4) references.

4. What are three of the common organizing strategies for a literature review? Provide a brief description of each strategy.

5. List the information you should include in your notes from a research article.

6. What is the difference between a scoping review and systematic review?

7. Which of the following statements is true?
   a. In APA style, you cite the source of an idea in a paraphrase by using a footnote at the end of your paper.
   b. In APA style, you cite the source of an idea by including the author and year in your paragraph.

8. What information do you usually include when listing a journal article in your reference list?

9. What is the role of a research proposal in an academic setting, such as when planning a thesis or dissertation?

Learning Activities

1. Choose one or more of the strategies for introducing the topic of a literature review (e.g., assertion, contrast, definition, diagnosis, issue, purpose, or prevalence). Write an example of an opening sentence for an article that illustrates the strategy.

2. Visit one of the online writing centers such as one of the two listed

below. Read the information about paraphrasing and citing information from another author's work.
   a. UW-Madison Writing Center https://writing.wisc.edu/handbook/
   b. Purdue Online Writing Lab (OWL) at https://owl.purdue.edu/owl/avoiding_plagiarism/index.html

3. Read a stand-alone literature review or the literature review in a research article. Find statements in the review that represent the author's/authors' critique and evaluation or the previous research.

4. Each of the following entries in a reference list has an error in format. Identify the error. A style reference such as the *Publication Manual of the American Psychological Association*, seventh edition (APA, 2020) would be helpful for this task.

   Baldner, E. F., Doll, E., & van Mersbergen, M. R. (2015). A review of measures of vocal effort with a preliminary study on the establishment of a vocal effort measure. *Journal of Voice*, 530–541. https://doi.org/10.1016/j.jvoice.2014.08.017

   Byiers, B. J., Reichle, J., & Symons, F. J. (2012). Single-Subject Experimental Design for Evidence Based Practice. *American Journal of Speech-Language Pathology, 21*, 397–414. https://doi.org/10.1044/1058-0360(2012/11-0036)

   Creswell, J. W. (2012). Qualitative inquiry & research design: *Choosing among five approaches, 3rd ed.* Sage Publications.

   Huber & Darling. (2011). Effect of Parkinson's disease on the production of structured and unstructured speaking tasks: Respiratory physiologic and linguistic considerations. *Journal of Speech, Language, and Hearing Research, 54,* 33–46. https://doi.org/10.1044/1092-4388(2010/09-0184)

   Lewis, D. E., Manninen, C. M., Valente, D. L., & Smith, N. A. (2014). Children's understanding of instructions presented in noise and reverberation. *American Journal of Audiology, 23*(3). https://doi.org/10.1044/2014_AJA-14-0020

   Lundberg et al. (2011). A randomized, controlled trial of the short-term effects of complementing an educational program for hearing aid users with telephone consultations. *Journal of the American Academy of Audiology, 22,* 654–662. https://doi.org/10.3766/jaaa.22.10.4

   Seeman, S., & Sims, R. (2015). Comparison of psychophysiological and dual-task measures of listening effort. *Journal of Speech, Language, and Hearing Research, 58,* 1781–1792. https://doi.org/10.1044/2015_JSLHR-H-14-0180

   Strand, E. A., McCauley, R. J., Weigand, S. D., Stoeckel, R. E., & Baas, B. S. (2013). A motor speech assessment for children with severe speech disorders: Reliability and validity evidence. *Journal of Speech, Language, and Hearing Research, 56:* 505–520. https://doi.org/10.1044/1092-4388(2012/12-0094)

   Strand, E. A., McCauley, R. J., Weigand, S. D., Stoeckel, R. E., & Baas, B. S. (2013). A motor speech assessment for children with severe speech disorders: Reliability and validity evidence. *Journal of Speech, Language, and Hearing Research, 56:* 505–520. https://doi.org/10.1044/1092-4388(2012/12-0094)

   Taylor, B., & Mueller, G. (2021). *Fitting and Dispensing Hearing Aids* (3rd ed.). Plural Publishing.

References

American Psychological Association. (2020). *Publication manual of the American Psychological Association* (7th ed.).

Aveyard, H. (2019). *Doing a literature review in health and social care: A practical guide*

(4th ed.). McGraw Hill Education/Open University Press.

Clark, J. H., Yeagle, J., Arbaje, A., Lin, F. R., Niparko, J. K., & Francis, H., W. (2012). Cochlear implant rehabilitation in older adults: Literature review and proposal of a conceptual framework. *The American Geriatrics Society*, *60*, 1936–1945. https://doi.org/10.1111/j.1532-5415.2012.04150.x

Cronin, P., Ryan, F., & Coughlan. M. (2008). Undertaking a literature review: A step-by step approach. *British Journal of Nursing*, *17*(1), 38–43. https://doi.org/10.12968/bjon.2008.17.1.28059

Donohue, C., Carnaby, G., & (Focht) Garand, K. L. (2021). Critically appraising systematic reviews in the field of speech-language pathology: A how-to guide for clinician readers. *American Journal of Speech-Language Pathology*, *31*(5), 664–677. https://doi.org/10.1044/2021_AJSLP-21-00004

Donohue, C., Carnaby, G., & (Focht) Garand, K. L. (2022). How to interpret and evaluate a meta-analysis in the field of speech-language pathology: A tutorial for clinicians. *American Journal of Speech-Language Pathology*, *31*(2), 664–677. https://doi.org/10.1044/2021_AJSLP-21-00267

Donohue, C., Carnaby, G., & (Focht) Garand, K. L. (2023). A clinician's guide to critically appraising randomized controlled trials in the field of speech-language pathology. *American Journal of Speech-Language Pathology*, *32*(2), 411–425. https://doi.org/10.1044/2022_AJSLP-22-00180

Fu, Q.-J., & Galvin, J. J., III. (2006). Recognition of simulated telephone speech by cochlear implant users. *American Journal of Audiology*, *15*, 127–132. https://doi.org/10.1044/1059-0889(2006/016)

Hart, C. (1998). *Doing a literature review: Releasing the social science research imagination*. Sage.

Hay, E., & Moran, C. (2005). Discourse formulation in children with closed head injury. *American Journal of Speech-Language Pathology*, *14*, 324–336. https://doi.org/10.1044/1058-0360(2005/031)

Imel, S. (2011). Writing a literature review. In T. S. Rocco & T. Hatcher (Eds.), *The handbook of scholarly writing and publishing* (pp. 145–160). Jossey-Bass/John Wiley & Sons.

Jones, K. (2007). Doing a literature review in health. In M. Saks & J. Allsop (Eds.), *Researching health: Qualitative, quantitative and mixed methods* (pp. 32–53). Sage.

Kramer, L. (2023, May 10). How to write a research proposal. *Grammarly Blog*. https://www.grammarly.com/blog/how-to-write-a-research-proposal/

Kuoppala, J., & Lamminpää, A. (2008). Rehabilitation and work ability: A systematic literature review. *Journal of Rehabilitation Medicine*, *40*(10), 796–804. https://doi.org/10.2340/16501977-0270

Leaman, M. C., & Edmonds, L. A. (2020). "By the way" . . . How people with aphasia and their communication partners initiate new topics of conversation. *American Journal of Speech-Language Pathology*, *29*, 375–392. https://doi.org/10.1044/2019_AJSLP-CAC48-18-0198

Mauszycki, S. C., & Wambaugh, J. L. (2020). Acquired apraxia of speech: Comparison of electropalatography treatment and sound production treatment. *American Journal of Speech-Language Pathology*, *29*, 511–529. https://doi.org/10.1044/2019_AJSLP-CAC48-18-0223

Munn, Z., Peters, M. D. J., Stern, C., Tufanaru, C., McArthur, A., & Aromataris, E. (2018). Systematic review or scoping review? Guidance for authors when choosing between a systematic or scoping review approach. *BMC Medical Research Methodology*, *18*(143), 1–7. https://doi.org/10.1186/s12874-0180611-x

Olin, A. R., Reichle, J., Johnson, L., & Monn, E. (2019). Examining dynamic visual scene displays: Implications for arranging and teaching symbol selection. *American Journal of Speech-Language Pathology*, *19*, 284–297. https://doi.org/10.1044/1058-0360(2010/09-0001)

Oliver, P. (2012). *Succeeding with your literature review: A handbook for students*. Open University Press/McGraw-Hill Education.

Pautasso, M. (2013). Ten simple rules for writing a literature review. *PLoS Computational Biol-*

ogy, *9*(7), e1003149. https://doi.org/10.1371/journal.pcbi.1003149

Purdue Online Writing Lab. (n.d.). *Academic proposals*. https://owl.purdue.edu/owl/graduate_writing/graduate_writing_genres/graduate_writing_genres_academic_proposals_new.html

Rojas, S., Kefalianos, E., & Vogel, A. (2020). How does our voice change as we age? A systematic review and meta-analysis of acoustic and perceptual voice data from healthy adults over 50 years of age. *Journal of Speech, Language, and Hearing Research, 63*, 533–551. https://doi.org/10.1044/2019_JSLHR-19-00099

Schmidt, R. K., Smyth, M. M., & Kowalski, V. K. (2008). *Lessons for a scientific literature review: Guiding the inquiry*. Libraries Unlimited/Greenwood Publishing Group.

Whittemore, R., & Knafl, K. (2005). The integrative review: Updated methodology. *Journal of Advanced Nursing, 52*, 546–553. https://doi.org/10.1111/j.1365-2648.2005.03621.x

Writing Center–University of North Carolina at Chapel Hill. (2020). *Literature reviews*. https://writingcenter.unc.edu/tips-and-tools/literature-reviews/

Ylvisaker, M., Turkstra, L., Coehlo, C., Yorkston, K., Kennedy, M., Sohlberg, M. M., & Avery, J. (2007). Behavioral intervention for children and adults with behaviour disorders after TBI: A systematic review of the evidence. *Brain Injury, 21*, 769–805. https://doi.org/10.1080/02699050701482470

6

Nonexperimental Research Design

Main Points

- The research design is your plan for how you are going to find the answer to your research question, including what, when, where, and how observations will be made.
- Survey research is a nonexperimental design that must carefully consider the types of questions, order of questions, and how responses will be summarized.
- Case studies are in-depth observations of an entity (a participant, a group, or a collective case study of several cases) that are frequently a mixed method of both qualitative and quantitative designs.
- Qualitative research designs tend to use verbal observation format, inductive reasoning, natural environment, and smaller sample sizes with more observations per participant.
- Observations in qualitative research may be influenced by the observer's knowledge or previous experience. Rigorous qualitative research will use approaches to minimize bias and provide descriptive and interpretive adequacy.

Identifying an interesting problem to study and turning that problem into an answerable research question are early steps in a process of systematic inquiry. If a literature search revealed only a few previous studies on the topic and none that finally answered the question, the next step is to gather original evidence. Before beginning this process, researchers decide on the best approach and then develop a detailed plan for conducting their research. This plan or *research design* might include information about identifying participants, assigning participants to groups, manipulating or measuring variables, and analyzing the findings (Trochim et al., 2016). In the design, you also might specify when you will make your observations and what the participants will do.

A research design is your plan for answering a research question or testing a research hypothesis. Researchers decide on the features of a design based on the nature of their study. Although research studies generally share at least one similarity—a question that needs an answer—the way a researcher obtains answers could vary broadly from making observations in an unobtrusive way to exposing participants to different experimental manipulations.

Nonexperimental Research Designs

Experimental studies are those in which researchers identify one or more factors that they will manipulate or control during the experiment; these research designs will be discussed in Chapter 8. Nonexperimental studies are those in which researchers investigate existing conditions or differences without manipulating them (Newhart & Patten, 2023). The designs for nonexperimental studies typically include plans to observe and describe behaviors, to determine relationships among measures of different skills, or to compare persons with different characteristics. Some examples of nonexperimental approaches include descriptive studies like surveys, opinion polls, case studies, and prevalence studies; relationship studies involving correlation and prediction; case-control studies and other comparisons of existing groups to identify differences by presence of a disorder, age, socioeconomic status, and so forth; and causal-comparative and cohort studies that examine the impact of possible causal factors over time (Newhart & Patten, 2023). In the next sections, we cover several common nonexperimental designs (survey, case study, longitudinal, correlation and regression, group comparison, and causal-comparative) and discuss their use in the field of communication sciences and disorders.

Survey Research

You might have personal experience with *survey research*. Perhaps a researcher has asked you to complete a paper-and-pencil, online, or telephone survey on some topic, such as your opinion on a certain product or on election issues. Survey research generally involves obtaining participants' responses to a series of questions, either through a written questionnaire or an interview (Trochim et al., 2016). Researchers might consider using a survey when they want to collect data that reflect opinions or reports of individual experiences and when they want to collect information from a relatively large number of participants (Writing@CSU, 1993–2024). Survey research may take a mixed-methods approach, incorporating both quantitative and qualitative analyses. When designing a survey, a researcher needs to decide on several components, such as those listed below:

1. Survey participants
2. Content of questions
3. Types of questions
4. Sequence of questions
5. Survey procedure (e.g., written or interview)

The subject matter of a survey is the most important factor to consider when deciding who should complete the survey. For example, if the survey focuses on consumer satisfaction with speech, language, or hearing services, the survey participants should be the persons who received those services rather than the audiologists and speech-language pathologists who provided the services. Sometimes researchers have choices regarding the most appropriate participants. For example, if a survey focuses on children's actions and attitudes toward peers with communication disorders, the survey participants could be the children or perhaps their teachers. Additionally, the researchers might decide to compare responses from different groups of participants. They might survey different age groups, different professions (audiologists, speech-language pathologists, speech-language-hearing scientists), persons in different geographic locations, and so forth.

The content of survey questions relates closely to the validity of the survey or the extent to which it covers the material professionals in the field would expect. Furthermore, survey researchers also need to consider if they are asking for information their respondents know, if the wording of the questions elicits appropriately specific information, and if the terminology in the questions is familiar to respondents (Trochim et al., 2016). A survey can include several types of questions, including yes/no, categorical response, rating scale, semantic differential, cumulative response, and open-ended formats (Trochim et al., 2016). Table 6–1 includes examples of each type of question.

In addition to making decisions about the kinds of questions to use, survey researchers also need to make decisions about the sequence of questions, as well as how to administer the questions to participants. Trochim et al. (2016) suggested that surveys should start with straightforward questions and present probing or difficult questions toward the end. In deciding whether to use a written survey or interview, researchers should consider the advantages and disadvantages of each approach. Advantages of written surveys include the possibility of displaying graphic or pictorial content, greater privacy for respondents, relatively low cost, and ability to recruit participants from a wider geographic area. Advantages of interviews include being able to explain the survey and answer participant questions, modify questions and ask follow-up questions, and include respondents who do not read or write (Trochim et al., 2016).

Although survey research is not the most common form of research in communication sciences and disorders, it does have an important role. For example, professional associations such as the American Speech-Language-Hearing Association conduct surveys on behalf of their membership (American Speech-Language-Hearing Association [ASHA], 2021, 2022, 2023). Surveys have also been published in professional journals on a variety of topics, and examples of these are described in Table 6–2. Examples of survey studies in communication sciences and disorders include surveying adults who stutter on quality of life, social support, and self-efficacy (Boyle, 2015); surveying ASHA-certified audiologists and speech-language pathologists on knowledge of, self-confidence in, and relevance of genetics for communication sciences and disorders (Peter et al., 2019); and surveying audiologists who fit hearing aids every month on strategies for fitting and fine-tuning hearing aids (Anderson et al., 2018).

Case Studies

Often audiologists and speech-language pathologists encounter unique and interesting cases in their clinical practice. For example, a speech-language pathologist might complete a speech and language evaluation of a child with a rare genetic disorder. Perhaps a search of the professional literature

Table 6–1. Examples of Five Different Types of Survey Questions

Type of Question	Example
Yes/No	1. Are you currently employed as an audiologists or speech-language pathologists? (Circle one) 　　Yes　　No
Categorical Response	2. What is your current class standing? (Place an X beside one) 　____ Freshman 　____ Sophomore 　____ Junior 　____ Senior 　____ Graduate
Rating Scale	3. Evidence-based practice will improve the quality of patient care in audiology and speech-language pathology. 　Strongly Agree　　　　　Neutral　　　　　Strongly Disagree 　　　1　　　　2　　　　3　　　　4　　　　5
Cumulative Response	4. In the past month, I provided speech, language, or hearing services to adults or children with: (Place an X beside all that apply.) 　____ articulation/phonological disorders 　____ auditory processing disorders 　____ conductive hearing loss 　____ fluency disorders 　____ language disorders 　____ sensorineural hearing loss 　____ voice disorders 　____ other (_____)
Open-Ended	5. In your opinion, what are the three most important issues facing the field of communication sciences and disorders?

revealed little if any information about the communication abilities of persons with this disorder. Hypothetically, an audiologist might complete hearing evaluations of workers and initiate a program to reduce industrial noise exposure at a manufacturing site. A search of the professional literature revealed very limited information on the unique challenges that emerged in this industrial setting. Both examples are situations that could lead to an interesting case study. Usually, when we think of case study research, we think of a descriptive study of an individual person. Case studies also can be descriptive studies of other "units," such as an individual classroom, a particu-

Table 6–2. A Sample of Recent Survey Research in the Field of Communication Sciences and Disorders

Author(s)	Groups Surveyed	Measure(s)
Anderson et al. (2018)	Audiologists who fit adults with hearing aids each month ($n = 248$)	Responses to questions regarding strategies for fitting and fine-tuning hearing aids
Blood et al. (2010)	School-based speech-language pathologists ($n = 475$)	Responses to questions about six scenarios that depicted bullying (three with specific mention of stuttering)
Boyle (2015)	Adults who stutter ($n = 249$)	Reponses to questions on quality of life, perceived social support, self-efficacy, and so forth
Brumbaugh and Smit (2013)	Speech-language pathologists working in pre-elementary settings ($n = 489$)	Responses to questions about treatment of speech sound disorders
Hyde and Punch (2011)	Teachers ($n = 151$) and parents ($n = 247$) of children who use cochlear implants	Survey responses to questions about the children's modes of communication
Larsen et al. (2012)	Parents of children with hearing loss ($n = 416$ returned surveys)	Survey responses to questions about when/how of early diagnosis
Peter et al. (2019)	Audiologists ($n = 233$) and speech-language pathologists ($n = 283$) with ASHA certification	Responses to questions assessing knowledge, self-confidence, and relevance of genetics in communication sciences and disorders
Schwartz and Drager (2008)	School-based speech-language pathologists ($n = 67$)	Responses to web-based survey covering knowledge and preparation for serving children with autism

lar acute care hospital, a specific industrial setting, and so forth. Also, researchers carrying out a case study could obtain either quantitative or qualitative data: Sometimes they choose both (Gillham, 2010; Hancock & Algozzine, 2011). For example, researchers might complete an in-depth evaluation using speech, language, and hearing tests that yield numerical scores. In addition, they could include interviews and direct observations. The data from the interviews and observations could be verbal in nature, such as direct quotes from those interviewed, or detailed field notes describing the person's behavior in different situations.

In designing a plan for a case study, researchers decide what measures, observations, and/or artifacts they want to collect. Two central features of most case studies are that the researchers use "multiple sources of evidence" (Gillham, 2010, p. 2) and that they study the case in typical, rather than experimental, settings (Gillham, 2010; Hancock & Algozzine, 2011). If the focus of a case study was a person with a communication disorder, you might gather information such as medical records and work samples (e.g., papers, drawings, other documents); you might administer a series of speech, language, and hearing tests; you would probably interview the client and/or family as appropriate; you also would observe the person in daily activities; and you almost always would obtain a spontaneous speech sample. If the focus of a case study was a unit such as a classroom or a medical facility, you could use many of the same methods, such as obtain records, review work samples, conduct interviews, or make observations. See, for example, a case study by Dupuis et al. (2019) evaluating medical comorbidities at one audiologic clinic. Data obtained for a unit case study might also include policy documents for the medical facility or the state's curriculum standards for that grade level. When studying a classroom, you probably would obtain work samples from many children, for instance, by collecting writing samples from them.

If you searched the professional literature in the field of communication sciences and disorders and specifically looked for case studies, you would find many examples. In audiology and speech-language pathology, case studies often focus on descriptions of the characteristics and/or treatment of persons with various disorders, such as Asperger's syndrome (Worth & Reynolds, 2008), children who use augmentative and alternative communication in a classroom setting (Ward et al., 2023), a young child who stutters (Santayana, 2023), cortical hearing impairment (Fowler et al., 2001), persistent horizontal semicircular canal benign paroxysmal positional vertigo (Moore, 2017), superior semicircular canal ampullae dehiscence (Ionescu et al., 2017), sudden sensorineural hearing loss (Kaul et al., 2019), and diagnosis of primary progressive aphasia in a multilingual individual (Utianski, 2023). Case studies may also provide insight on the interaction of multiple treatments/disorders. For example, variations in cochlear implant (CI) benefit or function have been reported in a case of a patient with a CI who received ototoxic chemotherapy (Harris et al., 2011) and in a case of a person with bilateral CIs with different hearing loss etiologies for each ear (McNeill & Eykamp, 2016).

Longitudinal Research

In *longitudinal research*, an individual or group is followed for some amount of time. Researchers often combine longitudinal observation with other approaches such as longitudinal case studies, a correlation study with the intent of predicting future capabilities or following different groups of children over time. Longitudinal research designs are common in studies of child development, including speech and language development. The amount of time covered in a longitudinal study varies considerably from relatively short studies of 1 to 2 years to very long-term studies of 25 or more years. Although longitudinal research often is nonexperimental, some experimental research does include long-term monitoring of treatment effects. Several of the case study examples identified above and some of the correlation/regression and group comparisons covered below are also longitudinal designs.

A cohort study is a special type of longitudinal research that allows researchers to study the emergence of disorders over time, the long-term effects of a disorder, or the long-term effects of treatment. One way to conduct a cohort study is to recruit a group of participants from the same birth or age group and following these individuals over time, periodically obtaining measures of the variables of interest, such as tests of speech, language, and hearing. Another way to conduct a cohort study is to identify a group of participants who share the characteristic of interest, such as children who received services for language disorders, or infants with hearing loss identified through an early detection program. At the time these individuals enter the study, they might not be experiencing any specific problems. The researchers might be interested, however, in determining if any problems emerge over time.

Two examples of large-scale longitudinal cohort studies are the Childhood Development after Cochlear Implantation (CDaCI) study (https://www.cdacistudy.org/; Fink et al., 2007) and the Outcomes of Children with Hearing Loss (OCHL) study (https://ochlstudy.org/; Moeller & Tomblin, 2015; Tomblin et al., 2015). With cohorts enrolled in a longitudinal research program, several studies of varying design and purpose are possible; a list of publications generated from the CDACI and OCHL studies are available at the respective websites. Two other examples of longitudinal research include a report on the incidence (i.e., new occurrence) and progression of tinnitus symptoms in a longitudinal study of hearing in a cohort of older persons (Gopinath et al., 2010) and a report on the long-term outcomes, into adulthood, associated with specific and nonspecific language impairment in a birth cohort in the United Kingdom (Law et al., 2009).

Another way to assess how a disorder progresses over time or characteristics at different ages/stages is to use a cross-sectional research design. Instead of observations of the same participants over a long period of time, cross-sectional designs make observations of different participants at different ages/stages over a shorter time frame. For example, Kumar and Sangamanatha (2011) recruited participants aged 20 to 85 years and assessed their performance, by decade of life, on temporal processing tasks. With a cross-sectional design, the authors did not have to wait for a 20-year-old to age to 85 but instead measured performance of different individuals at various ages. Cross-sectional techniques may also be used to assess prevalence; for example, Goman and Lin (2016) evaluated prevalence of hearing loss in the United States by decade of life in individuals aged 12 years to greater than 80 years, with data collection occurring over 10 years.

Correlation and Regression

Studies of relationships between two variables or among several variables and the kind of statistical analyses researchers perform are closely tied. If researchers are studying the relationship between two variables, then they usually perform a *correlation* analysis to determine strength of the relationship. If researchers are studying the relationship among several variables, they usually perform a *regression* analysis to determine the strength of the relationship and also which variables have the most predictive power. We will cover these statistical procedures in greater depth in Chapters 10 and 11. Our focus in this chapter is on the design of a study when the researcher's purpose is to investigate relationships.

Just as in designing other studies, researchers who are designing correlation and regression studies need to make decisions about who will participate, how to measure variables, and when to test the participants. In a correlation and regression study, a researcher recruits a group of participants and obtains two or more behavioral measures from each participant. This kind of study is nonexperimental because the researcher is measuring levels of performance that the participants have already achieved. The researcher is not training or manipulating the participants in any way to improve their performance. Usually, when researchers conduct correlation studies, they have reason to believe that two variables share some kind of relationship. The researchers might believe that both variables reflect the same underlying trait, or they might even suspect that the two variables share a causal relationship. Unfortunately, correlation research *cannot* establish causality, only that two variables relate to one another in some unknown way.[1]

Another decision you need to make when planning correlation and regression research is whether you are interested in the immediate relationship between the variables or the long-term relationship. If researchers are interested in an immediate relationship, they need to complete all their observations or testing within a relatively short time. For example, if some speech-language pathologists had developed a shorter, more efficient way to test children's expressive and receptive language abilities, they would want to compare their new approach to one or more existing and well-accepted tests. They would need to administer both tests within a relatively short time; otherwise, the children's expressive and receptive language abilities could improve to the point where the two tests no longer tapped the same underlying skills.

Sometimes researchers want to know how variables relate over time and conduct a longitudinal correlation or regression study. Often the goal of this type of research is to discover measures that will predict future performance. In designing a *prediction study*, researchers need to decide how long they should follow their participants. Do they want to predict performance 1 year in the future or longer? Researchers also need to decide how many measures they want to compare. They could design a study to investigate the relationship between just one predictor measure and one dependent measure (i.e., outcome measure). Researchers often obtain several predictor measures and determine which variable or combination of variables produced the best results. The research study may also be presented as identifying risk factors for development of a certain trait, disorder, or outcome. Some interesting examples of correlation or regression studies include several on the topic of predicting future academic achievement, literacy skills, or language abilities (Dale et al., 2020; Einarsdóttir et al., 2016; Pankratz et al., 2007; Reilly et al., 2007); a study to identify variables that predict communication participation in persons with multiple sclerosis (Baylor et al., 2010); an investigation of the relationship between verbal working memory and expressive vocabulary in 2-year-olds (Newbury et al., 2015); and a study evaluating predictors and/or risk factors for psychosocial development in children with hearing loss (Wong et al., 2018).

---

[1]Trochim et al. (2016) cited an interesting example that illustrates why the presence of a correlation is not evidence of a causal relationship. According to these authors, researchers have discovered a correlation between the number of infants born in the United States and the number of roads built in Europe. Trochim et al. pointed out that, although these two measures covary, there is no reason to assume a causal relationship. Rather, the two variables might both relate to a third unmeasured variable, such as the overall health of the world economy.

Group Comparisons

Group comparisons are another very common nonexperimental research approach in audiology and speech-language pathology. Although group comparisons can involve persons with normal communication, in communication sciences and disorders, group comparisons usually involve persons with some type of communication disorder, such as a developmental language disorder, phonological disorder, aphasia, voice disorder, stuttering, sensorineural hearing loss, and so forth. In research articles, you often see the term *case-control* for studies that involve a comparison of individuals with a disorder and a control group that is free of the disorder. When researchers design this type of study, they usually plan to test at least two different groups—for example, persons with hearing loss and those with normal hearing, or children with phonological delays and those with normal phonological development. The researchers also identify some skill(s) or characteristics they think will distinguish the two groups and decide on ways to measure those variables. Group comparisons have contributed to our understanding of the nature of speech, language, and hearing disorders; helped us better understand the impact of those disorders on development and participation; and provided clues into possible causes of communication disorders. Examples of nonexperimental group comparison studies in communication sciences and disorders include comparing adults with Parkinson's disease or multiple sclerosis to typical controls on measures of speech intelligibility (Stipancic et al., 2016); comparing adults with and without aphasia on measures of visual attention as recorded by eye tracking (Thiessen et al., 2016); comparing families with children who were deaf/hard of hearing, who had autism, or were both deaf/hard of hearing and had autism on questionnaires regarding family stress (Wiley et al., 2018); and comparing performance of older adults with and without probable mild cognitive impairment on an auditory processing test battery (Edwards et al., 2017). Table 6–3 includes a list of group comparison studies to illustrate the variety of topics addressed in the field of communication sciences and disorders.

Causal-Comparative Research

Identifying potential causal factors is an important avenue of study for audiologists and speech-language pathologists. Experimental research designs are the strongest designs for establishing cause-and-effect relationships, but experimenting on research participants to determine the causes of communication disorders would be entirely unethical. For example, if researchers hypothesized that inadequate nutrition during infancy caused developmental problems later in childhood, they should not conduct an experiment in which they randomly assigned some infants to a group that received an adequate diet and other infants to a group that received an inadequate diet. Such an experiment would violate the basic principles of protection of human participants and expose the infants to substantial harm. When conducting experimental research is inappropriate, researchers must identify an alternative approach for investigating the problem.

A *causal-comparative* study is one of the best alternatives for identifying potential causal factors. A causal-comparative study is similar to a prediction study but

Table 6–3. A Sample of Group Comparison Studies in the Field of Communication Sciences and Disorders

Author(s)	Groups Compared	Measure(s)
Blom and Paradis (2013)	Children with and without language impairment who were English language learners	A probe of past-tense use and a receptive vocabulary measure
Edwards et al. (2017)	Older adults with and without probable mild cognitive impairment	Auditory processing test battery
Fitzpatrick et al. (2015)	Children with normal hearing and children with mild unilateral or bilateral hearing loss	Direct audiological testing, parent reports, and vocabulary and language scores
Frizelle and Fletcher (2015)	Children with SLI, age-matched and younger children	Sentence repetition and scores on a test of working memory
Howell and Ratner (2018)	Adults who stutter and adults with typical speech	Ability to monitor phonemes in nouns and verbs and in different word positions
Jackson et al. (2020)	Children with a diagnosis of developmental language disorder and children with typical language development	Measures of short-term, verbal working, and visual-spatial memory
Lewis et al. (2015)	Adolescents with a history or speech sound disorder who did or did not have a language impairment	Tests of speech sound production, literacy, oral language, and oral motor abilities
Manheim et al. (2018)	Younger and older adults with normal hearing; older adults with hearing loss	Perception of time-compressed speech after brief exposure and after training
Moeller et al. (2007)	Infants with hearing loss and infants with normal hearing	Vocalizations
Stipancic et al. (2016)	Adults with Parkinson's disease or multiple sclerosis and typical controls	Speech intelligibility scores from listener transcriptions and analog scale judgments
Thiessen et al. (2016)	Adults with and without aphasia	Visual attention measured through eye tracking
Wiley et al. (2018)	Families with children who were deaf/hard of hearing, had autism spectrum disorder, or were both deaf/hard of hearing and had autism spectrum disorder	Questionnaires regarding family stress

incorporates a group comparison to investigate existing differences. One unique feature of causal-comparative studies is that researchers try to obtain several pieces of information about each participant. This feature is included to identify possible competing causal factors in the participants' background and thus to strengthen the evidence for the causal variable under study. Often potential causal factors covary with other factors that also could cause speech, language, and hearing disorders. For example, poor medical care, inadequate housing, and poor nutrition are all factors associated with living in poverty. If researchers wanted to study poor nutrition as a causal factor in developmental disorders, they would have to consider if other variables, such as poor medical care or inadequate housing, also could be causal factors. In a well-designed causal-comparative study, researchers obtain information about many variables, not just the variable under study, to control for possible alternative explanations of their findings.

Researchers interested in conducting a causal-comparative study might decide to conduct either a retrospective study or a prospective study. In a retrospective causal-comparative study, researchers identify persons who vary on some condition (Newhart & Patten, 2023). Usually, this variable is the presence or absence of a medical or behavioral disorder like a speech, language, or hearing disorder. After identifying their participants, they obtain an extensive amount of information about their participants' medical history and family and social background (Newhart & Patten, 2023). Frequently, this information will include the variable that is the focus of their study, as well as information about possible alternative causal explanations. For example, if the variable under study was poor nutrition, the researchers would also obtain information about other important factors such as medical complications at birth, number of siblings, parent income and/or occupation, maternal and paternal education, and so forth.

Prospective causal-comparative studies share some similarities with retrospective studies. Researchers identify a potential causal factor, identify groups of persons who vary on this factor, and then obtain an extensive amount of information about their participants. The difference is that researchers in a prospective study identify their participants at the onset of the potential causal factor and then follow them in a longitudinal research study. For example, if the causal factor was employment in an occupation where workers were exposed to environmental toxins, the researchers would identify the workers when they started their employment. They also would recruit a similar group who worked in an environment that was free of toxins. Over the course of their study, the researchers would periodically evaluate their participants to determine if any had developed a medical disorder or perhaps communication disorder, and then determine if the occurrence of disorders was greater in the group exposed to the environmental toxins.

The reasoning behind a causal-comparative study is, if a variable stands out as a potential cause after you control for many other variables, you have a strong argument for that variable as a cause of the disorder. Examples of causal-comparative research in communication sciences and disorders include studies of the developmental outcomes of low-birthweight infants (Imgrund et al., 2019; Nguyen et al., 2018), studies of the implications of recurrent otitis media for speech and language development (Brennan-Jones et al., 2020), and a retrospective study evaluating children with hearing loss, grouped according to vestibular loss presence/severity, and factors that might be associated with vestibular loss (Janky et al., 2018). Although evidence from nonexperimental research is not sufficient to establish cause-and-effect relationships, the evidence is stronger if the researchers control for other variables. Thus, in the research focusing on low birthweight and otitis media, the researchers needed to obtain information about other potential causal factors such as medical complications at birth, quality of prenatal care, number of siblings, parent income and/or occupation, and maternal and paternal education, among others.

Qualitative Research

Qualitative research is a term that encompasses a number of research approaches that share several characteristics. The most obvious characteristic is how researchers record and report their findings. In qualitative research, the data typically include verbal statements: direct quotes from participants, excerpts from writing samples, or detailed descriptions of behaviors (Gillham, 2010; Newhart & Patten, 2023; Trochim et al., 2016). In contrast, the data in quantitative research are numeric in nature.

Another characteristic is that qualitative researchers usually rely on *inductive reasoning* to formulate a theory (Newhart & Patten, 2023; Trochim et al., 2016). A qualitative researcher begins by gathering data in the form of oral or written statements, detailed descriptions, and so forth. After examining these specific forms of information, a qualitative researcher might identify trends or themes that emerged in the data and from these themes begin formulating a theory that fits the situation. That is, a qualitative researcher reasons from specific observations, to general trends, to overarching concepts. In contrast, quantitative researchers usually employ *deductive reasoning* and begin with one or more theories about possible outcomes. They develop a specific hypothesis or prediction that stems from theory. Quantitative researchers design a study that yields specific information that either supports or refutes their predictions. Thus, they reason from the general theory to a hypothesis or prediction, to gathering specific data to test their predictions.

Another important characteristic of qualitative research is that researchers study their participants in natural environments and situations. Qualitative researchers emphasize the need to understand the meaning of their participants' statements and behaviors and thus consider it vital to study participants in a natural, not artificial, context. In contrast, quantitative researchers usually set up an experimental or laboratory situation for their participants and ask their participants to perform activities they might not do in a typical day. Quantitative researchers emphasize the need to control the experimental situation so that all participants have very similar experiences during the study.

Qualitative researchers also tend to be responsive to their participants, be open-ended in their research approach, and adjust their procedures as a situation dictates. Thus, a qualitative researcher would use a set of questions as an interview guide but would follow the participants' lead regarding the topic of the interview. Similarly, they might plan to observe participants in certain situations but would be comfortable with a change in schedule and making observations in a different situation. In quantitative, group studies, the researchers' goal is to summarize findings across participants. Therefore, they need to obtain responses to the same questions from all participants and observe and test their participants in the same situations. Quantitative researchers have less freedom to modify their procedures to accommodate the unique needs of participants.

See Table 6–4 for a summary of general differences between quantitative and qualitative research, keeping in mind that specifics for a particular research question or problem may vary. Although considering how qualitative research compares to quantitative research is helpful, research often is neither purely qualitative nor purely quantitative (Chong & Plonsky, 2021; Damico & Simmons-Mackie, 2003; Gillham, 2010). In a study that is primarily qualitative, a researcher might count the number of statements that fit a certain theme; in a study that is primarily quantitative, a researcher might take detailed field notes regarding participants' behavior during a test situation. Furthermore, a quantitative researcher might obtain a series of specific observations before considering the theoretical bases for the study. An inductive approach is not exclusive to qualitative research. Some research may employ a mixed-methods research design, incorporating both quantitative and qualitative analyses. For example, to investigate how parents perceived the support they received when their child was diagnosed with hearing loss, researchers used a survey/questionnaire with a rating scale, cumulative response, and open-ended questions, in addition to semi-structured interviews with a smaller group of participants (Scarinci et al., 2018).

Because of their training and preferences, some researchers might consider themselves to be primarily qualitative researchers. Such persons would tend to approach most problems from a qualitative perspective. As we noted, however, qualitative and quantitative research are not exclusive approaches, and sometimes the decision to use a qualitative or quantitative approach is based on the nature of the problem rather than on researcher preferences (Gillham, 2010). Some problems might be inherently suited to a qualitative approach. If very little is known about a problem, if recruiting participants requires special care, if a problem is best understood through the viewpoint of an insider, or if a problem is best approached through long-term interaction and observation, researchers might favor a qualitative approach (Gillham, 2010; Newhart & Patten 2023). Qualitative research approaches are particularly valuable for understanding client perspectives on treatment and quality of life, and the reasons that clients fail to follow through with treatments (Curry, 2015b; Everard & Howell, 2018; Moorcroft et al., 2020).

Table 6–4. General Characteristics of Qualitative Versus Quantitative Research Designs

	Qualitative	*Quantitative*
Format	Verbal	Numeric
Reasoning	Inductive	Deductive
Environment	Natural	Controlled
Sample size	Smaller	Larger
Data per participant	More	Less

Sources and Analysis of Qualitative Data

Qualitative research is a grouping of research methodologies that share the characteristics presented above. Before discussing several of the most popular methodologies, we cover some general approaches to data collection and data analysis. The data sources for qualitative research could include one or more of the following:

- Interviews
- Open-ended surveys
- Focus groups
- Observations
- Documents or other artifacts
- Audio or video recordings of interactions

Qualitative researchers commonly employ more than one method to generate data (e.g., following a focus group with individual interviews, conducting interviews and then direct observations, or obtaining documents such as writing samples as well recordings of interactions or conversations). *Methods triangulation* is a term that refers to employing more than one approach to gathering data (Newhart & Pattern, 2023).

Qualitative researchers might choose one of several approaches when designing a study or even combine approaches (Trochim et al., 2016). Although qualitative research approaches apply to visual data (Rose, 2023), often data analysis starts with transcripts of spoken conversations or responses, written documents, written responses to questions, and/or detailed field notes. The process of data analysis begins with reading and rereading the transcripts, first to develop overall impressions of the content and eventually to code and interpret the content. Qualitative data analysis is an iterative process of coding, revising codes, and recoding data, as well as identifying the need to collect additional data (Bradley et al., 2007; Curry, 2015a). Codes are words or short phrases that the research team applies to segments of their transcripts (e.g., to conversational turns, sentences, or phrases) that capture the concept or real meaning that a participant was conveying (Bradley et al., 2007; Chong & Plonsky, 2021; Suter, 2012). Participant comments or statements that reflect the same underlying meaning would receive the same code. Through the process of reading and coding transcripts, qualitative researchers typically discover broad commonalities among some of their codes. Identifying commonalities leads to a code structure with overarching concepts or themes and subordinate concepts or subthemes or some other approach to categorization (Bradley et al., 2007; Curry, 2015a; Suter, 2012). Curry (2015a) noted that sometimes qualitative researchers start with a preliminary set of codes that they developed from their own experiences as well as from a review of literature on the topic. Having a preliminary set of codes does not lock the researcher into using the codes. Rather, researchers could still revise their codes as they read and reread transcripts in "an integrative approach" (Curry, 2015a). Reading, coding, and recoding transcripts is a lengthy process; qualitative researchers often employ software to manage the process. Readers might look for reviews online for tools such as NIVIVO, Atlas.ti, MAXQDA, and Dedoose, among others (Northwestern Libraries, 2022).

Many qualitative researchers utilize transcripts and some form of iterative coding in the initial stage of preparing their results. The way that the researchers ultimately report and discuss their findings in their final product, whether a research article or presentation, depends on the qualitative research method that guided their study. In the following section, we describe several of these approaches (e.g., ethnography, grounded theory, phenomenological analysis, conversation analysis, and case study) to illustrate some of the options available for qualitative studies.

Ethnography

Ethnographic research emerged from the field of anthropology and encompasses several methods of studying events or behaviors within their cultural context (Berg & Lune, 2012; Damico & Simmons-Mackie, 2003). Two concepts closely tied to ethnography are participant observation and field research (Trochim et al., 2016). Researchers using ethnographic methods spend considerable time in the situation or culture they are studying. That is, they spend time "in the field" initially to gain acceptance as a participant and eventually to gather information from persons within the culture. Methods used in participant observation include writing down detailed field notes, interviewing persons from the culture, and collecting cultural artifacts (Gillham, 2010; Miller et al., 2003).

Historically, anthropologists traveled to a remote geographic location to study a native culture. In contemporary applications of ethnographic methods, however, the notion of culture has a broader definition and might include the culture of a classroom, of a particular organization, of an event, and so forth (Hancock et al., 2009). One thing that sets scientific inquiry apart is its systematic nature. Miller et al. (2003) noted that researchers using ethnographic methods achieve scientific rigor through the number and extent of their observations, the detailed way they record or describe their observations, repeated review of their data, and ongoing revision of interpretations or conclusions.

When conducting an ethnographic study, the researcher identifies a cultural group that will be the focus of the inquiry (Creswell, 2013; Suter, 2012). This group might be relatively small, maybe a few audiologists or speech-language pathologists, but usually is fairly large, such as all personnel employed in a particular medical care facility. The key in defining a cultural group is that the members interact on a regular basis (Creswell, 2013). To study the group in question, researchers immerse themselves into the day-to-day activities of group members. Some of the challenges in ethnographic research are gaining access to the cultural group, identifying appropriate themes to study within the culture (e.g., relationship hierarchies, socialization and education practices), and then obtaining representative data from multiple sources, including direct observations of interactions, interviews, documents, and so forth (Creswell, 2013). Examples of settings for ethnographic research relevant to communication sciences and disorders include a residential school for the Deaf (O'Brien & Placier, 2015), a "social recreational group" for individuals with early-onset dementia (Phinney et al., 2016), and an Aboriginal community for culturally appropriate ways to evaluate children's narrative abilities (Peltier, 2014).

Grounded Theory

Qualitative researchers using a grounded theory approach have the goal of developing conceptual or theoretical models to account for observed behaviors, events, situations, and so forth. Trochim et al. (2016) described the product of grounded theory research as "an extremely well-considered explanation for some phenomenon of interest—the grounded theory" (p. 62). The data obtained to develop such a theory are similar to that collected in an ethnographic approach. Thus, a researcher will conduct interviews, make observations in the field, and collect documents for analysis.

The foundation of grounded theory research is a multifaceted approach to coding that begins with *open coding* as the researchers read and reread transcripts and documents, as well as create an initial set of codes to represent their data (Chong & Plonsky, 2021; Phillips et al., 2024). In this initial step, the codes emerge from the data rather than from preexisting expectations (Henwood & Pidgeon, 2003). *Axial coding* refers to examining the specific codes that the researchers created through open coding to identify commonalities and similarities among the codes. Qualitative researchers engage in *selective coding* when they identify a core or all-encompassing code that links to a theory or explanation that fits the data (Cohen et al., 2018; Henwood & Pidgeon, 2003; Phillips et al., 2024; Sybing, n.d.).

Although we discussed open, axial, and selective coding in order, grounded theory research often involves a recurring process of collecting data, examining, and coding. As concepts and theoretical notions emerge, additional data collection is more focused and designed to test these initial ideas. According to Henwood and Pidgeon (2003), researchers engage in data collection and coding until it is no longer productive, and no new "relevant insights" emerge (p. 136).

Ultimately, the adequacy of a grounded theory approach depends on how successful researchers were in generating a theory that fits their specific observations and provides explanatory power. Examples of research in communication sciences and disorders using a grounded theory approach include studies investigating effective ways to teach telepractice within a speech-language pathology program (Overby, 2018), the views of individuals who stutter with regard to psychological counseling (Lindsay & Langevin, 2017), shared decision-making for individuals with tinnitus and their clinicians (Pryce et al., 2018), understanding audiologists' perspectives on the ethics of working with industry (Ng et al., 2019), and explaining the parenting stress of mothers with children who are deaf/hard of hearing (Jean et al., 2018).

Phenomenological Analysis

The goal of researchers who adopt a *phenomenology* approach is to study a phenomenon or situation from the viewpoint of participants (Trochim et al., 2016). Researchers try to discover what participants perceive, how they interpret a situation, and what meanings they assign to events. "Lived experience" is a phrase commonly associated with phenomenology (Suter, 2012, p. 366). Giorgi and Giorgi (2003a) described an adaptation of phenomenology for scientific investigation in the field of psychology. In this version of phenomenology, researchers begin by obtaining "descriptions of experiences" from participants, often through interviews (Giorgi & Giorgi, 2003a, p. 247). In the next phase of the study, researchers read transcriptions of the interviews to gain an overall impression of the content and to discern the meanings being expressed by participants (Giorgi & Giorgi, 2003a). Once researchers have a transcript that is divided into a series of meaning units, the next step is to translate these meaning units into a few words that capture the "psychological meaning lived by P [the participant]" (Giorgi & Giorgi, 2003a, p. 254). Some examples of these interpretations include "feelings of emotional ambivalence" and "feelings of unsafety" (Giorgi & Giorgi, 2003a, p. 256). Giorgi and Giorgi (2003b) noted that the purpose of phenomenological research is to develop a clearer understanding of the situations people go through in their everyday lives. Phenomenological analyses have been applied to understanding speech-language pathologists' assessment procedures for children who use augmentative and alternative communication (Lund et al., 2017), perceptions of writing postinjury from adults with traumatic brain injury (Dinnes & Hux, 2022), and third-party disability of adult children of a parent with hearing loss (Preminger et al., 2015), among other topics.

Case Study

As noted previously, case study researchers might collect quantitative data, qualitative data, or a mixture of both (Hancock & Algozzine, 2011). When approached from a qualitative perspective, case study research methods have considerable overlap with other methods such as ethnography or phenomenology. Researchers spend time observing the case, conducting interviews, and reviewing various kinds of documents. What distinguishes case study research is the focus on an entity such as a person, event, classroom, or institution (Berg & Lune, 2012; Damico & Simmons-Mackie, 2003; Suter, 2012). Another common feature of a qualitative case study is that the researchers collect data in multiple ways, such as from interviews, observations in natural settings, and documents (Phillips et al., 2024). When designing a case study, researchers consider how broadly they want to investigate the case. Sometimes the scope of a study is all-inclusive: Researchers attempt to gather data from as many sources as possible, and they try to understand the influences that determine how the case functions within society (Berg & Lune, 2012). At other times, a case study is highly focused; researchers gather data only at a particular time, or they gather data regarding one of the case's many roles. When conducting a focused case study, researchers are trying to understand the influences that determined the case's actions and motivations at a particular time or when performing a particular role (Berg & Lune, 2012). The focus of data analysis in case study research is on the individual person or organization, but researchers might recruit more than one case that fits the topic of interest (Suter, 2012).

Berg and Lune (2012) noted that researchers have different goals when conducting case study research. In an *intrinsic* case study, the researchers' goal is to understand the particular entity they are studying, rather than to understand a larger context such as a culture or the organization of social behavior. In an *instrumental* case study, researchers identify a case that represents a phenomenon they want to study. They conduct a thorough investigation of this case by gathering data through various methods such as observation, multiple interviews, and examination of documents. The researchers' aim is to discover answers to questions of general interest in their field of study, rather than to gain insight into the behaviors and motivations of the individual case. Finally, in a *collective* case study, researchers identify several instrumental cases and gather data from all of them. A more extensive set of data should enhance researchers' ability to draw conclusions or gain insights that will generalize to other, similar entities (Berg & Lune, 2012). In fields such as communication sciences and disorders, case studies often focus on the perspectives of individuals with a communication or swallowing disorder. Two examples of qualitative case studies are parent perspectives on a cochlear implant when their child has cochlear nerve deficiency (Kotjan et al., 2013) and perspectives from the spouse of an individual with semantic variant primary progressive aphasia (Pozzebon et al., 2017).

Conversation Analysis

Conversation analysis (CA) is a qualitative approach that has been applied to many different conversational interactions, such as conversations between health care providers and their patients, parents and their children, counselors and their clients, and persons with communication disorders and their family members (Drew, 2008). CA focuses on interpersonal verbal communication, often with spoken language but also with American Sign Language. CA researchers focus on naturally occurring interactions from people's everyday experiences and not on research-specific interactions such as with focus groups or interviews (Sidnell, 2016). The data for CA usually are recordings of conversational interactions from which researchers study aspects such as turn taking, repair, actions that link to the goals of an interaction, and sequences of conversational actions (Sidnell, 2016). Specifically, the researcher might look at sequences of turns, or adjacency pairs, in which the actions of one speaker entail reciprocal expectations about the action of a conversational partner (Drew, 2008; Sidnell, 2016). That is, if you greet someone to initiate a conversation, you expect a response in turn; if you ask someone a question, you expect an answer.

In CA, speaker turns are viewed as actions that might suggest an appropriate response on the part of a listener. The response will show the speaker whether the partner appropriately understood the action (Drew, 2008). Depending on the partner's response, the speaker might either attempt a repair because of a misunderstanding or provide an appropriate response to the turn. Each participant's action or speaking turn is the basis for the partner's next turn, in a series of adjacent pairs. According to Drew (2008), the key features of CA are the researchers' use of data that emerge from natural situations in the form of audio or video recordings, use of actual statements rather than coded data, focus on "interactional properties" rather than quantifying turn types, and generating an explanation for how participants developed shared understanding of each other's conversational turns. In addition to an orthographic transcript of the conversation, CA researchers also use codes for prosodic features such as emphasis, pitch changes, duration of sounds, and codes for turn taking such as partial overlaps (see Drew, 2008).

The aim of CA is to determine ways that individuals organize conversation. Researchers who use CA collect many examples of conversation actions and partner responses, examine them for similarities, and thus discover phenomena that are common across actions and speakers. CA has been used to investigate conversational interactions in situations related to the field of communication sciences and disorders, such as investigations of communication with individuals with dementia (Hall et al., 2018), adults with aphasia (Barnes & Ferguson, 2015), and older adults with hearing impairment (Ekberg et al., 2017).

Overall, quantitative research approaches are far more common in the field of communication sciences and disorders than qualitative approaches. Nevertheless, several good examples of qualitative research are available in recent articles, as shown in Table 6–5.

One of the roles of a research design is to ensure that the results of a study accurately reflect the actual or real situation. Damico and Simmons-Mackie (2003, p. 133) noted that "interpretive adequacy" is the goal of qualitative research. One might think of interpretative adequacy as "describing and explaining" an experience in a way that reflects the participants' understanding of it and captures its meaning to society in general (Damico & Simmons-Mackie,

Table 6–5. A Sample of Studies in the Field of Communication Sciences and Disorders That Have Employed Qualitative Research Methods

Author(s)	Participants	Method
Barnes et al. (2023)	Two adults with cognitive communication disorders and verbosity following a traumatic brain injury and their conversational partners	Use conversation analysis to investigate how verbosity affected turn taking in interpersonal interactions
Ekberg et al. (2017)	Audiologists ($n = 26$) and older clients ($\geq$ age 55)	Used conversation analysis to investigate communication breakdowns and repairs with a focus on "other-initiated repair"
Gilbey (2010)	Parents/families of children with hearing losses; losses identified early in childhood ($n = 14$)	Conducted an analysis of themes on data from semi-structured interviews focusing on how the parents learned about their children's hearing losses
Hersh (2009)	Twenty-one persons with aphasia and 16 family members	A grounded theory approach was used to analyze participants' responses in an interview about their discharge from therapy
Hersh et al. (2012)	Thirty-four speech-language pathologists (SLPs)	Interpreted thematic analysis was used to analyze interviews to better understand how SLPs viewed the goals of aphasia therapy
Irizarry-Pérez et al. (2024)	Five Spanish-speaking mothers of bilingual children who were receiving school-based speech and language services	Used interpretative phenomenological analysis to identify themes from the mothers' responses in semi-structured interviews
Quinn et al. (2023)	Special education teachers ($n = 6$), speech-language pathologists ($n = 13$), and one assistant	Used coding and constant comparative method to identify themes related to children's use of augmentative and alternative communication in their classrooms

2003). In the following section, we discuss that ways that qualitative researchers provide evidence of interpretive adequacy and credibility.

Scientific Rigor in Qualitative Research

One of the functions of a research design is to establish the validity or credibility of the researchers' findings. In qualitative approaches, researchers might not use the term *validity*, but they do use other similar terms, such as *trustworthy*, *plausible*, or *credible* (Phillips et al., 2024; Newhart & Patten, 2023; Suter, 2012). Thus, when designing a qualitative study, researchers include procedures to demonstrate that their findings accurately portray the actual phenomenon or accurately interpret participants' experiences.

Some common issues that qualitative researchers need to address include researcher bias, descriptive adequacy, and interpretive adequacy. All persons have previous experiences, knowledge, and points of view that predispose them to act and to interpret new experiences in certain ways. In other words, all persons have sources of bias that influence their actions and thoughts. When researchers allow their previous experiences, knowledge, and points of view to influence their observation and interpretation of a phenomenon, the researcher is exhibiting *researcher* bias. In an extreme form, researchers might be selective in what they see, hear, and record due to this bias. The issue of researcher bias is crucial for qualitative approaches because the findings depend on the researchers' observations, field notes, interview questions, and interpretations. Eliminating the sources of bias—that is, the researchers' previous experiences, knowledge, and points of view—is unrealistic. Instead, qualitative researchers take steps to demonstrate that their data and interpretations were not unduly influenced by these pre-existing influences (Suter, 2012).

One strategy for minimizing bias is *reflexivity*. Researchers consider their previous experiences and beliefs associated with the topic of the study and reflect on how these experiences and beliefs might have influenced how they approached the research question, data collection, and interpretation (Jaye, 2002). Researchers sometimes overtly discuss their potential biases in their research notes or report. Another strategy researchers might use to address potential biases is *negative case sampling*. Given an awareness of how their prior experiences and beliefs could influence their findings, researchers might test their conclusions by a deliberate attempt to find instances in their data or perhaps to collect new data that are at odds with these conclusions (Bowen, 2005). Another strategy to address researcher bias is to use a triangulation strategy. In *researcher triangulation*, more than one person participates in developing the research question, collecting data, and analyzing and interpreting the findings (Newhart & Patten, 2013). If researchers with diverse backgrounds arrive at the same interpretations of the findings, the conclusions from the study are stronger.

To demonstrate *descriptive adequacy*, researchers need to show that they provided an accurate factual account of the events they observed and experiences participants reported. In addition, researchers try to demonstrate that they collected sufficient data to provide meaningful insights into the phenomenon under study. One strategy researchers use to enhance their descriptive adequacy is *prolonged engagement* in the field (Creswell & Miller, 2000). By spending more time in the field, researchers build greater rapport with participants, are more likely to observe significant events, and have opportunities to observe phenomena repeatedly. Researchers also use various forms of triangulation to increase descriptive adequacy. In *methods triangulation*, a researcher uses several different strategies to collect data, such as observation in the field, interview of participants, and review of documents (Newhart & Patten, 2023), and in *data triangulation*, a researcher collects data from several different participants using a similar strategy. For example, the researcher could interview a person with a communication disorder, interview one or more of their peers, interview family members, and perhaps interview an employer or teacher. A final strategy researchers might employ is *thick description*. A thick description is a highly detailed, specific description of a phenomenon (Suter, 2012). A researcher could prepare a factual account of a situation or event without achieving the level of a thick description. What sets a thick description apart is how thoroughly the researcher describes an event. For example, if researchers were describing an interaction between a parent and child, they would include details about the surroundings, what artifacts are present, and details about the behaviors of the participants.

The *interpretive adequacy* of qualitative research depends on how well the researchers captured and conveyed the meaning of an experience. When qualitative researchers focus on what an experience means to the participants, *participant feedback* is the primary strategy for establishing interpretive adequacy. The researchers might ask participants to read a factual description or an interpretation of an event, conversation, series of behaviors, and so forth. Then, the participants provide their views on the accuracy of the description or interpretation (Creswell & Miller, 2000).

Qualitative researchers might or might not use the term *validity* when referring to how well their findings represent an actual phenomenon. They almost always would include some of the above strategies or similar ones to demonstrate that their research was credible and trustworthy.

Summary

For some research questions, the best approach is to study an existing situation or phenomenon. Nonexperimental research, like experimental research, is a systematic form of inquiry with the goal of finding answers to relevant questions. Experimental research involves deliberate manipulation of the variable under investigation, however, and nonexperimental research involves studying a variable or difference that already is present. One might think of nonexperimental research as studying differences that are naturally occurring and experimental research as studying differences planned and created by the researchers. Researchers have many methods for investigating problems in a nonexperimental way. In the field of communication sciences and disorders, examples of nonexperimental research include surveys, case studies, prevalence studies, correlation and prediction studies, group comparisons, and causal-comparative studies. Although nonexperimental research approaches involve studying naturally occurring phenomena, they still include the features of systematic inquiry, such as a well-thought-out question, and a plan for collecting and analyzing data to answer that question.

Qualitative research encompasses a number of research approaches such as case studies, ethnography, grounded theory, and phenomenology. Qualitative researchers often gather data in the natural context of their participants' everyday lives, using methods such as observation in the field, collection and analysis of documents, and interviews. Usually, researchers collect, analyze, and report verbal data in the form of oral or written statements and detailed descriptions. Another characteristic is that researchers usually rely on inductive reasoning, beginning with specific forms of information and generating concepts and theories that fit that data. To enhance the credibility of their findings, qualitative researchers collect an extensive amount of data, often recruit more than one participant, use several data collection strategies, and check their observations and interpretations with other researchers as well as with the participants.

Review Questions

1. What is the primary difference between experimental and nonexperimental research designs?

2. Provide an example for each of the following types of nonexperimental research designs.
   a. Survey research
   b. Correlation study
   c. Case-control study
   d. Case study

3. Are case studies an example of qualitative or quantitative research? Explain your answer.

4. Do researchers conduct correlation studies to establish a cause-and-effect relationship between two variables? Explain your answer.

5. Explain how researchers test their participants when conducting a prediction study.

6. What kind of study is the best alternative for identifying potential cause-and-effect relationships when conducting a true experiment is not practical?

7. Identify the characteristics of qualitative research. Choose all that apply.
   a. Researchers using this approach rely on inductive reasoning.
   b. Researchers often use this research approach when very little is known about a topic.
   c. This research method usually yields a statistical report of results.
   d. The results might include quotes from the participants' statements.
   e. The researcher usually spends only a short time with each participant.

8. Which of the following research questions is most appropriate for a quantitative approach? Which is most appropriate for a qualitative approach? Explain your answers.
   a. What are the differences between the school interactions, with both peers and teachers, of fifth-grade students with communication disorders and fifth-grade students with typical communication behaviors?
   b. To what extent does parent education level predict the interaction skills of parents of 1-year-old infants with a history of very low birthweight and parents of 1-year-old infants with normal birthweight?

9. Which of the following are nonexperimental research approaches? Select all that apply.
   a. Randomly assigning participants to treatment and control groups
   b. Comparing scores on two tests in a correlation study
   c. Comparing children with communication disorders to age-matched peers
   d. Comparing baseline and treatment performance in a single-subject study
   e. Surveying a random sample of speech-language pathologists

10. What threat to credibility or validity might be occurring in the following scenario? A qualitative researcher was interested in studying how children with specific language impairment (SLI) communicated with their classroom teachers. The researcher believed that SLI would interfere with effective classroom communication. The researcher only wrote down instances in which communication breakdowns occurred between the children and their teachers.

11. List two strategies qualitative researchers use to address the issue of researcher bias.

12. How do qualitative researchers ensure that they have accurately portrayed the *meaning* of their participants' actions, statements, and beliefs?

Learning Activities

1. To learn more about the research designs covered in this chapter, read studies that exemplify that approach. See Appendix 6–1 for a list of example studies for each research design.

2. Select one of the following hypothetical research scenarios. Decide what research approach you would use. Provide some examples of the issues you need to consider in planning such a study.
   a. A graduate student wants to investigate the effects of communication disorders on the daily activities and participation patterns of persons with speech, language, or hearing disorders. Help the student develop a more detailed research question and research design. What research approach(es) should this student consider?
   b. A school-based speech-language pathologist (SLP) developed a procedure called *Rapid Spontaneous Speech Analysis*, which is a relatively quick way to assess preschool and school-aged children's spontaneous conversation. This SLP wants to conduct a study to determine if this new procedure is a valid measure of expressive language skills. Help the SLP develop a more detailed research question and research design. What research approach(es) should this SLP consider?

References

American Speech-Language-Hearing Association. (2021). *2021 audiology survey*. https://www.asha.org/research/memberdata/audiology-survey/

American Speech-Language-Hearing Association. (2022). *2022 schools survey.* https://www.asha.org/research/memberdata/schools-survey/

American Speech-Language-Hearing Association. (2023). *2023 SLP health care survey.* https://www.asha.org/research/memberdata/healthcare-survey/

Anderson, M. C., Arehart, K. H., & Souza, P. E. (2018). Survey of current practice in the fitting and fine-tuning of common signal processing features in hearing aids for adults. *Journal of the American Academy of Audiology, 29*(2), 118–124. https://doi.org/10.3766/jaaa.16107

Barnes, S., Bransby-Bell, J., Gallagher-Beverley, Z., Mullay, J., McNeil, R., & Taylor, C. (2023). Verbosity, traumatic brain injury, and conversation: A preliminary investigation, *Aphasiology, 37*(1), 1–24. https://doi.org/10.1080/02687038.2021.1977233

Barnes, S., & Ferguson, A. (2015). Conversation partner responses to problematic talk produced by people with aphasia: Some alternatives to initiating, completing, or pursuing, repair. *Aphasiology, 29*(3), 315–336. https://doi.org/10.1080/02687038.2013.874547

Baylor, C., Yorkston, K., Bamer, A., Britton, D., & Amtmann, D. (2010). Variables associated with communicative participation in people with multiple sclerosis: A regression analysis. *American Journal of Speech-Language Pathology, 19*, 143–153. https://doi.org/10.1044/1058-0360(2009/08-0087)

Berg, B. L., & Lune, H. (2012). *Qualitative research methods for the social sciences* (8th ed.). Pearson.

Blom, E., & Paradis, J. (2013). Past tense production by English second language learners with and without language impairment. *Journal of Speech, Language, and Hearing Research, 56*, 281–294. https://doi.org/10.1044/1092-4388(2012/11-0112)

Blood, G. W., Boyle, M. P., Blood, I. M., & Nalesnik, G. R. (2010). Bullying in children who stutter: Speech-language pathologists' perceptions and intervention strategies. *Journal of Fluency Disorders, 35*(2), 92–109. https://doi.org/10.1016/j.jfludis.2010.03.003

Bowen, G. A. (2005). Preparing a qualitative research-based dissertation: Lessons learned. *The Qualitative Report, 10*, 208–222. https://nsuworks.nova.edu/tqr/vol10/iss2/2/

Boyle, M. P. (2015). Relationships between psychosocial factors and quality of life for adults who stutter. *American Journal of Speech-Language Pathology, 24*, 1–12. https://doi.org/10.1044/2014_AJSLP-14-0089

Brennan-Jones, C. G., Whitehouse, A. J. O., Calder, S. D., Da Costa, C., Eikelboom, R. H., Swanepoel, D. W., & Jamieson, S. E. (2020). Does otitis media affect later language ability? A prospective birth cohort study. *Journal of Speech, Language, and Hearing Research, 63*(7), 2441–2452. https://doi.org/10.1044/2020_JSLHR-19-00005

Brumbaugh, K. M., & Smit, A. B. (2013). Treating children ages 3–6 who have speech sound disorder: A survey. *Language, Speech, and Hearing Services in Schools, 44*, 306–319. https://doi.org/10.1044/0161-1461(2013/12-0029)

Chong, S. W., & Plonsky, L. (2021). A primer on qualitative research synthesis in TESOL. *TESOL Quarterly, 55*(3), 1024–1034. https://doi.org/10.1002/tesq.3030

Cohen, L., Manion, L., & Morrison, K. (2018). *Research methods in education* (8th ed.). Routledge.

Creswell, J. W. (2013). *Qualitative inquiry and research design: Choosing among five approaches* (3rd ed.). Sage.

Creswell, J. W., & Miller, D. L. (2000). Determining validity in qualitative inquiry. *Theory Into Practice: Getting Good Qualitative Data to Improve Educational Practice, 39*(3), 124–130. http://www.jstor.org/journal/theointoprac

Curry, L. (2015a). *Fundamentals of qualitative research methods: Data analysis (Module 5).* YouTube. https://www.youtube.com/watch?v=opp5tH4uD-w&list=PLqHnHG5X2PXCsCMyN3_EzugAF7GKN2poQ&index=5

Curry, L. (2015b). *Fundamentals of qualitative research methods: Developing a qualitative research question.* YouTube. https://www.youtube.com/watch?v=_0HxMpJsm0I&list=PLqHnHG5X2PXCsCMyN3_EzugAF7GKN2poQ&index=2

Dale, P. S., von Stumm, S., Selzam, S., & Hayiou-Thomas, M. E. (2020). Does the inclusion of a genome-wide polygenic score improve early risk prediction for later language and literacy delay? *Journal of Speech, Language, and Hearing Research, 63*(5), 1467–1478. https://doi.org/10.1044/2020_JSLHR-19-00161

Damico, J. S., & Simmons-Mackie, N. N. (2003). Qualitative research and speech-language pathology: A tutorial for the clinical realm. *American Journal of Speech-Language Pathology, 12*, 131–143. https://doi.org/10.1044/1058-0360(2003/060)

Dinnes, C. R., & Hux, K. (2022). Perceptions about writing by adults with moderate or severe traumatic brain injury. *American Journal of Speech-Language Pathology, 31*(2), 838–853. https://doi.org/10.1044/2021_AJSLP-21-00212

Drew, P. (2008). Conversation analysis. In J. A. Smith (Ed.), *Qualitative psychology: A practical guide to research methods* (2nd ed., pp. 132–157). Sage.

Dupuis, K., Reed, M., Bachmann, F., Lemke, U., & Pichora-Fuller, M. K. (2019). The circle of care for older adults with hearing loss and comorbidities: A case study of a geriatric audiology clinic. *Journal of Speech, Language, and Hearing Research, 62*, 1203–1220. https://doi.org/10.1044/2018_JSLHR-H-ASCC7-18-0140

Edwards, J. D., Lister, J. J., Elias, M. N., Tetlow, A. M., Sardina, A. L., Sadeq, N. A., Brandino, A. D., & Harrison Bush, A. L. (2017). Auditory processing of older adults with probable mild cognitive impairment. *Journal of Speech, Language, and Hearing Research, 60*, 1427–1435. https://doi.org/10.1044/2016_JSLHR-H-16-0066

Einarsdóttir, J. T., Björnsdóttir, A., & Símonardóttir, I. (2016). The predictive value of preschool language assessments on academic achievement: A 10-year longitudinal study of Icelandic children. *American Journal of Speech-Language Pathology, 25*, 67–79. https://doi.org/10.1044/2015_AJSLP-14-0184

Ekberg, K., Hickson, L., & Grenness, C. (2017). Conversation breakdowns in the audiology clinic: The importance of mutual gaze. *International Journal of Language & Communication Disorders, 52*(3), 346–355. https://doi.org/10.1111/1460-6984.12277

Everard, R, A., & Howell, P. (2018). We have a voice: Exploring participants' experiences of stuttering modification therapy. *American Journal of Speech-Language Pathology, 27*(3S), 1273–1286. https://doi.org/10.1044/2018_AJSLP-ODC11-17-0198

Fink, N. E., Wang, N.-Y., Visaya, J., Niparko, J. K., Quittner, A., Eisenberg, L. S., & Tobey, E. A. (2007). Childhood Development after Cochlear Implantation (CDaCI) study: Design and baseline characteristics. *Cochlear Implants International, 8*(2), 92–116. https://doi.org/10.1002/cii.333

Fitzpatrick, E. M., Durieux-Smith, A., Gaboury, I., Coyle, D., & Whittingham, J. (2015). Communication development in early-identified children with mild bilateral and unilateral hearing loss. *American Journal of Audiology, 24*, 349–353. https://doi.org/10.1044/2015_AJA-15-0003

Fowler, C. G., Kile, J. E., & Hecox, K. E. (2001). Electrical status epilepticus in slow wave sleep: Prospective case study of a cortical hearing impairment. *Journal of the American Academy of Audiology, 12*(4), 174–182.

Frizelle, P., & Fletcher, P. (2015). The role of memory in processing relative clauses in children with specific language impairment. *American Journal of Speech-Language Pathology, 24*, 47–59. https://doi.org/10.1044/2014_AJSLP-13-0153

Gilbey, P. (2010). Qualitative analysis of parents' experience with receiving the news of the detection of their child's hearing loss. *International Journal of Pediatric Otorhinolaryngology, 74*(3), 265–270. https://doi.org/10.1016/j.ijporl.2009.11.017

Gillham, B. (2010). *Case study research methods.* Continuum Research Methods. Bloomsbury Publishing.

Giorgi, A. P., & Giorgi, B. M. (2003a). The descriptive phenomenological psychological method. In P. M. Camic, J. E. Rhodes, & L. Yardley (Eds.), *Qualitative research in psychology: Expanding perspectives in methodology and design* (pp. 243–259). American Psychological Association.

Giorgi, A. P., & Giorgi, B. M. (2003b). Phenomenology. In J. A. Smith (Ed.), *Qualitative psychology: A practical guide to research methods* (pp. 25–50). Sage.

Goman, A. M., & Lin, R. R. (2016). Prevalence of hearing loss by severity in the United States. *American Journal of Public Health, 106,* 1820–1822. https://doi.org/10.2105/AJPH.2016.303299

Gopinath, B., McMahon, C. M. Rochtchina, E., Karpa, M. J., & Mitchell, P. (2010). Incidence, persistence, and progression of tinnitus symptoms in older adults: The Blue Mountains Hearing Study. *Ear and Hearing, 31,* 407–412.

Hall, K, Lind, C., Young, J. A., Okell, E., & van Steenbrugge, W. (2018). Familiar communication partners' facilitation of topic management in conversations with individuals with dementia. *International Journal of Language & Communication Disorders, 53*(3), 564–575. https://doi.org/10.1111/1460-6984.12369

Hancock, B., Ockleford, E., & Windridge, K. (2009). *An introduction to qualitative research.* National Institute for Health Research. https://www.academia.edu/6790109/An_Introduction_to_Qualitative_Research

Hancock, D. R., & Algozzine, B. (2011). *Doing case study research: A practical guide for beginning researchers* (2nd ed.). Teachers College Press.

Harris, M. S., Gilbert, J. L., Lormore, K. A., Musunuru, S. A., & Fritsch, M. H. (2011). Cisplatin ototoxicity affecting cochlear implant benefit. *Otology & Neurotology, 32*(6), 969–972. https://doi.org/10.1097/MAO.0b013e3182255893

Henwood, K., & Pidgeon, N. (2003). Grounded theory in psychological research. In P. M. Camic, J. E. Rhodes, & L. Yardley (Eds.), *Qualitative research in psychology: Expanding perspectives in methodology and design* (pp. 131–155). American Psychological Association.

Hersh, D. (2009). How do people with aphasia view their discharge from therapy? *Aphasiology, 23,* 331–350. https://doi.org/10.1080/02687030701764220

Hersh, D., Sherratt, S., Howe, T., Worrall, L., Davidson, B., & Ferguson, A. (2012). An analysis of the "goal" in aphasia rehabilitation. *Aphasiology, 26*(8), 971–984. https://doi.org/10.1080/02687038.2012.684339

Howell, T. A., & Ratner, N. B. (2018). Use of a phoneme monitoring task to examine lexical access in adults who do and do not stutter. *Journal of Fluency Disorders, 57,* 65–73. https://doi.org/10.1016/j.jfludis.2018.01.001

Hyde, M., & Punch, R. (2011). The modes of communication used by children with cochlear implants and the role of sign in their lives. *American Annals of the Deaf, 155,* 535–549. https://doi.org 10.1353/aad.2011.0006

Imgrund, C. M., Loeb, D. F., & Barlow, S. M. (2019). Expressive language in preschoolers born preterm: Results of language sample analysis and standardized assessment. *Journal of Speech, Language, and Hearing Research, 62*(4), 884–895. https://doi.org/10.1044/2018_JSLHR-L-18-0224

Ionescu, E. C., Al Tamami, N., Neagu, A., Ltaief-Boudrigua, A., Gallego, S., Hermann, R., Truy, E., & Thai-Van, H. (2017). Superior semicircular canal ampullae dehiscence as part of the spectrum of the third window abnormalities: A case study. *Frontiers in Neurology, 8,* 683. https://doi.org/10.3389/fneur.2017.00683

Irizarry-Pérez, C. D., Bell, L. M., Rodriguez, M. N., & Vanessa Viramontes, V. (2024). Spanish-speaking mothers' experiences of school-based speech therapy. *Language, Speech, and Hearing Services in Schools.* Advance online publication. https://doi.org/10.1044/2024_LSHSS-23-00043

Jackson, E., Leitão, S., Claessen, M., & Boyes, M. (2020). Working, declarative, and procedural memory in children with developmental language disorder. *Journal of Speech, Language, and Hearing Research, 63*(12), 4162–4178. https://doi.org/10.1044/2020_JSLHR-20-00135

Janky, K. L., Thomas, M. L. A., High, R. R., Schmid, K. K., & Ogun, O. A. (2018). Predictive factors for vestibular loss in children with hearing loss. *American Journal of Audiology, 27,* 137–146. https://doi.org/10.1044/2017_AJA-17-0058

Jaye, C. (2002). Doing qualitative research in general practice: Methodological utility and engagement. *Family Practice, 19,* 557–562.

Jean, Y. Q., Mazlan, R., Ahmad, M., & Maamor, N. (2018). Parenting stress and maternal coherence: Mothers with deaf or hard-of-hearing children. *American Journal of Audiology, 27*, 260–271. https://doi.org/10.1044/2018_AJA-17-0093

Kaul, V. F., Kidwai, S., Lupicki, A., & Cosetti, M. (2019). An unusual case of sudden sensorineural hearing loss after cycling class. *American Journal of Otolaryngology, 40*, 605–608. https://doi.org/10.1016/j.amjoto.2019.04.016

Kotjan, H., Purves, B., & Small, S. A. (2013). Cochlear implantation for a child with cochlear nerve deficiency: Parental perspectives explored through narrative. *International Journal of Audiology, 52*, 776–782. https://doi.org/10.3109/14992027.2013.820000

Kumar, A. U., & Sangamanatha, A. V. (2011). Temporal processing abilities across different age groups. *Journal of the American Academy of Audiology, 22*, 5–12. https://doi.org/10.3766/jaaa.22.1.2

Larsen, R., Muñoz, K., DesGeorges, J., Nelson, L., & Kennedy, S. (2012). Early hearing detection and intervention: Parent experiences with the diagnostic hearing assessment. *American Journal of Audiology, 21*, 91–99. https://doi.org/10.1044/1059-0889(2012/11-0016)

Law, J., Rush, R., Schoon, I., & Parsons, S. (2009). Modeling developmental language difficulties from school entry into adulthood: Literacy, mental health, and employment outcomes. *Journal of Speech, Language, and Hearing Research, 52*, 1401–1416. https://doi.org/10.1044/10924388(2009/08-0142)

Lewis, B. A., Freebairn, L., Tag, J., Ciesla, A. A., Iyengar, S. K., Stein, C. M., & Taylor, H. G. (2015). Adolescent outcomes of children with early speech sound disorders with and without language impairment. *American Journal of Speech-Language Pathology, 24*, 150–163. https://doi.org/10.1044/2014_AJSLP-14-0075

Lindsay, A., & Langevin, M. (2017). Psychological counseling as an adjunct to stuttering treatment: Clients' experiences and perceptions. *Journal of Fluency Disorders, 52*, 1–12. https://doi.org/10.1016/j.jfludis.2017.01.003

Lund, S., K., Quach, W., Weissling, K., McKelvey, M., & Dietz, A. (2017). Assessment with children who need augmentative and alternative communication (AAC): Clinical decisions of AAC specialists. *Language, Speech, and Hearing Services in Schools, 48*, 56–68. https://doi.org/10.1044/2016_LSHSS-15-0086

Manheim, M., Lavie, L., & Banai, K. (2018). Age, hearing, and the perceptual learning of rapid speech. *Trends in Hearing, 22*, 1–18. https://doi.org/10.1177/2331216518778651

McNeill, C., & Eykamp, K. (2016). Cochlear implant impedance fluctuation in Ménière's disease: A case study. *Otology & Neurotology, 37*(7), 873–877. https://doi.org/10.1097/MAO.0000000000001061

Miller, P. J., Hengst, J. A., & Wang, S-H. (2003). Ethnographic methods: Applications from developmental cultural psychology. In P. M. Camic, J. E. Rhodes, & L. Yardley (Eds.), *Qualitative research in psychology: Expanding perspectives in methodology and design* (pp. 219–242). American Psychological Association.

Moeller, M. P., Hoover, B., Putnam, C., Arbataitis, K., Bohnenkamp, G., Peterson, B., Wood, S., Lewis, D., Pittman, A., & Stelmachowicz, P. (2007). Vocalizations of infants with hearing loss compared with infants with normal hearing. Part I: Phonetic development. *Ear and Hearing, 28*, 605–627. https://doi.org/10.1097/AUD.0b013e31812564ab

Moeller, M. P., & Tomblin, J. B. (2015). An introduction to the outcomes of children with hearing loss study. *Ear and Hearing, 36*, 4S–13S. https://doi.org/10.1097/AUD.0000000000000210

Moorcroft, A., Scarinci, N., & Meyer, C. (2020). "We were just kind of handed it and then it was smoke bombed by everyone": How do external stakeholders contribute to parent rejection and the abandonment of AAC systems? *International Journal of Language & Communication Disorders, 55*(1), 59–69. https://doi./10.1111/1460-6984.12502

Moore, B. M. (2017). Clinical decision-making to address poor outcomes in persistent horizontal semicircular canal benign paroxysmal positional vertigo: A case study. *Physiotherapy Theory and Practice, 33*(5), 429–438.

https://doi.org/10.1080/09593985.2017.1318426

Newbury, J., Klee, T., Stokes, S. F., & Moran, C. (2015). Exploring expressive vocabulary variability in two-year-olds: The role of working memory. *Journal of Speech, Language, and Hearing Research, 58*, 1761–1772. https://doi.org/10.1044/2015_JSLHR-L-15-0018

Newhart, M., & Patten, M. L. (2023). *Understanding research methods: An overview of the essentials* (11th ed.). Routledge Taylor & Francis Group.

Ng, S. L., Crukley, J., Kangasjarvi, E., Poost-Foroosh, L., Aiken, S., & Phelan, S. K. (2019). Clinician, student and faculty perspectives on the audiology-industry interface: Implications for ethics education. *International Journal of Audiology, 58*(9), 576–586. https://doi.org/10.1080/14992027.2019.1602737

Nguyen, T.-N.-N., Spencer-Smith, M., Haebich, K. M., Burnett, A., Scratch, S. E., Cheong, J. L. Y., Doyle, L. W., Wiley, J. F., & Anderson, P. J. (2018). Language trajectories of children born very preterm and full term from early to late childhood. *The Journal of Pediatrics, 202*, 86–91. https://doi.org/10.1016/j.jpeds.2018.06.036

Northwestern Libraries. (2022, April). *QDA software guides and tutorials.* https://libguides.northwestern.edu/c.php?g=114906&p=9075213

O'Brien, C. A., & Placier, P. (2015). Deaf culture and competing discourses in a residential school for the Deaf: "Can do" versus "can't do." *Equity & Excellence in Education, 48*(2), 320–338. https://doi.org/10.1080/10665684.2015.1025253

Overby, M. S. (2018). Stakeholders' qualitative perspectives of effective telepractice pedagogy in speech-language pathology. *International Journal of Language & Communication Disorder, 53*, 101–112. https://doi.org/10.1111/1460-6984.12329

Pankratz, M. E., Plante, E., Vance, R., & Insalaco, D. M. (2007). The diagnostic and predictive validity of the Renfrew Bus Story. *Language, Speech, and Hearing Services in Schools, 38*, 390–399. https://doi.org/10.1044/0161-1461(2007/040)

Peltier, S. (2014). Assessing Anishinaabe children's narratives: An ethnographic exploration of elders' perspectives. *Canadian Journal of Speech-Language Pathology and Audiology, 38*(2), 174–193. https://www.cjslpa.ca/files/2014_CJSLPA_Vol_38/No_02/CJSLPA_Summer_2014_Vol_38_No_2_Paper_3_eltier.pdf

Peter, B., Dougherty, M. J., Reed, E. K., Edelman, E., & Hanson, K. (2019). Perceived gaps in genetics training among audiologists and speech-language pathologists: Lessons from a national survey. *American Journal of Speech-Language Pathology, 28*, 408–423. https://doi.org/10.1044/2018_AJSLP-18-0069

Phillips, K. M., Tichavakunda, A. A., & Sedaghat, A. R. (2024). Qualitative research methodology and applications: A primer for the otolaryngologist. *Laryngoscope, 134*(1), 27–31. https://doi.org/10.1002/lary.30817

Phinney, A., Kelson, E., Baumbusch, J., O'Connor, D., & Purves, B. (2016). Walking in the neighbourhood: Performing social citizenship in dementia. *Dementia, 15*(3), 381–394. https://doi.org/10.1177/1471301216638180

Pozzebon, M., Douglas, J., & Ames, D. (2017). "It was a terrible, terrible journey": An instrumental case study of a spouse's experience of living with a partner diagnosed with semantic variant primary progressive aphasia. *Aphasiology, 31*(4), 375–387. https://doi.org/10.1080/02687038.2016.1230840

Preminger, J. E., Montano, J. J., & Tjørnhøj-Thomsen, T. (2015). Adult-children's perspectives on a parent's hearing impairment and its impact on their relationship and communication. *International Journal of Audiology, 54*, 720–726. https://doi.org/10.3109/14992027.2015.1046089

Pryce, H., Hall, A., Marks, E., Culhane, B.-A., Swift, S., Straus, J., & Shaw, R. L. (2018). Shared decision-making in tinnitus care—an exploration of clinical encounters. *British Journal of Health Psychology, 23*, 630–645. https://doi.org/10.1111/bjhp.12308

Quinn, E. D., Atkins, K., & Cook, A. (2023). Exploring classroom factors and augmentative and alternative communication use in qualitative interviews. *American Journal of Speech-Language Pathology, 32*(5), 2158–2177. https://doi.org/10.1044/2023_AJSLP-23-00041

Reilly, W., Wake, M., Bavin, E. L., Prior, M., Williams, J., Bretherton, L., Eadie, P., Barrett, Y., & Ukoumunne, O. C. (2007). Predicting language at 2 years of age. A prospective community study. *Pediatrics, 120*(6), e1441–e1449. https://doi.org/10.1542/peds.2007-0045

Rose, G. (2023). *Visual methodologies: An introduction to researching with visual materials* (5th ed.). Sage.

Santayana, G. (2023). Problem-solving in the Lidcombe program: A single case report. *Perspectives of the ASHA Special Interest Groups, 8*(5), 925–931. https://doi.org/10.1044/2023_PERSP-22-00184

Scarinci, N., Erbasi, E., Moore, E., Ching, T. Y. C., & Marnane, V. (2018). The parents' perspective of the early diagnostic period of their child with hearing loss: Information and support. *International Journal of Audiology, 57*(Suppl. 2), S3–S14. https://doi.org/10.1080/14992027.2017.1301683

Sidnell, J. (2016). Conversation analysis. In M. Aronoff (Ed.), *Oxford research encyclopedias: Linguistics*. Oxford University Press. https://doi.org/10.1093/acrefore/9780199384655.013.40

Stipancic, K. L., Tjaden, T., & Wilding, G. (2016). Comparison of intelligibility measures for adults with Parkinson's disease, adults with multiple sclerosis, and healthy controls. *Journal of Speech, Language, and Hearing Research, 59*, 230–238. https://doi.org/10.1044/2015_JSLHR-S-15-0271

Sutter, W. N. (2012*). Introduction to educational research: A critical thinking approach.* Sage.

Sybing, R. (n.d.). Understanding selective coding in qualitative research. *ATLAS.ti*. https://atlasti.com/research-hub/selective-coding?_gl=1*17mbcv7*_up*MQ..*_ga*NzU1ODEwMTEzLjE3MDkxNjk1NTU.*_ga_K459D5HY8F*MTcwOTE2OTU1NC4xLjEuMTcwOTE3MDY0OC4wLjAuMA

Thiessen, A., Beukelman, D., Hux, K., & Longenecker, M. (2016). A comparison of the visual attention patterns of people with aphasia and adults without neurological conditions for camera-engaged and task-engaged visual scenes. *Journal of Speech, Language, and Hearing Research, 59*, 290–301. https://doi.org/10.1044/2015_JSLHR-L-14-0115

Tomblin, J. B., Walker, E. A., McCreery, R. W., Arenas, R. M., Harrison, M., & Moeller, M. P. (2015). Outcomes of children with hearing loss: Data collection and methods. *Ear and Hearing, 36*, 14S–23S. https://doi.org/10.1097/AUD.0000000000000212

Trochim, W. M. K., Donnelly, J. P., & Arora, K. (2016). *Research methods: The essential knowledge base* (2nd ed.). Cengage Learning.

Utianski, R. L. (2023). Differential diagnosis of primary progressive apraxia of speech in a nonnative English-speaking patient: A clinical case study. *Perspectives of the ASHA Special Interest Groups, 8*(5), 834–846. https://doi.org/10.1044/2023_PERSP-23-00043

Ward, H., King, M., & Soto, G. (2023). Augmentative and alternative communication services for emergent bilinguals: Perspectives, practices, and confidence of speech-language pathologists. *American Journal of Speech-Language Pathology, 32*(3), 1212–1235. https://doi.org/10.1044/2023_AJSLP-22-00295

Wiley, S., Meinzen-Derr, J., Hunter, L., Hudock, R., Murphy, D., Bentley, K., & Williams, T. (2018). Understanding the needs of families of children who are deaf/hard of hearing with an autism spectrum disorder. *Journal of the American Academy of Audiology, 29*, 378–388. https://doi.org/10.3766/jaaa.16139

Wong, C. L., Ching, T. Y. C., Leigh, G., Cupples, L., Button, L., Marnane, V., Whitfield, J., Gunnourie, M., & Martin, L. (2018). Psychosocial development of 5-year-old children with hearing loss: Risks and protective factors. *International Journal of Audiology, 57*(Suppl. 2), S81–S92. https://doi.org/10.1080/14992027.2016.1211764

Worth, S., & Reynolds, S. (2008). The assessment and identification of language impairment in Asperger's syndrome: A case study. *Child Language Teaching and Therapy, 24*, 55–71.

Writing@CSU. (1993–2024). *Writing guide: Survey research*. https://writing.colostate.edu/guides/guide.cfm?guideid=68

APPENDIX 6–1

Examples of Research Designs

Note that studies may be more complex and incorporate multiple or mixed designs in addition to the referenced design.

Survey

Anderson, M. C., Arehart, K. H., & Souza P. E. (2018). Survey of current practice in the fitting and fine-tuning of common signal processing features in hearing aids for adults. *Journal of the American Academy of Audiology, 29*(2), 118–124. https://doi.org/10.3766/jaaa.16107

Boyle, M. P. (2015). Relationships between psychosocial factors and quality of life for adults who stutter. *American Journal of Speech-Language Pathology, 24*, 1–12. https://doi.org/10.1044/2014_AJSLP-14-0089

Peter, B., Dougherty, M. J., Reed, E. K., Edelman, E., & Hanson, K. (2019). Perceived gaps in genetics training among audiologists and speech-language pathologists: Lessons from a national survey. *American Journal of Speech-Language Pathology, 28*, 408–423. https://doi.org/10.1044/2018_AJSLP-18-0069

Schwartz, H., & Drager, K. D. R. (2008). Training and knowledge in autism among speech-language pathologists: A survey. *Language, Speech, and Hearing Services in Schools, 39*, 66–77. https://doi.org/10.1044/0161-1461(2008/007)

Stark, B. C., Dutta, M., Murray, L. L., Fromm, D., Bryant, L., Harmon, T. G., Ramage, A. E., & Roberts, A. C. (2021). Spoken discourse assessment and analysis in aphasia: An international survey of current practices. *Journal of Speech, Language, and Hearing Research, 64*(11), 4366–4389. https://doi.org/10.1044/2021_JSLHR-20-00708

Case Study

Craig, H. K., & Telfor, A. S. (2005). Hyperlexia and autism spectrum disorder: A case study of scaffolding language growth over time. *Topics in Language Disorders, 25*, 364–324.

Dupuis, K., Reed, M., Bachmann, F., Lemke, U., & Pichora-Fuller, M. K. (2019). The circle of care for older adults with hearing loss and comorbidities: A case study of a geriatric audiology clinic. *Journal of Speech, Language, and Hearing Research, 62*, 1203–1220. https://doi.org/10.1044/2018_JSLHR-H-ASCC7-18-0140

Kaul, V. F., Kidwai, S., Lupicki, A., & Cosetti, M. (2019). An unusual case of sudden sensorineural hearing loss after cycling class. *American Journal of Otolaryngology, 40*, 605–608. https://doi.org/10.1016/j.amjoto.2019.04.016

Kotjan, H., Purves, B., & Small, S. A. (2013). Cochlear implantation for a child with cochlear nerve deficiency: Parental perspectives explored through narrative. *International Journal of Audiology, 52*, 776–782. https://doi.org/10.3109/14992027.2013.820000

Pozzebon, M., Douglas, J., & Ames, D. (2017). "It was a terrible, terrible journey": An instrumental case study of a spouse's experience of living with a partner diagnosed with semantic variant primary progressive aphasia. *Aphasiology, 31*(4), 375–387. https://doi.org/10.1080/02687038.2016.1230840

Worth, S., & Reynolds, S. (2008). The assessment and identification of language impairment in Asperger's syndrome: A case study. *Child Language Teaching and Therapy, 24*, 55–71.

Correlational and Regression

Baylor, C., Yorkston, K., Bamer, A., Britton, D., & Amtmann, D. (2010). Variables associated with communicative participation in people with multiple sclerosis: A regression analysis. *American Journal of Speech-Language Pathology, 19*, 143–153. https://doi.org/10.1044/10580360(2009/08-0087)

Einarsdóttir, J. T., Björnsdóttir, A., & Símonardóttir, I. (2016). The predictive value of preschool language assessments on academic achievement: A 10-year longitudinal study of Icelandic children. *American Journal of Speech-Language Pathology, 25*, 67–79. https://doi.org/10.1044/2015_AJSLP-14-0184

Erb, J., Ludwig, A. A., Kunke, D., Fuchs, M., & Obleser, J. (2019). Temporal sensitivity measured shortly after cochlear implantation predicts 6-month speech recognition outcome. *Ear and Hearing, 40*(1), 27–33. https://doi.org/10.1097/AUD.0000000000000588

Newbury, J., Klee, T., Stokes, S. F., & Moran, C. (2015). Exploring expressive vocabulary variability in two-year-olds: The role of working memory. *Journal of Speech, Language, and Hearing Research, 58*, 1761–1772. https://doi.org/10.1044/2015_JSLHR-L-15-0018

Wong, C. L., Ching, T. Y. C., Leigh, G., Cupples, L., Button, L., Marnane, V., Whitfield, J., Gunnourie, M., & Martin, L. (2018). Psychosocial development of 5-year-old children with hearing loss: Risks and protective factors. *International Journal of Audiology, 57*(Suppl. 2), S81–S92. https://doi.org/10.1080/14992027.2016.1211764

Group Comparison

Edwards, J. D., Lister, J. J., Elias, M. N., Tetlow, A. M., Sardina, A. L., Sadeq, N. A., Brandino, A. D., & Harrison Bush, A. L. (2017). Auditory processing of older adults with probably mild cognitive impairment. *Journal of Speech, Language, and Hearing Research, 60*, 1427–1435. https://doi.org/10.1044/2016_JSLHR-H-16-0066

Helmstaedter V., Buechner, A., Stolle, S., Goetz, F., Lenarz, T., & Durisin, M. (2018). Cochlear implantation in children with meningitis related deafness: The influence of electrode impedance and implant charge on auditory performance—a case control study. *International Journal of Pediatric Otorhinolaryngology, 113*, 102–109. https://doi.org/10.1016/j.ijporl.2018.07.034

Stipancic, K. L., Tjaden, T., & Wilding, G. (2016). Comparison of intelligibility measures for adults with Parkinson's disease, adults with multiple sclerosis, and healthy controls. *Journal of Speech, Language, and Hearing Research, 59*, 230–238. https://doi.org/10.1044/2015_JSLHR-S-15-0271

Thiessen, A., Beukelman, D., Hux, K., & Longenecker, M. (2016). A comparison of the visual attention patterns of people with aphasia and adults without neurological conditions for camera-engaged and task-engaged visual scenes. *Journal of Speech, Language, and Hearing Research, 59*, 290–301. https://doi.org/10.1044/2015_JSLHR-L-14-0115

Wiley, S., Meinzen-Derr, J., Hunter, L., Hudock, R., Murphy, D., Bentley, K., & Williams, T. (2018). Understanding the needs of families of children who are deaf/hard of hearing with an autism spectrum disorder. *Journal of the American Academy of Audiology, 29*, 378–388. https://doi.org/10.3766/jaaa.16139

Causal-Comparative

Janky, K. L., Thomas, M. L. A., High, R. R., Schmid, K. K., & Ogun, O. A. (2018). Predictive factors for vestibular loss in children with hearing loss. *American Journal of Audiology, 27*, 137–146. https://doi.org/10.1044/2017_AJA-17-0058

Kilbride, H. W., Thorstad, K., & Daily, D. K. (2004). Preschool outcome of less than 801gram preterm infants compared with full-term siblings. *Pediatrics, 113*, 742–747.

Lampi, K. M., Lehtonen, L., Tran, P. L., Suominen, A., Lehti, V., Banerjee, P. N., Gissler, M., Brown, A. S., & Sourander, A. (2012). Risk of autism spectrum disorders in low birth weight and small for gestational age infants. *Journal of Pediatrics, 161*, 830–836. https://doi.org/10.1016/j.jpeds.2012.04.058

Shriberg, L. D., Flipsen, P., Jr., Thielke, H., Kwiatkowski, J., Kertoy, M. K., Katcher, M. L., Nellis, R. A., & Block, M. G. (2000). Risk for speech disorder associated with early recurrent otitis media with effusion: Two retrospective studies. *Journal of Speech, Language, and Hearing Research, 43*, 79–99. https://doi.org/10.1044/jslhr.4301.79

Ethnographic

O'Brien, C. A., & Placier, P. (2015). Deaf culture and competing discourses in a residential school for the Deaf: "Can do" versus "can't do." *Equity & Excellence in Education, 48*(2), 320–338. https://doi.org/10.1080/10665684.2015.1025253

Peltier, S. (2014). Assessing Anishinaabe children's narratives: An ethnographic exploration of elders' perspectives. *Canadian Journal of Speech-Language Pathology and Audiology, 38*(2), 174–193. https://www.cjslpa.ca/files/2014_CJSLPA_Vol_38/No_02/CJSLPA_Summer_2014_Vol_38_No_2_Paper_3_Peltier.pdf

Phinney, A., Kelson, E., Baumbusch, J., O'Connor, D., & Purves, B. (2016). Walking in the neighbourhood: Performing social citizenship in dementia. *Dementia, 15*(3), 381–394. https://doi.org/10.1177/1471301216638180

Grounded Theory

Jean, Y. Q., Mazlan, R., Ahmad, M., & Maamor, N. (2018). Parenting stress and maternal coherence: Mothers with deaf or hard-of-hearing children. *American Journal of Audiology, 27*, 260–271. https://doi.org/10.1044/2018_AJA-17-0093

Lindsay, A., & Langevin, M. (2017). Psychological counseling as an adjunct to stuttering treatment: Clients' experiences and perceptions. *Journal of Fluency Disorders, 52*, 1–12. https://doi.org/10.1016/j.jfludis.2017.01.003

Ng, S. L., Crukley, J., Kangasjarvi, E., Poost-Foroosh, L., Aiken, S., & Phelan, S. K. (2019). Clinician, student and faculty perspectives on the audiology-industry interface: Implications for ethics education. *International Journal of Audiology, 58*, 576–586. https://doi.org/10.1080/14992027.2019.1602737

Overby, M. S. (2018). Stakeholders' qualitative perspectives of effective telepractice pedagogy in speech–language pathology. *International Journal of Language & Communication Disorder, 53*, 101–112. https://doi.org/10.1111/1460-6984.12329

Pryce, H., Hall, A., Marks, E., Culhane, B.-A., Swift, S., Straus, J., & Shaw, R. L. (2018). Shared decision-making in tinnitus care—an exploration of clinical encounters. *British Journal of Health Psychology, 23*, 630–645. https://doi.org/10.1111/bjhp.12308

Phenomenological

Lund, S., K., Quach, W., Weissling, K., McKelvey, M., & Dietz, A. (2017). Assessment with children who need augmentative and alternative communication (AAC): Clinical decisions of AAC specialists. *Language, Speech, and Hearing Services in Schools, 48*, 56–68. https://doi.org/10.1044/2016_LSHSS-15-0086

Preminger, J. E., Montano, J. J., & Tjørnhøj-Thomsen, T. (2015). Adult-children's perspectives on a parent's hearing impairment and its impact on their relationship and communication. *International Journal of Audiology, 54*, 720–726. https://doi.org/10.3109/14992027.2015.1046089

Conversation Analysis

Barnes, S., Bransby-Bell, J., Gallagher-Beverley, Z., Mullay, J., McNeil, R., & Taylor, C. (2023). Verbosity, traumatic brain injury, and conversation: A preliminary investigation, *Aphasiology, 37*(1), 1–24. https://doi.org/10.1080/02687038.2021.1977233

Barnes, S., & Ferguson, A. (2015). Conversation partner responses to problematic talk produced by people with aphasia: Some alternatives to initiating, completing, or pursuing, repair. *Aphasiology, 29*(3), 315–336. https://doi.org/10.1080/02687038.2013.874547

Hall, K, Lind, C., Young, J. A., Okell, E., & van Steenbrugge, W. (2018). Familiar communication partners' facilitation of topic management in conversations with individuals with dementia. *International Journal of Language & Communication Disorders, 53*(3), 564–575. https://doi.org/10.1111/1460-6984.12369

7

Research on Assessments and Diagnostic Approaches

Main Points

- Assessments are frequently used as diagnostics in clinical environments and as outcome measures in research. However, assessments must first be investigated themselves to ensure their accuracy (*validity*) and consistency (*reliability*).
- Different types of validity and reliability measures may be appropriate depending on the characteristics and goals of the assessment.
- Item response theory is a relatively newer approach that evaluates items of an assessment in relation to an individual's traits, such as ability level.

A fundamental concern in research, as well as in clinical assessment, is to assess or measure in a way that is trustworthy and meaningful. One of the challenges for the field of communication sciences and disorders is that the characteristics we want to measure seldom are directly observable. Although audiologists and speech-language pathologists measure some variables that are physical in nature (e.g., air pressure, fundamental frequency, muscle action potentials, durations), many variables of interest are like psychological variables and measured with samples of behavior (Urbina, 2014). Measurements, even physical ones, are inherently inexact and clinicians and researchers need to keep that in mind (Urbina, 2014).

Researchers and clinicians need to understand the construction of rigorous measurement tools, either to choose appropriate published tests or to develop their own measures (Lester et al., 2014). Thus, this chapter focuses on the design of research that demonstrates the quality of assessments, whether for a published instrument or for a novel measure in an individual study.

Key Concepts in Measurement

To demonstrate that measurement tools are assessing abilities and characteristics in a way that is trustworthy and meaningful, researchers and test developers conduct studies on the tools. Often these studies employ nonexperimental research designs. Research that focuses on the development and improvement of measurement tools such as tests, questionnaires, checklists, and so forth fall under the branch of psychology called *psychometrics* (American Psychological Association, 2018; El-Den et al., 2020; Loewenthal & Lewis, 2021; Vitoratou et al., 2023). To better understand research on tests and other assessment approaches, we first need to consider a few key concepts about measurement.

Nearly all the assessment tools in audiology and speech-language pathology have the purpose of measuring some underlying *construct*, and often the construct is not something that we can directly observe. A construct is an underlying ability or trait that those who develop and use assessment tools want to infer from a set of observable behaviors or responses (Urbina, 2014). In a concrete way, the observable behaviors are answers to test items and the inferred underlying ability of receptive vocabulary, use of grammatical forms, ability to perceive tones or speech sounds, and so forth. Another related concept is that the answers to test items represent a *sample of behaviors* that represent the underlying construct and not all possible behaviors. As with any sample, the particular responses to the items on the day of a test may or may not be a good representation of the individual's underlying abilities or traits. An individual might perform differently on another day or with a slightly different set of test items. Potential variability in performance on a test means that researchers and clinicians might obtain test results that have some level of error in representing the underlying construct. If error in measurement is a possibility, we would benefit from knowing how much error we might expect. Thus, researchers and test developers conduct studies to provide evidence that the tools they created provide an adequate sample of behaviors to represent the construct of interest and that the tools also measure those behaviors in a way that minimizes error.[1]

Researchers and test developers who are planning studies for new measurement tools often operate from one of two theoretical perspectives. The first, and most common in the field of communication sciences and disorders, is *classical test theory*. Classical test theory encompasses assessment approaches that utilize a total score to estimate an individual's level of ability, knowledge, or trait (López-Pina & Veas, 2024). In conducting psychometric studies from the perspective of classic test theory, researchers and test developers acknowledge the fact that the obtained test is an imperfect estimate of the underlying construct. Thus, the obtained score on a test is a combination of the hypothetical true score plus measurement error, where the measurement error might impact the true score in a positive or negative way.

The other theoretical perspective, *item response theory*, is becoming more common in the development of audiology and speech-language pathology assessment tools. Item response theory considers the relationship between test performance and the underlying construct in a somewhat different way. As the name might imply, item response theory involves examining an individual's response to a particular item and determining how that item response related to the individual's level of ability, knowledge, or trait (Baylor et al., 2011; Fergadiotis et al., 2023; Urbina, 2014). The result of an item response analysis typi-

---

[1]You might wonder why we did not say "eliminates" error. Although eliminating error would be a desirable outcome, in real life, we cannot completely eliminate error because our assessments always involve a sample of behavior.

cally is a mathematical model that captures the relative difficulty of a test item and its power to differentiate among test takers on an ability or trait being measured (Urbina, 2014). For example, a test developer might test a group of individuals who possess different levels of an ability from low to high. Items on the test might range from least to most difficult. In a well-constructed set of test items, individuals with high ability should have the best chance of getting the most difficult items correct, whereas most test takers would get the easiest items correct. Analyses within item response theory provide evidence about how responses to individual items relate to levels of the underlying construct that the test developers intend to measure.

In the sections that follow, we discuss the kinds of research that test developers conduct to demonstrate the adequacy of their new assessment procedure. One additional notion to keep in mind is that any discussion of the adequacy of a test or other measurement links to the stated purpose of the tool (Brink & Louw, 2011). Thus, in the discussion of psychometric research in the following sections, we need to keep in mind the intended purpose of the measurement procedure and the degree to which the research supports that purpose.

Measurement Accuracy

A crucial consideration in developing tests and other measures is the extent to which the instrument provides an accurate and meaningful assessment of the underlying construct. The term *validity* refers to how well a test or measurement accomplishes its purpose. Research on validity provides evidence that scores from a test or measure represent an ability, behavior, or trait in an accurate way. The American Educational Research Association (AERA) et al. (2014) linked validity to the intended interpretations of test scores and indicated that validation research should "provide a sound scientific basis for the proposed score interpretations" (AERA et al., 2014, p. 11).

Research to support the validity of a particular use of a test or other measurement typically includes more than one type of validity, listed below.

- Judgmental
  - Face validity
  - Content validity
- Empirical—Criterion
  - Concurrent validity
  - Predictive validity
- Empirical—Theoretical
  - Construct

As we discuss these various types of validity, keep in mind that a test or procedure is valid for a specific purpose. Clinical and research interpretations of test scores are only meaningful when we use the test for its intended purpose. For example, administering a test of vocabulary comprehension is appropriate if you want to assess word knowledge, but not if you want to assess higher-order language use such as drawing inferences or recognizing word relationships.

Face and Content Validity

Both face and content validity involve judgments of test content and procedures; the difference lies in who makes the judgments. Professionals in various fields have ideas about the areas they usually assess or measure. A person who is reasonably well trained in the content of their field should have an informed opinion regarding what should be measured to document abilities such as language comprehension, speech sound production, speech recognition, and so forth. We use the term *face validity* to refer to validity based on a person's judgment of how well a test appears to accomplish its purpose. When professionals in communication sciences and disorders examine a test or other instrument and decide that it appears to have appropriate content, we could say that the test has face validity. Face validity might be regarded as a rather informal approach to establishing validity because it is based on individual ideas regarding appropriate content or procedures. Persons examining a test use their own internal standards when judging face validity rather than some type of empirical evidence. In some applications of face validity, the judges are untrained persons rather than professionals such as audiologists or speech-language pathologists. The notion of obtaining the opinions of untrained persons makes sense when you consider that the persons who take speech, language, or hearing tests usually are not trained in the fields of audiology or speech-language pathology. The persons who take tests might be more likely to maintain high motivation and attention to the task if they perceive that the test they are taking is an appropriate and meaningful way to assess their knowledge or skills. In a way, face validity might be thought of as the validity established by consumers. The consumers for speech, language, and hearing tests are the audiologists and speech-language pathologists who purchase the tests and their clients who take the tests.

The term *content validity* refers to another way of establishing validity using judgment. Demonstrating the content validity of a test usually involves a comparatively formal approach, however. Rosenthal and Rosnow (2008, p. 113) noted that a test with good content validity includes the "kinds of material (or content areas)" an expert in the field would expect. Another aspect of content validity is that authors base their testing approach on a model or theory that is well known. For example, tests of language abilities generally address components of language such as syntax, morphology, and semantics. Tests of word recognition usually include words that represent the phonological system of the target language.

To establish content validity, test developers might engage in all or most of the following: (1) define the purpose of the test; (2) conduct a thorough review of the literature and current tests on the construct of interest; (3) develop a bank of possible items to include on the test; (4) recruit a panel of experts to review the proposed items, (5) review the expert input and add, eliminate, or modify possible items; (6) conduct a pilot study with a group of test takers; (7) analyze the group's responses to items and make modifications; and (8) conduct validation research on the final version of the test with a larger group (AERA et al., 2014; Polit & Beck, 2006; Steiner et al., 2015).

One way that test developers could utilize a panel of experts is to host one or more focus groups and conduct a qualitative study. Focus group participants might respond to questions about the value of the proposed test items, how well the items represent the domain, and possible item bias on factors such as gender, culture, socioeconomic status, and so forth.

Panel members base their judgments on how well the test represents the underlying model or theory and how broadly it samples the expected content. The judges may also consider whether or not the test employs appropriate response modes, provides material in a motivating and attractive format, and addresses different skill levels such as recalling basic facts and definitions or drawing inferences.

Test developers might also obtain quantitative data from expert judges. A quantitative study might yield expert ratings on the value of each test item often using a 4-point rating scale with anchors such as highly relevant to not relevant or essential to unnecessary (Polit & Beck, 2006; Yusoff, 2019). A simple way to utilize the experts' rating is to calculate an average rating for each test item and then to retain items with the highest average ratings and eliminate or modify items with the lowest ratings. Polit and Beck (2006) and Ayre and Scally (2014) described two additional numerical analyses that test developers might use, the content validity index (CVI) and content validity ratio (CVR). The calculation of these indices is beyond the scope of this text. However, clinicians and researchers who are choosing measures should recognize that CVI and CVR reflect expert judgments on how well test items represent the intended content of a test.

Test developers in the field of communication sciences and disorders might recruit a panel of judges who are highly respected in the field of audiology or speech-language pathology. These individuals will draw on their knowledge of the field of audiology or speech-language pathology, on the information the test authors provide about the construct and theory underlying the test, and on their knowledge of the characteristics of better-quality tests. Often, test authors revise the original version of a test based on the feedback they receive from this panel of experts.

Keeping in mind that a test is valid for a specific purpose with certain people and test situations (Steiner et al., 2015), test developers often extend the items analysis to examine how different subgroups perform on test items, such as persons of different genders, cultural and linguistic backgrounds, socioeconomic backgrounds, or geographic locations. The purpose of examining subgroup performance is to determine if any of the items exhibit bias toward persons of any of the subgroups (AERA et al., 2014; López-Pina & Veas, 2024). Urbina (2014) described in detail how to conduct a study to determine item fairness.

Criterion Validity

Criterion validity is an empirical approach to validity that involves comparing a new test or measure to an existing one with a similar purpose that serves as the standard of comparison (Kurpius & Stafford, 2006; Lester et al., 2014; Urbina, 2014). One way to establish criterion validity is to recruit a group of participants and administer both the new test and the standard, comparison test to these participants. When you administer the new test and the criterion measure relatively close together, you are establishing the *concurrent validity* of your test. That is, you determine that the new test measures a content area in a way that is similar to the existing test, when the participants take the tests at approximately the same time.

Another form of criterion validity is when you administer the new test to a group of participants and determine how they perform on a criterion measure in the future. This latter type of criterion validity is sometimes called *predictive validity*. When scores on a test are valuable for predicting success in a future activity, such as career success, graduate school performance, or reading achievement, the test is said to have predictive validity. To establish predictive validity, test developers conduct a longitudinal study in which they administer their new assessment approach to a group of participants and then follow those participants over time, often a year or more later. The participants are reevaluated at the later time to determine if scores on the new test successfully predicted their future performance. An example of predictive validity is when educators or speech-language pathologists administered phoneme awareness tasks to children at approximately age 4 or 5 to determine if phonemic awareness abilities predicted future reading achievement. When the children were older, perhaps in first or second grade, the researchers assessed their reading skills and compared their reading scores with their earlier scores on the phonemic awareness tasks.

To conduct a study to provide evidence of criterion validity, whether concurrent or predictive, test developers and researchers need to recruit a group of participants and administer the new test as well as at least one additional measure called the *reference standard* (Brink & Louw, 2011; Center for Evidence Based Medicine [CEBM], 2024; Critical Appraisal Skills Programme, 2024; Scottish Intercollegiate Guidelines Network [SIGN], 2006). The reference standard should relate to the purpose of the new test and be a meaningful and accurate way to assess the underlying construct. The reference standard could be another well-developed test or a nontest variable such as success in graduate school or future success in the field of communication sciences and disorders (Urbina, 2014). The reference standard also could be a diagnosis (e.g., fluency disorder or sensorineural hearing loss) that stemmed from a battery of tests that together resulted in the diagnosis. Whether the researchers administer the new test and the reference standard within a relatively close time frame or administer the reference standard at some point in the future depends on the purpose of the validation study—to demonstrate concurrent validity with the reference standard or predictive validity with the reference standard.

When authors want to compare scores on a new test with scores on an existing standard of comparison, they might choose to compute a *validity coefficient*. A validity coefficient is similar to a correlation coefficient and ranges from 0.0 to 1.00. If a new test has no relationship to the standard of comparison, the validity coefficient will be low (e.g., approaching 0.0), but if the new test has a strong relationship to the standard of comparison, the validity coefficient will be high (e.g., approaching 1.0). Ideally, test developers want to obtain relatively high coefficients when they compute validity coefficients. Guidelines for interpreting correlation coefficients suggest that a correlation of approximately 0.75 or higher would be a strong correlation (Newhart & Patten, 2023); similarly, a validity coefficient of 0.75 or higher would indicate a strong relationship between new and comparison tests. Somewhat lower coefficients would be acceptable in some situations. This would be true when examining predictors of activities or achievements that have multiple influences, such as performance at work or school achievement. A single predictor, such as a test of discipline-specific knowledge, would only capture some of the influences on future job performance. Another caution to keep in mind is that a strong validity coefficient only has value if test developers have confidence that the standard of comparison was itself a valid assessment tool. For example, if the goal was to develop a measure that would predict future success as an audiologist or speech-language pathologist, the standard of comparison probably should be some measure of future performance in a clinical setting. Grades in graduate-level courses would not be a meaningful standard of comparison when the goal is to predict clinical skill.

In clinical fields such as audiology and speech-language pathology, accuracy is an essential characteristic of tests when the stated purpose is to diagnose individuals with communication disorders. To document diagnostic accuracy, test developers often obtain data on sensitivity and specificity (Steiner et al., 2015). *Sensitivity* encompasses how well a test identifies individuals who actually have the underlying trait or disorder and is expressed as a proportion of individuals accurately identified. *Specificity* encompasses how well a test identifies those who do not have the underlying trait or disorder. Sensitivity indicates how well the test identifies the presence of a condition and specificity how well it identifies that absence of a condition (Urbana, 2014).

To conduct research on sensitivity and specificity, test developers need to accurately determine the presence or absence of a condition in a study group. Typically, accurate diagnosis involves administering a highly regarded test or battery of tests that comprise the "gold standard" for diagnosis. The test developers then compare the results of their new test and the gold standard. Table 7–1 illustrates a hypothetical outcome for a study of test sensitivity and specificity. The desirable outcome is for the new test to identify the same individuals as the gold standard (i.e., test positive on both tests or negative on both tests). In this example, sensitivity was 90%. The new test identified 36 out of 40 individuals who actually had the condition. The specificity was 81%. The new test correctly identified 130 out of 160 individuals who did not have the condition.

Test developers could calculate two additional measures from sensitivity and specificity results. *Positive predictive value* refers to the percentage of individuals who test positive and actually have a condition and reflects the extent to which a measure overidentified individuals. For the example in Table 7–1, positive predictive value is 36 ÷ (36 + 30) * 100 or 55%. *Negative predictive value* refers to the percentage of individuals who test negative and actually are free of the condition. Negative predictive value in the example in Table 7–1 is 130 ÷ 134 * 100 or 97%.

One might wonder about the logic of comparing a new test with one that serves as a standard of comparison. If a test is available that audiologists or speech-language

Table 7–1. Illustration of Test Specificity and Sensitivity

	Positive for Condition on the "Gold Standard"	Negative for Condition on the "Gold Standard"
Positive for condition on the new test	36[a]	30
Negative for condition on the new test	4	130[a]
TOTALS	40	160

Note: Sensitivity is 36 ÷ 40 * 100 or 90%. Specificity is 130 ÷ 160 * 100 or 81%; [a]Positive on both tests or negative on both tests.

pathologists regard as the standard way of assessing a particular communication behavior, why would you need to develop a new test? Authors might have several reasons for developing a new assessment procedure. One reason could be to develop a shorter version of a test that takes less time to administer. A "short form" of an assessment might be published as a stand-alone test or as a subtest within a comprehensive assessment tool. An example of this would be when authors of a language test include a subtest to assess vocabulary comprehension. In this situation, test authors might compare their new subtest to the Peabody Picture Vocabulary Test–Fourth Edition, which could serve as the standard of comparison for vocabulary comprehension tests. Another example of this is when audiologists explored the use of shorter word lists to assess word recognition abilities of persons with hearing loss (Runge & Hosford-Dunn, 1985). In this case, the researchers compared their participants' performance on the short form of the test with the full test to determine if the two versions yielded similar results. Other reasons to develop a new test procedure and compare it with an existing test are when test authors believe the existing test has weaknesses that they have eliminated in their new test and when test authors are developing a series of tests that assess various aspects of speech, language, or hearing.

Construct Validity

Construct validity, the final type of measurement validity, might be the most challenging to understand. As noted earlier, a construct is an underlying ability or trait. The purpose of a test or measure might be to assess a single underlying ability of trait; alternately, a test might assess multiple constructs that have some meaningful association (Newhart & Patten, 2023). Test developers typically operate from the perspective of a particular theory or model that guides their choices of what behaviors to sample and how to design questions to test those behaviors. To establish construct validity, test developers analyze patterns of performance on test items to determine if they reflect the underlying theory or model.

To establish construct validity, test developers or researchers conduct a study in which they administer the new test to a reasonably large group of age-appropriate individuals. In one approach, the study participants complete only the new test, and the test developers look at patterns or relationships among test items. In another approach, the study participants complete two or more measures, which allows for examining relationships between test items and external standards of comparison.

One kind of relationship that provides support for a behavioral construct is *convergence* (López-Pina & Veas, 2024; Urbina, 2014). When a person performs in a similar way on test items, the items might be said to exhibit convergence. Similarly, when a person performs similarly on two different tests that appear to test the same construct, the two tests might be said to exhibit convergence. Another kind of relationship that is important for establishing the validity of a behavioral construct is a *divergent* relationship (López-Pina & Veas, 2024; Urbina, 2014). A divergent relationship might emerge when a researcher compares a person's performance on tests that represent two different behavioral constructs. For example, one test might assess an individual's motor skills, and a second test might assess cognitive abilities. A person could have very good cognitive abilities and relatively poorer motor skills, and, thus, scores from the test that taps cognitive abilities could be quite different from scores on a test that taps motor skills. A meaningful behavioral construct, as represented by performance on a set of test items, should exhibit both patterns of convergence and divergence, and analyzing patterns of convergent and divergent relationships between tests is one way to establish construct validity.

A second way that test developers study construct validity is to analyze patterns of relationships among items on a single test. Some tests and measures are built to assess a single underlying construct, whereas others are built to assess multiple, related constructs. An analysis of the correlations or relationships among scores on test items could confirm whether a test actual fits the theorized model. *Factor analysis* is an advanced set statistical methods for identifying one or more dimensions that underlie a large set of measurements (i.e., item responses; López-Pina & Veas, 2024; Urbina, 2014). In test development research, the measurements are the test item responses from a relatively large number of test takers, perhaps 100 to 200. The factor analysis provides test developers with data to either confirm the underlying dimensions predicted from the test's theoretical model, called confirmatory factor analysis, or possibly discover underlying dimensions, called exploratory factor analysis (López-Pina & Veas, 2024; Urbina, 2014).

Let's consider an example from the field of speech-language pathology. Oral language is a construct that speech-language pathologists frequently assess. A hypothetical model of oral language skills might include language components such as phonology, syntax, morphology, and semantics, as well as expressive and receptive language skills.

The behavioral constructs for such a model might be areas such as syntax in expressive language and receptive language, semantics in expressive language and receptive language, and so forth. When conducting a study to analyze how well a test samples these constructs, a researcher would expect to find the closest relationships among test items that sample the same behavioral construct. Thus, a strong relationship or convergence should emerge among items that sample syntax in expressive language, but these items should show a weak relationship or divergence compared with items that sample a different behavioral construct such as semantics in receptive language. Similarly, if researchers compared performance on the new test items with performance on an external standard, they would expect to find convergence when the two tests sample similar behavioral constructs (e.g., a subtest that samples expressive morphology compared with an established test of expressive morphology) but divergence when the two tests sample different behavioral constructs (e.g., the subtest that samples expressive morphology compared with an established test of receptive vocabulary).

Professionals who are developing a test for publication or trying to document the appropriateness of a measurement approach for an empirical study have a number of choices regarding how to demonstrate the validity of their procedures, including face validity, criterion validity, content validity, and construct validity. In addition to knowing that tests and measures provide valid information about underlying construct(s) linked to their intended purpose, clinicians and researchers in the field of communication sciences and disorders need to know that their assessment tools also measure in a consistent way. The next section of this chapter covers measurement consistency.

Measurement Consistency

The term *reliability* refers to the extent to which a test yields consistent and repeatable results (Newhart & Patten, 2023; Rosenthal & Rosnow, 2008). Like the options available for establishing validity, researchers and test developers also have several options for determining the extent to which their assessment procedures yield results that are consistent and repeatable. Research to support the validity of a particular use of a test or other measurement typically includes more than one type of validity, listed below.

- Reliability across raters
  - Interrater reliability
  - Intrarater reliability
- Reliability across time
  - Test-retest reliability
  - Alternate or parallel forms reliability
- Internal consistency reliability
  - Split-half reliability

As we discuss these various approaches, keep in mind that a test or procedure is reliable for specific purposes and under certain circumstances. Thus, a test might be a reliable measure when the client is attentive and focused on the task, but not when the client is inattentive or focused on some extraneous environmental stimulus. A test might be a reliable way to identify characteristics or traits but might not be a reliable way to measure change in those characteristics or traits over time. Decisions about the validity or reliability of a test are not dichotomous (e.g., a valid or invalid test; a reliable or unreliable test). Rather, these decisions reflect the degree to which a test is valid or the degree to which it is reliable. When reviewing research, we also need to remember that the research is meaningful for individuals from the same population as the sample that took part in the reliability study and not for all possible test takers (Steiner et al., 2015).

Rater Reliability

Rater reliability encompasses comparisons of scores from two different raters or from the same rater at two different instances. If a measurement procedure has *interrater reliability*, the procedure is one that yields consistent results when two different examiners or raters use the procedure to test the same persons. For *intrarater reliability*, the one examiner or rater readministers or rescores tests from individuals they tested previously, maybe about 2 weeks ago. To establish interrater reliability, researchers and test developers usually recruit a group of participants and then ask different examiners to score or test these participants using the same administration or scoring procedures. The different examiners could test the participants separately, usually at about the same time (such as both test administrations within 2 weeks of each other), or the examiners could individually score the same test sessions. The procedures to establish intrarater reliability are similar except the same examiner or rater would readminister or rescore the test a second time.

A couple of methods are available to establish rater reliability. One option is to compute a correlation coefficient to determine the strength of the relationship between two scores for each test taker, either from two examiners or raters or from the same examiner at different times. A strong correlation means that the two sets of scores yielded similar results. Persons who scored high when initially tested also scored high when tested a second time; conversely, persons who scored low when initially tested also scored low when tested a second time.

If test scores represent a continuous construct, test developers and researchers could compute a Pearson product-moment correlations coefficient as long as the data are consistent with the assumptions of normal distribution (Stemler, 2019). If test scores represent rank-ordered data, the test developers could compute a Spearman rank-ordered correlation coefficient. Both of these correlations are covered in Chapter 11 of this text. The Pearson and Spearman correlation coefficients range from 0 to 1.0, with values closer to 0 being low and values close to 1.0 being high. Readers might also see other options such as an interclass correlation coefficient or Cohen's kappa coefficient in studies of measurement reliability (Kurpius & Stafford, 2006). For more detailed descriptions of the latter options, readers might consult either Steiner et al. (2015) or Stemler (2019). Kurpius and Stafford (2006) suggested that a reliability coefficient of .70 would be adequate for research purposes when the comparisons are between or among groups, but reliability coefficients should be .80 or .90 and above for clinical purposes.

Stemler (2019) noted that percent agreement can be preferrable to calculating a correlation between test scores. Percent agreement captures information about the extent to which two or more raters score each test item the same way. Percent agreement can be a straightforward calculation as in the number of agreements ÷ (number of agreements + disagreements). Stemler also described a modified percent agreement (e.g., agreement if ratings fall within ± 1) and a procedure using Cohen's kappa statistic in which the calculation accounts for the level of agreement that would occur by chance alone. Generally, numerical estimates of agreement tend to be higher when looking at relative agreement as represented in the correlation between two raters compared to absolute agreement as represented by the item-by-item percent agreement between raters.

The example in Table 7–2 illustrates the difference between a correlation between two raters and percent agreement across items. The test in the example had 50 items; each rater independently scored the responses from 20 participants. Thus, the total number of responses across items was 1,000. The Pearson correlation coefficient between the scores from Examiner 1 and Examiner 2 was .99, indicating a strong level of agreement. However, the examiners actually differed on 10 of the 20 test scores. This occurred because the examiners scored 28 test responses differently, which resulted in a percent agreement of 97% (972/1,000 × 100). Stemler noted that calculating percent agreement in this simple way does not account for chance levels of agreement. Therefore, Cohen's kappa statistic, which provides a correction for chance agreement, is included in Table 7–2 as well. The kappa statistic was 94%. In our example, each calculation yielded a level of interrater agreement that would be acceptable for research or clinical purposes, but this might not be the case in all interrater studies.

Brink and Louw (2011) noted that individuals who develop and use tests and measurements need to consider some quality control aspects of studies of rater reliability. When investigating interrater reliability, the test researchers should keep the scores of other raters concealed. Similarly, when

Table 7–2. Illustration of Correlation and Absolute Agreement Between Two Raters

Participant ID	Examiner 1	Examiner 2
1	32	32
2	**29**	**30**
3	13	13
4	11	11
5	43	43
6	4	4
7	**14**	**15**
8	11	11
9	**28**	**32**
10	9	9
11	**28**	**31**
12	37	37
13	**23**	**28**
14	**16**	**18**
15	**21**	**25**
16	**31**	**32**
17	**27**	**31**
18	11	11
19	50	50
20	**19**	**22**

Note: Pearson correlation coefficient between the scores from Examiner 1 and Examiner 2 was .99. Bolded rows indicate instances when the two examiners differed in scoring items resulting in score differences. The percent of agreement for the two examiners across items was 97%. Cohen's kappa, which provides a correction for chance level agreement, was 94%.

studying intrarater reliability, the researchers should keep the raters' prior scores concealed.

Reliability Across Time

Another form of research on test reliability addresses the stability of scores across time. Both test-retest reliability and alternate forms reliability reflect the stability of scores over time, but in different ways. To establish *test-retest reliability*, the researchers recruit a group of participants and test them at two different times. With test-retest reliability, the same examiner usually administers both tests. If a measurement procedure has strong test-retest reliability, the measure yields consistent results from one time to the next when administered by the same person. As with interobserver reliability, you can compute a correlation coefficient to determine the degree of test-retest reliability once you obtain two scores for each participant. Selecting a measure with strong test-retest reliability is an important consideration when conducting a study of treatment outcomes because you need a measure that yields stable results from one test administration to the next. In that way, it is more likely that the changes you observe from the beginning to end of the study relate to the treatment received and not to measurement instability.

You might wonder how test-retest reliability is different from intrarater reliability because both types of studies involve two sets of scores from the same test takers. The two forms of reliability can be linked but are subtly different and can be studied separately. For example, test developers and researchers might ask raters to rescore a recorded test administration resulting in intrareliability estimates based on a single test administration (Harvey, 2021). Also, some tests and measures are self-report instruments that do not involve a rater. Test developers might recruit a group of test takers to complete the self-assessment at two different times to provide test-retest reliability data that did not involve an examiner or rater (Harvey, 2021).

Alternate forms reliability is a variation that test developers choose as an alternative to test-retest reliability (Urbina, 2014). In *alternate forms reliability*, the researchers or test developers construct two different, but one hopes equivalent, forms of a measure. The two forms include comparable test items and measurement of the same behavioral construct(s). Researchers conduct a study similar to the ones described above to determine if two different versions of a measure are alike and yield similar test scores. However, in this case, researchers administer one form to the participants first and then administer the second form a short time later. Again, because you have two scores from each participant, you can compute a correlation coefficient to determine the degree of reliability between the two alternate forms.

Urbina (2014) distinguished alternate forms and parallel forms of tests. Both alternate and parallel forms involve two or more test versions that cover the same content, have the same test structure, and use the same administration procedures. When test developers create parallel forms, the developers conduct research to show that the two versions also have statistical similarity on characteristics such as means and standard deviations (Urbina, 2014).

Internal Consistency Reliability

A final type of reliability is *split-half reliability*. To determine this type of reliability, you administer a test once to your participants. Following test administration, you split the test items into two equivalent forms and then compare the participants' scores for each form. One simple way to divide a test into equivalent halves is to split it into odd-numbered and even-numbered items. Rosenthal and Rosnow (2008) noted that obtaining two equivalent forms can be problematic depending on how the test is constructed and how it is divided. Generally, a measure that samples a single behavioral construct with a set of similar items would be easier to divide into equal halves than a measure that samples several behavioral constructs with different types of items. Because you obtain two scores from each participant, you can compute a correlation coefficient between the two halves of the test. Split-half reliability is regarded as a measure of internal consistency (Trochim et al., 2016). That is, the correlation between two halves of a test reflects the extent to which items on the test measure the same behavioral construct. Although the split-half reliability procedure has some limitations, one advantage is that you can determine this type of reliability from a single test administration. This could be an advantage for a researcher who wants to establish the reliability and internal consistency of a novel assessment procedure.

Simply dividing a test into odd and even numbers is a basic way of obtaining a split-half reliability coefficient, but the method has some weaknesses. One issue is that the two halves have fewer items and thus underrepresent the actual reliability of the entire test because the magnitude of a reliability coefficient is influenced by the number of items on a test (Trochim et al., 2016). Test developers often adopt a more sophisticated approach, the Spearman-Brown formula, for estimating the reliability of an entire test based on the split-half correlation (Lester et al., 2014; Trochim et al., 2016). Another issue is that a split into odd and even items does not necessarily create two equivalent versions of the test. Cronbach's alpha is a procedure that many test developers use to evaluate internal consistency.[2] Although an oversimplification, one can conceptualize Cronbach's alpha as the average correlation from all possible combinations when a test is split in half (Kurpius & Stafford, 2006; Lester et al., 2014). For example, an eight-item test would have 70 different combinations of 4 and 4. A test with more items will have many more combinations. The specific details of the Spearman-Brown formula and Cronbach's alpha are beyond the scope of this text, but audiologists and speech-language pathologists who have an interest in developing a new test or measure should be familiar with these options.

Once test developers or researchers complete studies that provide information about reliability of scores, they can go a step further and calculate additional statistics such as the standard error of measurement (see Chapter 11). As noted previously, determining reliability of an assessment procedure is a matter of degree. Computing correlation coefficients for interobserver, test-retest, or other forms of reliability provides quantitative information about the level of reliability. The level of reliability you need depends on how you plan to use the scores. Audiologists and speech-language pathologists who are testing individual clients and making decisions based on the client's test scores have a need for measures with high reliability. Higher reliabilities are necessary when individual scores will be interpreted. However, if you are going to base your conclusions on mean group scores, somewhat lower reliability coefficients are tolerable. This would be the case for a researcher who has tested many participants with the intention of comparing the scores of different groups.

Item Response Theory

Thus far, the research approaches that we have covered reflect the perspectives of classical test theory with a focus on establishing the reliability and validity of total test or subtest scores. Classical test theory has been the dominant approach for development of tests and measurements in the field of communication sciences and disorders. However, test developers and research have another option for studying the validity of a new measure called item response theory (Baylor et al., 2011). Con-

---

[2] The Kuder-Richardson 20 procedure is an alternative to Cronbach's alpha that is appropriate for tests with dichotomous response options such as yes/no responses (Kurpius & Stafford, 2006; Urbina, 2014).

sistent with its name, *item response theory* is an approach to research on tests and measurements that focuses on "the functional relationship between performance on a test item, the test item's characteristics, and the test taker's standing on the construct being measured" (Urbina, 2014, p. 3).

When conducting studies from the perspective of classical test theory, test developers need to administer the same items to all participants in the study's sample for analysis of total test scores. Using item response theory (IRT) when developing a test has some advantages compared to the classical procedures. One advantage is that the research provides information about item difficulty and how individuals with different levels of ability or trait respond to the item. Understanding item characteristics such as item difficulty means that you can compare the performance levels of different test takers even when the test takers respond to different items. You also can more easily compare test taker responses across different tests if the two tests measure the same underlying construct.

The basis of item response theory is a group of mathematical models that capture the relationship between status on an underlying construct, or level of ability, knowledge, or trait, and observed responses to test items (Urbina, 2014). Some mathematical models are relatively simple such as a model that relates an individual's level of ability to the difficulty of an item. Besides item difficulty, item research might focus on the discrimination parameters of an item or its ability to distinguish among low, moderate, and high ability levels, and item fairness or the degree to which the item functions differently for subgroups representing differences in gender, socioeconomic status, or race. An item response study requires that researchers identify and define the construct of interest, create a relatively large set of possible test items, administer possible test items to a large sample of appropriate individuals, and complete mathematical analyses of item responses relative to the test taker standing on the construct of interest (Baylor et al., 2011). Information from the item analyses might guide decisions about what items to keep, revise, or discard (Baylor et al., 2011).

One of the outcomes of an IRT mathematical analysis is an "item characteristic curve" (Baylor et al., 2011, p. 247). Figure 7–1 is an illustration of a relatively straightforward item characteristic curve depicting the probability of a correct response relative to one's level of ability. Level of an ability or trait often is represented by a scale of −3.0 to +3.0 with −3.0 representing lower ability, 0.0 representing moderate ability, and 3.0 representing high ability. In Figure 7–1, Item 1 is relatively easier and individuals with an ability level of approximately −1.0 have a 0.50 probability of getting the item correct; individuals with high ability, a level of 2.0 or higher, have a 1.0 probability of getting Item 1 correct. Item 2 is relatively more difficult and individuals with an ability of approximately 1.0 have a 0.50 probability of getting the item correct, and even individuals with the highest ability (e.g., 3.0) did not reach a 1.0 probability of getting the item correct. Item characteristics curves can represent other relationships such as the item's discrimination parameters or the probability of chance success due to a correct guess (Baylor et al., 2011; Fergadiotis et al., 2023; Urbina, 2014).

Using an item response theory approach provides test developers and researchers with some valuable options for developing new tests and measures. IRT models allow for the development of shorter tests that are still reliable. One of the applications of IRT models is in computer-based adaptive testing. With these types of tests, the items a test taker completes depend on their prior responses. Ultimately, an adaptive test can

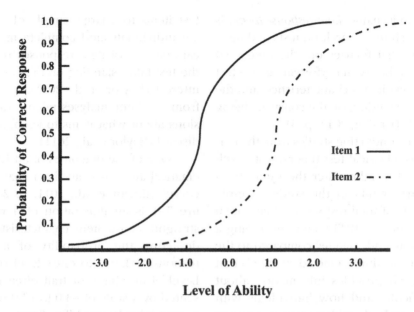

Figure 7–1. Illustration of item response curves for two items with different levels of difficulty.

determine the test taker's level of ability, knowledge, or trait and adjust the test items to achieve the most accurate estimate of that level. Even though test takers have different versions of the test, the scores are still comparable because the prior test research established item parameters such as difficulty, discrimination parameters, and so forth.

As consumers of test development research, we should expect to see more applications of item response theory in the field of communication sciences and disorders. We also need to be aware of some cautions related to IRT applications. The current IRT mathematical models work best for tests and measures that focus on a single underlying construct. Also, test items should exhibit "local independence," meaning that you cannot have questions that relate to one another, such as multiple comprehension questions on the same reading passage (Fergadiotis et al., 2023). Additionally, researchers might apply the wrong mathematical model to their item data, which can produce misleading results. Ideally, test developers and researchers will include information about their research analyses and discuss trialing alternate item parameter models to make sure they identify the model that is a best fit. Some underlying constructs are challenging to model, particularly when the construct scales from low to moderate to high ability. Reise and Waller (2009) discussed several examples from clinical assessment in the field of psychology that do not follow typical patterns. Readers who desire more detail regarding test development using IRT approaches and some of the challenges might read the articles by Baylor et al. (2011) and Reise and Waller.

Most published tests in audiology and speech-language pathology include information in their test manuals about the research to establish validity and reliability, and to determine item characteristics. On occasion, the most appropriate outcome measures for a study, however, might be novel or unpublished procedures. In these situations, researchers usually include information in the methods section of the research report about how they established the reliability of the measurements. Audiologists and speech-language pathologists also might find research articles that focus on the properties of tests and measures. Table 7–3 has some example articles that represent both research from the perspective of classical test theory and item response theory.

Summary

Speech-language pathologists and audiologists require tests and measures that provide information about our clients that is trustworthy and meaningful. Similarly, researchers need to choose measurement procedures or tests that assess in an accurate and consistent way to ensure that the findings of a study are worthwhile. To achieve these goals, test developers and researchers conduct studies from the perspective of classical test theory or item response theory.

Studies within classical test theory have objectives such as determining whether or not a new assessment tool is valid and reliable for its intended purpose. Validity refers to how accurately a measure or procedure represents an actual behavioral construct. Reliability refers to the extent to which a measure or procedure yields consistent or repeatable results. The options for establishing validity of a measure include face, criterion, content, and construct validity. Face validity could be established in a relatively informal way, but researchers and test developers conduct specific kinds of studies to establish the other forms of validity. Researchers also have several options for establishing reliability, including interobserver reliability, test-retest reliability, alternate forms reliability, and internal consistency reliability. The best measures and procedures for answering researchers' questions are those that have both high validity and reliability.

Studies within item response theory have objectives related to determining item characteristics and how individuals who represent different levels of an ability or trait respond to individual items. These studies yield information about item difficulty, item discrimination parameters, and differential item functioning related to membership in subgroups (i.e., item bias or fairness). Audiologists and speech-language pathologists as consumers of tests and measures should expect to see research on how well our tools accomplish their intended purposes.

Table 7–3. Examples of Studies in the Field of Communication Sciences and Disorders That Have Included Analyses from Classical Test Theory or Item Response Theory

Author(s)	*Participants*	*Method*
Boeschen Hospers et al. (2016)	Adults aged 18 to 70 years who participated in the Netherlands Longitudinal Study on Hearing ($n = 2{,}352$)	Applied item response theory (IRT) analyses to a self-report instrument, the Amsterdam Inventory for Auditory Disability and Handicap; determined that the inventory was appropriate for IRT analysis; reported on item characteristics such as item difficulty and item discrimination

continues

Table 7–3. *continued*

Author(s)	Participants	Method
Brackenbury et al. (2017)	Preschool children who represented a range of articulatory abilities as measured by the Goldman-Fristoe Test of Articulation–Second edition (GFTA-2) ($n = 154$)	Conducted item response theory analyses of subsets of items from the GFTA-2 to identify smaller sets of items that could function as a screening measure and adequately predict full test scores
Castilla-Earls and Fulcher-Rood (2018)	Children from ages 4 to 6 ($n = 100$) and three raters	Raters completed the Grammaticality and Utterance Length Instrument from the children's narrative retells; the researchers evaluated convergent validity through comparisons to other language measures and divergent validity through a comparison to a cognitive assessment
De Anda et al. (2022)	Children with dual English-Spanish exposure from three separate studies (total $n = 87$)	Conducted studies on an expressive language inventory for dual English-Spanish language learners to investigate several forms of validity
Fergadiotis et al. (2023)	Individuals with aphasia ($n = 107$) who had taken the Verb Naming Test (VNT)	Conducted item response theory analyses of items from the VNT; explored fit of different IRT models and concluded that IRT analyses were feasible for this test
Hornsby et al. (2022)	Multiphase study with 907 participants in Phase 3, including 7- to 17-year-old children ($n = 211$), parents ($n = 392$), and school professionals ($n = 304$), and 1,200 participants in Phase 4 also including children ($n = 225$), parents ($n = 532$), and school professionals ($n = 542$)	Administered preliminary version of self-report fatigue scale to participants in Phase 3; conducted exploratory factor analysis and item response theory analyses to identify items for the final version of the scale; administered final version of the scale to participants in Phase 4 and repeated the analyses from Phase 3; also conducted studies of test-retest reliability and construct validity
McRackan et al. (2019)	Adults aged 19 to 88 who had received a cochlear implant ($n = 371$)	Followed test development guidelines to generate and test a set of 81 items that met requirements for item response theory analyses; from the larger set of questions, created a 35-item domain-specific self-report instrument and a 10-item global instrument; selected items to represent a range of difficulty and the best discrimination parameters

Review Questions

1. _____ is a branch of psychology that focuses on the development and improvement of measurement tools such as tests, questionnaires, and checklists.

2. Explain how the concept of an *underlying construct* relates to observable behaviors or responses. Provide an example.

3. What is the most important difference between *classical test theory* and *item response theory?* Which is more dominant in the field of communication sciences and disorders?

4. Is it appropriate to say that a test is valid measure? Explain your answer.

5. A validity coefficient often is based on what statistic? Given the nature of this statistic, a validity coefficient would range from _____ to _____.

6. Provide a brief definition of test *sensitivity* and *specificity.*

7. _____ refers to the extent to which a test yields consistent and repeatable results.

8. What type of reliability is important for measuring the outcomes of a treatment study? How do you establish this type of reliability?

9. Identify the most accurate statement:
   a. A speech, language, or hearing test with high reliability might have low validity.
   b. A speech, language, or hearing test with high validity might have low reliability.

10. Describe each of the following forms of reliability:
    a. Interobserver reliability
    b. Test-retest reliability
    c. Parallel forms reliability
    d. Split-half reliability

11. Which statement is true?
    a. We test our subjects at two different times to establish split-half reliability.
    b. We test our subjects at two different times to establish test-retest reliability.

12. In item response theory, what is the usual relationship between the difficulty of an item and the test taker's level of ability or knowledge?

13. In item response theory, what is the difference between a test item's discrimination parameters and its fairness?

14. Identify three correct statements about research conducted from the perspective of item response theory (IRT).
    a. To conduct an IRT study, all test takers must answer the same test items.
    b. IRT research typically focuses on the pattern of responses to individual test items.
    c. An IRT study might yield an item characteristic curve showing item difficulty.
    d. In IRT research, you cannot compare test takers who complete different versions.

e. IRT studies might focus on item difficulty, discrimination parameters, or fairness.

Learning Activities

1. Select a published test or measure from the field of communication sciences and disorders. Review the test manual and look for answers for the following questions.
   a. What is the purpose of the test or measure?
   b. What general approach to test development did the authors take? Classical test theory? Item response theory? Both?
   c. What research studies did the authors conduct?
      i. Types of validity
      ii. Types of reliability
      iii. Item parameters (e.g., difficulty, discrimination, differential function or fairness)

2. Visit the following website to learn more about the research and the development of tests and measures.
   a. National Council on Measurement in Education–Digital Module Library (https://www.ncme.org/itemsportal/digital-modules)

References

American Educational Research Association, American Psychological Association, & National Council on Measurement in Education Joint Committee on the Standards for Educational and Psychological Testing. (2014). *Standards for educational and psychological testing.* American Educational Research Association.

American Psychological Association (2018, April 19). Psychometrics. *APA dictionary of psychology.* https://dictionary.apa.org/psychometrics

Ayre, C., & Scally, A. J. (2014). Critical values for Lawshe's content validity ratio: Revisiting the original methods of calculation. *Measurement and Evaluation in Counseling and Development, 47*(1), 79–86. https://doi.org/10.1177/0748175613513808

Baylor, C., Hula, W., Donovan, N. J., Doyle, P. J., Kendall, D., & Yorkston, K. (2011). An introduction to item response theory and Rasch models for speech-language pathologists. *American Journal of Speech-Language Pathology, 20*, 243–259. https://doi.org/10.1044/1058-0360(2011/10-0079)

Boeschen Hospers, J. M., Smits, N., Smits, C., Stam, M., Caroline B. Terwee, C. B., & Kramer, S. E. (2016). Reevaluation of the Amsterdam Inventory for Auditory Disability and Handicap using item response theory. *Journal of Speech, Language, and Hearing Research, 59*, 373–383. https://doi.org/10.1044/2015_JSLHR-H-15-0156

Brackenbury, T., Zickar, M. J., Munson, B., & Storkel, H. L. (2017). Applying item response theory to the development of a screening adaptation of the Goldman-Fristoe Test of Articulation–Second edition. *Journal of Speech, Language, and Hearing Research, 60*, 2672–2679. https://doi.org/10.1044/2017_JSLHR-L-16-0392

Brink, Y., & Louw, Q. A. (2011). Clinical instruments: Reliability and validity critical appraisal. *Journal of Evaluation in Clinical Practice, 18*(2012), 1126–1132. https://doi.org/10.1111/j.1365-2753.2011.01707.x

Castilla-Earls, A., & Fulcher-Rood, K. (2018). Convergent and divergent validity of the grammaticality and utterance length instrument. *Journal of Speech, Language, and Hearing Research, 61*, 120–129. https://doi.org/10.1044/2017_JSLHR-L-17-0152

Center for Evidence Based Medicine. (2024). *Critical appraisal tools: Diagnostics.* Nuffield Department of Primary Care Health Sciences.

https://www.cebm.ox.ac.uk/resources/ebm-tools/critical-appraisal-tools

Critical Appraisal Skills Programme. (2024). *CASP checklists: CASP diagnostic study checklist.* https://casp-uk.net/casp-tools-checklists/

De Anda, S., Cycyk, L, M., Moore, H., Huerta, L., Larson, A. L., & King, M. (2022). Psychometric properties of the English–Spanish vocabulary inventory in toddlers with and without early language delay. *Journal of Speech, Language, and Hearing Research*, 65(2), 672–691. https://doi.org/10.1044/2021_JSLHR-21-00240

El-Den, S., Schneider, C., Mirzaei, A., & Carter, S. (2020). How to measure a latent construct: Psychometric principles for the development and validation of measurement instruments. *International Journal of Pharmacy Practice*, 28, 26–336. https://doi.org/10.1111/ijpp.12600

Fergadiotis, G., Casilio, M., Dickey, M. W., Steel, S., Nicholson, H., Fleegle, M., Swiderski, A., & Hula, W. D. (2023). Item response theory modeling of the Verb Naming Test. *Journal of Speech, Language, and Hearing Research*, 66, 1718–1739. https://doi.org/10.1044/2023_JSLHR-22-00458

Harvey, N. D. (2021). A simple guide to interrater, intra-rater and test-retest reliability for animal behaviour studies. *OSF Preprints.* https://doi.org/10.31219/osf.io/8stpy

Hornsby, B. W. Y., Camarata, S., Cho, S.-J., Davis, H., McGarrigle, R., & Bess, F. H. (2022). Development and evaluation of pediatric versions of the Vanderbilt Fatigue Scale for Children with hearing loss. *Journal of Speech, Language, and Hearing Research*, 65, 2343–2363. https://doi.org/10.1044/2022_JSLHR-22-00051

Kurpius, S. E. R., & Stafford, M. E. (2006). *Testing and measurement: A user-friendly guide.* Sage.

Lester, P. E., Inman, D. & Bishop, L. K. (2014). *Handbook of tests and measurement in education and the social sciences* (3rd ed.). Rowman & Littlefield Publishers.

Loewenthal, K. M., & Lewis, C. A. (2021). *An introduction to psychological tests and scales* (3rd ed.). Taylor & Francis Group.

López-Pina, J.-A., & Veas, A. (2024). Validation of psychometric instruments with classical test theory in social and health sciences: A practical guide. *Annals of Psychology*, 40(1), 163–170. https://doi.org/10.6018/analesps.583991

McRackan, T. R., Hand, B. N., Cochlear Implant Quality of Life Development Consortium, Velozo, C. A., & Dubno, J. R. (2019). Cochlear Implant Quality of Life (CIQOL): Development of a profile instrument (CIQOL-35 Profile) and a global measure (CIQOL-10 Global). *Journal of Speech, Language, and Hearing Research*, 62, 3554–3563. https://doi.org/10.1044/2019_JSLHR-H-19-0142

Newhart, M., & Patten, M. L. (2023). *Understanding research methods: An overview of the essentials* (11th ed.). Routledge Taylor & Francis Group.

Polit, D. F., & Beck, C. T. (2006). The Content Validity Index: Are you sure you know what's being reported? Critique and recommendations. *Research in Nursing & Health*, 29, 489–497. https://doi.org/10.1002/nur

Reise, S. P., & Waller, N. G. (2009). Item response theory and clinical measurement. *Annual Review of Clinical Psychology*, 5, 27–48. https://doi.org/10.1146/annurev.clinpsy.032408.153553

Rosenthal, R., & Rosnow, R. L. (2008). *Essentials of behavioral research: Methods and data analysis* (3rd ed.). McGraw-Hill.

Runge, C. A., & Hosford-Dunn, H. (1985). Word recognition performance with modified CID W-22 word lists. *Journal of Speech and Hearing Research*, 28, 355–362.

Scottish Intercollegiate Guidelines Network (SIGN). (2006). *Methodology checklist 5: Diagnostic studies.* https://www.sign.ac.uk/what-we-do/methodology/checklists/

Steiner, D. L., Norman, G. R., & Cairney, J. (2015). *Health measurement scales: A practical guide to their development and use* (5th ed.). Oxford University Press.

Stemler, S. E. (2019). A comparison of consensus, consistency, and measurement approaches to estimating interrater reliability. *Practical Assessment, Research, and Evaluation*, 9, Article 4. https://doi.org/10.7275/96jp-xz07

Trochim, W. M. K., Donnelly, J. P., & Arora, K. (2016). *Research methods: The essential knowledge base* (2nd ed.). Cengage Learning.

Urbina, S. (2014). *Essentials of psychological testing* (2nd ed.). Wiley.

Vitoratou, S., Uglik-Marucha, N., Hayes, C., & Pickles, A. (2023). *A comprehensive guide for assessing measurement tool quality: The Contemporary Psychometrics (ConPsy) Checklist.* https://osf.io/t2pbj/download?format=pdf

Yusoff, M. S. B. (2019). ABC of content validation and content validity index calculation. *Education in Medicine Journal, 11*(2), 49–54. https://doi.org/10.21315/eimj2019.11.2.6

8

Experimental Research and Levels of Evidence

Main Points

- Researchers control independent variables, which have multiple levels (conditions, degrees). Researchers measure dependent variables (outcomes) for each level of the independent variable.
- True experimental research designs consist of at least one variable controlled by the researchers and true random assignment of participants to groups.
- Within-subject comparisons evaluate multiple measures made on the same participant. Between-subject comparisons evaluate the same measure made on different participants.
- A switching replications design allows for different groups to serve as controls without denying treatment to anyone; different groups receive the treatment at different times.
- Consider factors other than independent variable(s) when interpreting results, such as maturation and learning effects.

An important step in conducting empirical research is to develop a plan or design for making observations and collecting data. The particular features of this design will depend on the nature of the problem you are investigating. One of the initial decisions is whether to design a study that uses experimental or nonexperimental procedures. For example, do you need to change a situation in some way, perhaps by providing an experimental treatment, to answer your question? Or can you answer your question simply by making observations and measurements of existing phenomena? If researchers intend to obtain evidence to support a cause-and-effect relationship, an experimental research design is nearly always the best approach[1] (Trochim et al.,

---

[1] In Chapter 6, we discussed instances when researchers would be interested in cause-and-effect relationships, such as the cause of a particular speech, language, or hearing disorder, but experimental manipulation of the causal variable would be inappropriate. Research in which persons are deliberately exposed to a variable that could cause a communication disorder would be unethical.

2016). In an *experimental research design*, researchers identify one or more factors that they will manipulate or control during the experiment. The variables that researchers manipulate are called *independent variables*. Researchers also identify one or more ways that they will measure the outcomes of the experiment. That is, they measure the effects of their experimental manipulation on the participants' behavior. These outcome measures are called *dependent variables*. The point of experimental research is to establish that the experimental manipulation is the reason for any differences observed in the participants' performance on the outcome measures.

Audiologists and speech-language pathologists usually think of the term *treatment* as referring to the actions we take to improve our clients' speech, language, and/or hearing. Meanwhile, researchers use the term *treatment* in a broader sense. The term *treatment* in experimental research refers to the conditions you manipulate or the independent variable(s). Certainly, the experimental manipulation might be a comparison of two treatments in the therapeutic sense. That is, the researcher might be interested in which of two treatments leads to the most improvement at the end of a study. The experimental manipulation might be something that does not have a lasting therapeutic effect, however. For example, researchers might study persons with normal communication abilities to determine how two different presentation modes affect their performance on a task. This experimental manipulation would not produce a lasting improvement in the participants' abilities but would still be considered a treatment effect when discussing the results of such a study.

Researchers make a number of decisions in planning an experimental study. They decide on the different treatments or experiences participants will receive during the study and how to measure the outcomes associated with those different treatments. In addition, they make decisions about recruiting participants and when to obtain outcome measures. The procedures for recruiting and selecting participants are covered in another chapter. When to obtain outcome measures is a characteristic of the research designs we cover in this chapter. In some research approaches, participants are tested only once at the end of a study. In other approaches, they might be tested both at the beginning and at the end of the study or even a couple of times after the end of the study.

An additional decision that researchers make during the planning phase relates to the number of different treatments they will compare. When discussing the number of treatments, researchers sometimes use a phrase such as *levels of the independent variable or levels of treatment*. Previously, we considered examples in which researchers compared two different treatments or manipulations. Researchers could design a study, however, in which they compared three or more different treatments, depending on what comparisons were logical as well as practical. What is logical depends on the nature of the problem the researchers are investigating and the answers available from previous research. What is practical depends primarily on the number of participants you can recruit for the study. For example, some types of communication disorders have a relatively low prevalence, and recruiting enough participants to divide into even two treatment groups could be a challenge.

In the following sections on research design, we make a distinction between *true experimental designs* (i.e., experimental research designs) and *quasi-experimental designs*. Both experimental and quasi-experimental research designs incorporate one feature: researcher manipulation of a variable. The researcher creates different conditions or experiences for the participants by manipulating one or more factors during the study (Newhart & Patten, 2023; Trochim et al., 2016). Only a true experimental design incorporates the second feature of random assignment of participants to different experimental groups. Generally speaking, a study that incorporates both features, experimental manipulation and random assignment, provides stronger evidence than a quasi-experimental study. Thus, in the discussion that follows, those research designs that are true experimental designs provide a stronger or higher level of evidence than those that are classified as quasi-experimental.

Experimental Research Designs

In this section, we describe several experimental research designs (posttest-only randomized group designs, pretest-posttest randomized control group designs, Solomon randomized four-group design, switching replications design, and factorial designs). To illustrate each of the designs, we use a common system of notation to represent the various steps in the research design (e.g., Newhart & Patten, 2023; Trochim et al., 2016). For example, one of the things researchers must do is observe and obtain measures of their participants' behavior. In the notation system, the letter O represents an observation and measurement step. Another step in experimental research is to implement a treatment or manipulation of some variable. The letter X represents application of the experimental treatment. Finally, in a true experimental design, the participants are randomly assigned to the various treatment groups at the beginning of the study. The letter R represents the step of random assignment to groups.

Posttest-Only Designs

The most basic example of a true experimental design is a *posttest-only randomized control group design* (Newhart & Patten, 2023; Trochim et al., 2016). In this design, the researchers randomly assign participants to different treatment groups, implement the different treatments, and then observe and measure their participants' behavior. This design is considered a posttest-only design because the participants are tested only after they complete the treatment step. The notation for this type of design is as follows:

Example 1

Posttest-Only Randomized Control Group
    R   X   O
    R   O

In this design, the two rows beginning with R illustrate random assignment of participants to two different groups. The sequence R X O means that one group received treatment and then completed a posttest observation and measurement step. The other group, represented by the sequence R O, completed only the posttest test measurement step. The control group in this example is a *no-treatment control* rather than an alternative treatment control.

Researchers often want to compare two different treatments or experimental manipulations rather than treatment and no-treatment conditions. The notation for a posttest-only design in which the researcher compares two treatments is slightly different, as shown below.

Example 2

Posttest-Only Randomized Treatment Groups
  R X_1 O
  R X_2 O

Researchers could vary this basic design in several ways. For example, they might want to compare two alternative treatments as well as a no-treatment control group, as in Example 3, or they might compare three different treatments, as in Example 4.

Example 3

Posttest-Only Randomized Treatment and Control Groups
  R X_1 O
  R X_2 O
  R   O

Example 4

Posttest-Only Randomized Treatment Groups (with three treatments)
  R X_1 O
  R X_2 O
  R X_3 O

Another option researchers might consider is to have a second posttest observation and measurement step (e.g., an R X O O sequence). A second posttest would provide information about the long-term effects of treatment. Audiologists and speech-language pathologists almost always obtain measures of their clients' performance before treatment and again after treatment to document progress, so you might wonder why researchers would design a study in which they test their participants only once at the end of the study. One reason to use a posttest-only design is when the researchers have reason to think giving a pretest could falsify their findings.

For example, participants could learn something from the pretest that enables them to perform better on the posttest. The term *pretest sensitization or reactive effect of testing* refers to learning from a pretest or changing one's behavior due to taking a pretest. Newhart and Patten (2023) used the example of students taking a pretest over course content. These students might learn something about the topics covered in the course and focus more study time on those topics. Another possible reason to use a posttest-only design is when giving a pretest would not be feasible. An example of this might be research conducted with some type of emergency medical procedure. Perhaps medical researchers have reason to believe a certain drug could improve recovery of persons with traumatic injuries, if the patients receive the drug as soon as they enter the hospital. They design a study in which patients receive either standard emergency room care or the drug plus the standard care. However, the researchers decided they could not take time to pretest their patients before initiating treatment. Therefore, they planned to use a posttest-only randomized control group design.

Pretest-Posttest Randomized Control Group Design

When considering true experimental designs, perhaps the most frequently used type is a *pretest-posttest randomized control group design* (Newhart & Patten, 2023). In a pretest-posttest design, researchers observe and measure their participants' behavior twice: at the beginning of the study before participants receive treatment and again at the end of the study after participants complete the treatment step. Thus, the sequence of steps for this design is random assignment of participants to different groups, pretest observation and measurement of both groups, implementation of treatment for one of the groups, and posttest observation and measurement of both groups. Example 5 illustrates the notation for this type of design.

Example 5

Pretest–Posttest Randomized Control Group
R O X O
R O O

The various options that we discussed for the posttest-only design also apply to a pretest-posttest design. For example, researchers could investigate changes associated with two different treatments rather than comparing a treatment group and a no-treatment control group (e.g., two treatment sequences such as R O X_1 O and R O X_2 O). They also could compare two alternative treatments as well as a no-treatment control group, or they might compare three different treatments, as in Examples 6 and 7.

Example 6

Pretest–Posttest Randomized Treatment and Control Groups
R O X_1 O
R O X_2 O
R O O

Example 7

Pretest–Posttest Randomized Treatment Group (with three treatments)
R O X_1 O
R O X_2 O
R O X_3 O

Pretest-posttest designs are sometimes called *mixed-model* designs. The pretest-posttest comparison involves repeated measures of the same participants, sometimes described as a *within-subjects* factor. The treatment/no-treatment comparison involves measures from different participants, or a *between-subjects* factor. Mixed designs combine within-subjects and between-subjects factors and are well suited to investigations of treatment effects.

One of the major advantages of a pretest-posttest design is that the pretest provides evidence that the two groups were not significantly different before you initiated treatment. Thus, any group differences observed at the end of the study can be attributed to the treatment. Although random assignment of participants to groups is a way to avoid systematic variation between treatment and control groups, it is not a way to ensure that the two groups are equivalent. By chance, researchers could create two groups that varied on a relevant skill at the beginning of the study. If the control group started the study with greater skill on the outcome measure, the preexisting difference could mask a treatment effect. On the other hand, if the treatment group started the study with greater skill on the outcome measure, the preexisting difference could create a false treatment effect. Thus, when choosing a posttest-only or a pretest-posttest design, researchers need to weight the relative merits of identifying any preexisting differences against the possibility that learning from the pretest could contaminate their findings.

Solomon Randomized Four-Group Design

One of the most sophisticated true experimental designs is a *Solomon randomized four-group design* (Newhart & Patten, 2023). This design combines features of a posttest-only design and a pretest-posttest design. By using features of both designs, researchers have a way to check for pretest learning effects as well as to determine if treatment and control groups were different before the researchers initiated treatment. Example 8 illustrates the structure of a Solomon four-group design.

Example 8

Solomon Randomized Four-Group Design
```
R    O    X    O
R    O         O
R         X    O
R              O
```

A Solomon four-group design has two treatment groups represented by the R O X O and R X O sequences, as well as two control groups represented by the R O O and R O sequences. In interpreting this design, researchers would identify treatment effects if the participants in the two treatment groups improved more on the posttest than participants in the control groups. On the other hand, if both pretest groups, represented by R O X O and R O O, improved more than the posttest-only groups, that would mean participants were learning something from the pretest that enabled them to perform better on the posttest. A Solomon four-group design is a robust design for investigating treatment effects because a researcher has ways to evaluate both pretest learning and pretreatment group differences. The major disadvantage of this design is that researchers must recruit a much larger number of participants than in a posttest-only design or a pretest-posttest design. Cohen et al. (2018) described a variation on this design that tested for pretest sensitization by including one treatment group (R O X O) and two control groups, only one of which received the pretest (R O O and R O).

Switching Replications Design

Trochim et al. (2016) described one additional design that is of interest for conducting intervention research. In a *switching replications* design, the participants are randomly assigned to treatment and control groups to start the study. After the first posttest, the participants switch roles: The treatment group becomes the control group, and the control group becomes the treatment group for the second phase of the study. Trochim et al. noted that this design is an important one to consider when conducting treatment research because this design addresses an important issue in the pretest-posttest randomized control group designs—denying treatment to persons in the control group. Trochim et al. (p. 250) diagrammed this design as follows:

Example 9

Switching Replications Design
```
R    O    X    O         O
R    O         O    X    O
```

Factorial Designs

The final type of true experimental design that we cover is a *factorial design*. In a factorial design, the researchers plan to manipulate two or more independent variables simultaneously (e.g., Rosenthal & Rosnow, 2008; Trochim et al., 2016). When describing factorial designs, we could say that each of the independent variables is a factor, and each factor has two or more levels. By using a factorial design, researchers can determine how more than one independent variable impacts a dependent variable, plus they can determine how the two independent variables work together or influence one another.

Factorial designs actually are like a family of research designs with many possible variations. The following examples illustrate some of the options. The simplest factorial design is one with two independent variables and two levels for each of these variables. This simple design is often referred to as a 2-by-2 factorial design. An example of this design would be a treatment study in which speech-language pathologists (SLPs) investigate two different intervention approaches as well as two different intervention schedules. Let's assume that the SLPs compare a traditional intervention with a new intervention they created. In addition, the SLPs want to determine if different intervention schedules would affect how much the participants improve. They plan to compare two different treatment schedules. In one schedule, participants would receive intervention twice a week in 1-hour sessions. In the other schedule, participants would receive intervention four times a week in 30-minute sessions. Thus, all the participants would receive the same total amount of treatment. In this example, the two independent variables are intervention approach and schedule, the two levels of the intervention variable are the traditional and new approaches, and the two levels of the schedule variable are four 30-minute sessions and two 1-hour sessions.

To illustrate this factorial design, we are going to use a table rather than our notation system. The 2-by-2 intervention we described above is shown in Table 8–1. In the example, the SLPs recruited 40 individuals with speech and language disorders as participants and randomly assigned them to four different treatment options. One group received traditional intervention four times per week in 30-minute sessions, a second group received traditional intervention two times per week in 1-hour sessions, a third group received the new intervention four times per week in 30-minute sessions, and the fourth group received the new intervention two times per week in 1-hour sessions.

In this 2-by-2 factorial design, the researchers obtain information about the effects of two different independent variables. The effects associated with each of the independent variables are called *main effects*. In our example, if the participants who received the new intervention improved more than those who received traditional intervention, no matter how the intervention was scheduled, you could describe the finding as a main effect of intervention. If the participants

Table 8–1. An Illustration of a 2 By 2 Factorial Design

	Type of Intervention	
Schedule	Traditional Approach	New Approach
Four 30-minute sessions	Ten randomly assigned participants receive the traditional approach in four 30-minute sessions	Ten randomly assigned participants receive the new approach in four 30-minute sessions.
Two one-hour sessions	Ten randomly assigned participants receive the traditional approach in two one-hour sessions.	Ten randomly assigned participants receive the new approach in two one-hour sessions.

who received intervention in four 30-minute sessions per week improved more than those who received intervention in two 1-hour sessions per week, no matter what intervention approach they received, you could describe the finding as a main effect of schedule.

An important advantage of factorial designs is that researchers can investigate not only the effect of each independent variable but also how independent variables work together or influence one another. The effects associated with the way the independent variables work together are called *interaction effects*. Interaction effects occur in a factorial research design when the outcomes associated with one independent variable are different depending on the level of the other independent variable. An example of an interaction in our hypothetical study would be if the 30-minute sessions produced more improvement than the two 1-hour sessions, but only for the participants who received the new intervention approach. Let's make this example more concrete by using some numerical values in our illustration. For instance, both the group that received traditional intervention in 30-minute sessions and the group that received traditional intervention in 1-hour sessions improved by an average of 10 points at the end of the study. The group that received the new intervention in 1-hour sessions also improved by an average of 10 points at the end of the study; however, the group that received the new intervention in 30-minute sessions improved by 20 points. The presence of an interaction influences how you interpret your findings. In the above example, the SLPs would not be able to say that their new approach was significantly better overall; rather, their new approach was significantly better when delivered in four 30-minute sessions per week.

Like other true experimental designs, researchers have many options when creating a factorial design. For example, they could devise an independent variable with three or more levels, such as in a 2-by-3 factorial design. This type of design is illustrated in Table 8–2. In this example, the independent variables are speech recognition task and hearing aid orientation program. A group of audiologists wanted to investigate how well listeners with new hearing aid prescriptions performed on

Table 8–2. An Illustration of a 2 By 3 Factorial Design

Speech Recognition Task	Type of Orientation Program	
	Regular Orientation	Extended Orientation
Task One	Ten randomly assigned participants complete task one after a regular orientation.	Ten randomly assigned participants complete task one after an extended orientation.
Task Two	Ten randomly assigned participants complete task two after a regular orientation.	Ten randomly assigned participants complete task two after an extended orientation.
Task Three	Ten randomly assigned participants complete task three after a regular orientation.	Ten randomly assigned participants complete task three after an extended orientation.

different speech recognition tasks. They also wanted to determine if an extended orientation program would improve the listeners' performance on any or all of the tasks. The speech recognition task variable had three levels, and the orientation program had two levels. With this design, the researchers will be able to investigate two main effects, speech recognition task and orientation program, as well as the interaction between speech recognition task and orientation program.

Our next example is a factorial design with three independent variables. To illustrate this design, we return to our first example, investigating the effects of intervention approach and schedule. However, the SLPs who conducted the study decided to add a third variable, provision of a home program. This variable also has two levels: no home program and home program. The design shown in Table 8–3 is a 2-by-2-by-2 factorial design.

Although a factorial design provides a way to investigate several independent variables at the same time, one of the disadvantages of these designs is the need to recruit a relatively large number of participants. In our 2-by-2-by-2 factorial design, the researchers would need to recruit 80 participants to randomly assign 10 individuals to each of the possible treatment,

Table 8–3. An Illustration of a 2 By 2 By 2 Factorial Design

	Provision of Home Program			
	No Home Program		Home Program	
	Type of Intervention		Type of Intervention	
Schedule	Traditional Approach	New Approach	Traditional Approach	New Approach
Four 30-minute sessions	Ten randomly assigned participants receive the traditional approach in four 30-minute sessions with no home program.	Ten randomly assigned participants receive the new approach in four 30-minute sessions with no home program.	Ten randomly assigned participants receive the traditional approach in four 30-minute sessions with a home program.	Ten randomly assigned participants receive the new approach in four 30-minute sessions with a home program.
Two one-hour sessions	Ten randomly assigned participants receive the traditional approach in two one-hour sessions with no home program.	Ten randomly assigned participants receive the new approach in two one-hour sessions with no home program.	Ten randomly assigned participants receive the traditional approach in two one-hour sessions with a home program.	Ten randomly assigned participants receive the new approach in two one-hour sessions with a home program.

schedule, and home program combinations. This is twice the number of participants in the basic 2-by-2 factorial design in our first example (see Table 8–1). In addition, the interaction effects become quite complex each time you add another independent variable. In the 2-by-2-by-2 design, the researchers created eight different combinations of treatment approach, schedule, and home program. A three-way interaction would arise if just one of these combinations stood out as the most effective. For our basic 2-by-2 example, we described an interaction effect in which the group that received the new intervention in 30-minute sessions improved by 20 points, as compared to a 10-point improvement for all of the other treatment and schedule combinations. To illustrate a possible three-way interaction, let's consider those participants who received the new treatment approach scheduled in 30-minute sessions four times per week. The 2-by-2-by-2 design includes two groups with this combination. One group received a home program and the other did not. Perhaps, the group that received the combination of new treatment approach scheduled in 30-minute sessions four times per week plus a home program performed the best at the end of the study, gaining an average of 30 points on the posttest. In comparison, the group that received the combination of new treatment approach scheduled in 30-minute sessions four times per week with no home program gained 20 points. This would be an example of a three-way interaction, because both schedule and the provision of a home program interacted with the treatment approach.

Deciding how many independent variables to investigate is one of the major decisions that researchers make when planning a study with a factorial design. However, they need to consider other features too, such as whether to use a posttest-only design or a pretest-posttest design. They also might decide to conduct a long-term follow-up and include a second posttest observation in their research plan. Another possibility is to use a factorial design that combines experimental and nonexperimental variables. That is, researchers might decide to investigate one or more variables that they manipulate during the study and other variables that are preexisting conditions. One example of this would be to investigate an experimental variable such as intervention approach and a nonexperimental variable such as severity of disorder. This example is illustrated in Table 8–4 and is a modification of the example presented in Table 8–1. In Table 8–4, the researchers plan to inves-

Table 8–4. An Illustration of a 2 By 2 Factorial Design with Experimental and Nonexperimental Independent Variables

	Type of Intervention	
Level of Severity	**Traditional Approach**	**New Approach**
Mild-to-Moderate Disorders	Ten participants with mild-to-moderate disorders randomly assigned to receive the traditional approach.	Ten participants with mild-to-moderate disorders randomly assigned to receive the new approach.
Severe Disorders	Ten participants with severe disorders randomly assigned to receive the traditional approach.	Ten participants with severe disorders randomly assigned to receive the new approach.

tigate the effectiveness of the traditional and new intervention approaches with participants who have mild-to-moderate or severe speech and language disorders. The researchers can still assign participants to the intervention approaches on a random basis, but the severity levels involve preexisting conditions that cannot be assigned at random.

Each design we covered in this section is a true experimental design. The designs are true experiments as long as the researchers manipulate at least one of the independent variables, exercising experimental control over this variable, and randomly assign participants to the different levels of this variable. These two criteria, random assignment to groups and experimental manipulation of an independent variable, are essential for investigating cause-and-effect relationships. If researchers want to demonstrate that a new intervention approach led to significant improvement for their participants, they need to design a study in which they randomly assign participants to this new intervention and to at least one other group, such as a no-treatment control group or an alternate treatment group. Their experimental manipulation will be the type of treatment the participants receive. When researchers combine experimental and nonexperimental variables in a factorial study, they will be able to demonstrate a cause-and-effect relationship only for the experimental variable. The results from the nonexperimental comparison do not support conclusions about cause and effect, although information about the nonexperimental variable and how it interacts with the experimental manipulation could be important.

Research using true experimental designs is crucially important to professionals in audiology and speech-language pathology who provide treatment for individuals with communication disorders. Any clinical field that provides treatment services needs evidence to demonstrate the effectiveness of those services, and the strongest evidence for cause-and-effect relationships comes from true experimental research. The research base for audiology and speech-language pathology certainly includes a number of studies with both experimental manipulation of treatment variables and random assignment of participants to two or more groups. Table 8–5 includes a brief description of several studies from the field of communication sciences and disorders that used some variation on a randomized treatment and control design.

Importance of Experimental Control

Given the challenges of implementing a true experimental design, potential researchers might wonder about its importance. One reason researchers try to implement a true experimental design is to increase the validity of their conclusions regarding cause-and-effect relationships. If a study lacks a control group or the participants were not randomly assigned, the case for a cause-and-effect relationship between the independent variable and observed changes in the dependent variable is weak. The reason is that a number of alternative explanations, called *threats to internal validity*, could be the source of the changes in the dependent measure. Internal validity refers to the extent to which researchers' conclusions about cause-and-effect relationships are accurate (Newhart & Patten, 2023; Trochim et al., 2016). For example, if some researchers observed that their participants scored significantly higher on a posttest outcome measure compared to the pretest scores, the researcher would like to conclude that this improvement occurred because of the

Table 8–5. A Sample of Studies in the Field of Communication Sciences and Disorders with Randomized Treatment-Control Group Designs

Author(s)	Participants	Comparison
Arnott et al. (2014)	Recruited 54 children with stuttering who were between the ages of 3;0 and 5;11	Children randomly assigned to group or individual versions of the Lidcombe treatment program
Beukes et al. (2018)	146 adults with tinnitus	Randomly assigned to an experimental group receiving internet-based cognitive behavior therapy ($n = 73$) or a control group receiving standard monitoring ($n = 73$)
Doesborgh et al. (2003)	46 persons with aphasia after having a stroke who actually completed treatment	23 participants randomly assigned to a semantic treatment approach and 23 randomly assigned to a phonological treatment approach
Hesketh et al. (2007)	42 four-year-old children with speech disorders	Participants randomly assigned to phonological awareness ($n = 22$) or language stimulation treatment ($n = 20$)
Humes et al. (2017)	154 adults with mild to moderate hearing loss	Randomly assigned to groups receiving standard hearing aid service-delivery ($n = 53$), a placebo device treatment ($n = 50$), or a "consumer-decides" over-the-counter device service delivery ($n = 51$)
Lundberg et al. (2011)	69 adults, ages 60 to 75, who were fit with hearing aids at least one year prior to the study	Participants randomly assigned to a follow up with a book, weekly reading assignments, and telephone calls ($n = 33$), or a control group that only received the book ($n = 36$)
Mendel et al. (2003)	128 kindergarten children with normal hearing	Participants randomly assigned to one of six classrooms, three of which had sound field amplification ($n = 64$) and three of which did not ($n = 64$)
Murray et al. (2015)	26 children, ages 4 to 12 with a diagnosis of childhood apraxia of speech	Participants randomly assigned to either Rapid Syllable Transition treatment ($n = 13$) or the Nuffield Dyspraxia Programme–Third Edition ($n = 13$)
Spencer et al. (2015)	22 children from three Head Start classrooms qualified for the study based on Narrative Language Measure scores	Children randomly assigned to small group treatment ($n = 12$) or control conditions ($n = 10$)

treatment provided during their experiment. If the study lacked a control group, however, other possible causes of the improvement might exist that were unknown to the researchers. To illustrate these possible alternative explanations, several of the most common threats to internal validity are described in the following sections.

History

The threat of *history* means that some outside influence occurred during the course of your study, and this outside influence could account for the changes in outcome you observed at the end of your study. This threat might occur if researchers tried to conduct an intervention or training study using a single group of participants. For instance, the researchers might conduct their study with a group of students randomly selected from the same classroom. During the course of their study, the classroom teacher implemented some changes in their teaching methods and these changes addressed the same skills as the experimental training program the researchers were investigating. Because of this historical threat, the researchers would not know if their participants' improvements were due to the experimental manipulation or the classroom teacher's new methods. This alternate explanation for why the participants improved weakens any claims the researchers might make about the benefits of their experimental training program.

Maturation

The threat of *maturation* refers to increases in performance that are due to the participants' growth and development over time. This threat is particularly important when conducting research with children. Audiologists and speech-language pathologists might consider the possibility of recovery over time as a special form of the maturation threat. Both growth and development and recovery mean that participants make improvement from pretest to posttest even without treatment. As with most threats to internal validity, the primary way to control for the maturation threat is to include a control group as well as an experimental treatment group in your design. If the treatment group improves more than the control group from pretest to posttest, researchers have evidence that growth and maturation alone cannot account for their results.

Statistical Regression

In some experimental research, researchers recruit and select participants because they performed very poorly on some prestudy selection measure. This selection measure might also serve as the pretest measure for those participants who complete the study. A phenomenon called *statistical regression* occurs when persons who scored very high or very low on a test are retested (Newhart & Patten, 2023). Those who received extreme scores when first tested tend to score closer to the mean when retested. Any individual who takes a test repeatedly will exhibit some variability in their scores. If the person scored close to the mean to begin with, then the scores can vary up or down. Trochim et al. (2016) noted, however, that persons who score either extremely high or extremely low have a strong probability of scoring closer to the mean because that is the only direction their scores can move. If you already had an extremely low score on a test, the possibility of achieving an even lower score on retest is remote, but the possibility of achieving a higher score is relatively good. Those who are extremely low will tend to score higher just based on statistical averages, and those who score extremely high would tend to score lower. The threat of statistical regression is important for treatment studies because one of the selection criteria is that participants exhibit some deficiency on the skill that is the focus of the study. On average, the participants would tend to score higher on a posttest due to the phenomenon of statistical regression toward the mean, even if they received no benefit from the experimental treatment. This is why including a control group or an alternate treatment group in intervention research is extremely important.

Instrumentation

An *instrumentation* threat is possible in any pretest-posttest design. This threat encompasses both physical equipment used to elicit, record, and analyze responses as well as human "instruments" who observe and record behaviors. An instrumentation threat is operating in a study when the instrument changes in some way between the pretest and posttest. Thus, any differences in the participants' scores occur because of the instrumentation change rather than a treatment effect. Changes in how human observers score or measure behaviors could occur because of learning from pretest to posttest or because of fatigue or boredom with the task. If observers learn over the course of the study and become more accurate in identifying relevant behaviors, participants' scores might be higher at the end of the study due to observer changes rather than due to a real treatment effect. If observers become fatigued or bored, then they could become less accurate or vigilant from pretest to posttest. Failure to properly maintain calibration of a piece of equipment and an undiscovered equipment defect that occurred between the pretest and posttest also are examples of the instrumentation threat. The inadequate calibration or equipment defect could either create a false treatment effect or mask a treatment effect that actually existed. The best way to control for an instrumentation threat is to choose a research design with a control or alternative treatment group because the instrumentation problem will affect both the treatment and control groups. Additionally, researchers generally are careful about the calibration and maintenance of any physical instruments used in their studies, and include strategies such as assessing interobserver reliability to address the issue of changes in observer behavior over the course of the study.

Selection

A selection threat occurs when two or more groups differ in a systematic way, rather than in a random way, prior to a study (Newhart & Patten, 2023). Groups might differ in a systematic way if the researchers select their treatment and control groups in a nonrandom way. For example, researchers might want to conduct a study that involves a classroom intervention or even a community intervention (Trochim et al., 2016). Randomly assigning children to classrooms or individuals to communities is not practical. In these cases, researchers often work with the existing or "intact groups" when conducting a study (Newhart & Patten, 2023). One of the existing groups receives the experimental treatment and the other serves as a control. Studies of this type are not true experiments, and the findings might be shaped by group differences unrelated to the study. Any conclusions about cause-and-effect relationships are weakened because of possible alternate explanations for the findings. For example, a selection threat might co-occur with maturation differences (Trochim et al., 2016). One of the groups might have a different learning or growth rate prior to the study. Over the course of the study, this group will continue to improve at a faster rate than the other group. This difference in rate of improvement would be an alternate explanation for group differences observed at the end of the study. A selection threat might also co-occur with differences in group history. If researchers conduct a study with intact classrooms, differences in how the teachers teach their classes over the course of the study could be an alternative explanation. Thus, whenever it is feasible, researchers employ a true experimental design and randomly assign their participants to the treatment and control groups.

Mortality

Some threats to the internal validity of experimental research cannot be eliminated through random assignment of participants to groups. A *mortality* threat occurs when some participants drop out before the end of a study. This could occur whether the researchers used random assignment to form groups or worked with preexisting groups. If participants dropped out of the study on a random basis, mortality would be less of a threat. Sometimes participants have a reason for dropping out of a study, and this reason could distort the findings in some way. For example, participants who receive low scores on the pretest might withdraw from the study because they perceive themselves as doing poorly. In a treatment study, participants who experience less benefit from the treatment might be more likely to withdraw than those who perceive themselves as improving. If participants drop out in a systematic way, such as those who score low on the pretest or those who are making less improvement, then the results of the study might misrepresent the true effectiveness of the treatment. If only the high scorers or those who make the most progress remain in the study for the posttest, the treatment would seem more successful than it actually is. Trochim et al. (2016) suggested one way to investigate the impact of participant mortality is to compare the pretest scores of those who withdraw from the study and those who remain. If these scores are similar, then pretest differences probably are not a factor. Still, pretest scores would not be a way to control for different treatment experiences.

Quasi-Experimental Approaches

For some kinds of research, randomly assigning participants to treatment and control groups would be impractical. In the social sciences, researchers sometimes investigate the effectiveness of an intervention program provided to an entire community or organization (Trochim et al., 2016). In the field of education, researchers often implement and study innovative teaching and learning practices at the classroom level.[2] In these instances, randomly assigning participants to groups is not feasible.

---

[2]In some educational research, many classrooms participate in the research and the investigators randomly assign several classrooms to the experimental and control conditions. These types of studies are true experimental research. In a sense, the classrooms are a variable in the study and the students are described as being "nested" within the classrooms (Salkind, 2010). These sophisticated designs are beyond the scope of this chapter.

Researchers interested in community-, organization-, or classroom-based interventions still have ways to conduct their studies, but they often do so with preexisting groups of participants. If researchers design a study in which they create different conditions or experiences for the participants by manipulating some factor, but use existing groups rather than randomly formed groups, the design is a *quasi-experimental design*. Quasi-experimental designs have one of the features of a true experiment, researcher manipulation of a variable, but lack the second feature of random assignment of participants to different experimental groups (Newhart & Patten, 2023; Trochim et al., 2016). Quasi-experimental designs are valuable for investigating cause-and-effect relationships but are more susceptible to threats to internal validity, and particularly to the selection threat. This means that conclusions regarding cause-and-effect relationships drawn from quasi-experimental research are weaker than those drawn from true experimental research. In the sections that follow, we discuss some of the options researchers use when a true experimental design is impractical (nonequivalent control group designs, repeated measures group design, and single-subject designs).

Nonequivalent Control Group Designs

When the plan of a study involves identifying two preexisting or intact groups, assigning one of the groups to an experimental treatment condition and assigning the other to a control or alternative treatment condition, the design is a *nonequivalent control group design*. When using this design, researchers sometimes randomly assign one of the groups to the experimental condition and the other to the control condition. Randomly assigning intact groups does not eliminate the problems associated with using intact groups, however, and is not the same as randomly assigning individual participants to groups, although it might reduce researcher bias in deciding who receives the experimental treatment. A nonequivalent control group design is usually a pretest-posttest design rather than a posttest-only design. The reason for this is that the researchers have a greater need to determine if the groups were similar on the relevant variables before treatment. Unlike groups formed at random, intact groups might be systematically different before the study due to different prior experiences, different learning and maturation rates, and so forth. Thus, researchers usually administer a pretest to demonstrate that the groups were not significantly different before the study, at least on the tested variables.

The design notation for a quasi-experimental study is similar to that for a pretest-posttest randomized control study, except that use of an R to designate random assignment is inappropriate. In the design notation, the R for group assignment might be omitted (Patten, 2013), or an N might be used for nonrandom assignment of participants to groups (Trochim et al., 2016), as we do in the examples that follow. Example 10 illustrates a basic nonequivalent control group design, and Example 11 illustrates a design with both an alternate treatment group and a no-treatment control group. The primary difference between these designs and their true experimental counterparts is that the researchers are working with existing groups that were formed prior to the study for other purposes.

Example 10

Pretest–Posttest Nonequivalent Control Group
    N   O   X   O
    N   O   O

Example 11

Pretest–Posttest Nonequivalent Treatment and Control Groups

    N   O X_1 O
    N   O X_2 O
    N   O   O

A nonequivalent control group design could be combined with the switching replications design described in Trochim et al. (2016). As with any intervention study, researchers are often hesitant to withhold an innovative teaching practice that has the potential to genuinely improve student learning. In the switching replications design, both groups eventually have an opportunity to experience the innovative method; if the approach works both during the initial implementation and during the replication, the researchers have stronger evidence for a cause-and-effect relationship. A nonequivalent control group design with switching replications is illustrated in Example 12.

Example 12

Switching Replications Design With Nonequivalent Control Group

    N   O   X   O   O
    N   O   O   X   O

One additional quasi-experimental design to consider, particularly when conducting an intervention study, is a *double pretest* design (Trochim et al., 2016). In this design, the researchers select two existing groups of participants. One group of participants receives an experimental intervention, whereas the other group participates in a no-treatment control condition or receives an alternative intervention. Example 13 provides an illustration of a double pretest design with nonrandom assignment of participants to groups (Trochim et al., 2016, p. 270).

Example 13

Double Pretest–Posttest Nonequivalent Control Group

    N   O   O   X   O
    N   O   O   O

The primary advantage of a double pretest design is that it provides some control over the selection threat associated with different rates of maturation or learning. If the rates of learning of two groups differed, the groups might not be significantly different at the time of the first pretest but could be significantly different at the time of the posttest. If the researchers had only obtained the first pretest, they might have assumed the two groups were similar and the differences they observed after the experimental intervention were due to the intervention. Having the second pretest could provide evidence that the scores of the two groups were diverging before the experimental intervention occurred. On the other hand, if the groups were not significantly different on either the first or the second pretest, the researchers have a stronger basis for concluding that differences observed at the end of the study were due to their experimental intervention.

Repeated Measures Group Design

Another option researchers might consider is to design an experimental study with only one group of participants. In a *repeated measures design*, researchers obtain two or more measurements from the same participants. Sometimes repeated measures designs are nonexperimental in nature, and researchers obtain a series of measurements across time to observe participants' maturation or learning in an area of interest. Repeated measures designs can be experimental designs as well. In a repeated measures experimental design, participants serve as their own controls and experience all levels of the independent variable. Thus, we classify this design as a quasi-experimental rather than a true experimental design because participants are not randomly assigned to treatment and control groups. The advantages of using a repeated measures design, compared to randomized pretest-posttest designs, are that researchers do not need to recruit as many participants and the experimental and control groups are well matched because participants serve as their own controls. A repeated measures experimental design is only feasible, however, in situations where the order of the experimental and control conditions will not affect outcomes. Furthermore, researchers need to be aware of challenges in analyzing the findings from repeated measures experiments, particularly when participants are observed and measured three or more times (Max & Onghena, 1999).

Previously, we noted that some experimental manipulations are actual interventions designed to increase participants' abilities and skills. Other experimental manipulations are task manipulations designed to increase participants' performance at that moment but not necessarily to increase the performance in a permanent way. A repeated measures design could work quite well with the latter type of independent variable but probably is not well suited to actual intervention research. For example, researchers in audiology might want to compare two different amplification approaches for persons with hearing losses. They could randomly assign participants to the two amplification conditions, but this might not be practical if the number of participants who fit the researchers' criteria for participation was small. As an alternative, the researchers could test each of the participants twice, giving each participant an opportunity to try both amplification approaches. As another example, researchers might be interested in an interaction variable that might alter children's communication in a temporary way, perhaps promoting greater fluency or more talkativeness. The researchers might design a study in which the children participated for part of the time in the experimental condition and part of the time in the control condition. Even if the children participated in the experimental condition first, the expectation is that their conversational participation or fluency would return to typical levels in the control condition. Example 14 shows the simplest form of a repeated measures design with one group of participants who experience both the experimental (X_1) and control conditions (X_2).

Example 14

Repeated Measures Experimental Design
X_1 O X_2 O

Often, researchers increase the experimental control in repeated measures studies by counterbalancing the order of experimental and control conditions. Counterbalancing works well when the independent variable has two levels. Half of the participants complete the experimental condition first, followed by the control condition, whereas the remaining half complete the control condition followed by the experimental condition. Counterbalancing provides the researchers with a way to identify any order effects in their outcomes. Example 15 is an illustration of a repeated measures design with counterbalancing and random assignment to order of experimental and control experiences. In the example below, half of the participants undergo experimental treatment first, followed by an alternative treatment control condition; the other half undergo the alternative treatment first, followed by the experimental treatment. The R designates random assignment to order of treatment, but not to treatment or control conditions, because all participants experience both treatment options.

Example 15

Repeated Measures Experimental Design with Counterbalancing

    R X_1 O X_2 O
    R X_2 O X_1 O

Repeated measures designs are also referred to as within-subject designs. This means that individual participants experience the different levels of the independent variable or treatment and control conditions (Shearer, 1997). Repeated measures designs are a viable option for investigating some questions in the field of communication sciences and disorders as demonstrated in studies including the following: Antonucci and MacWilliam (2015), Baker et al. (2014), Chapman et al. (2006), Gordon-Salant et al. (2007), McArdle et al. (2012), Salorio-Corbetto et al. (2019), Sandage et al. (2014), and Spratford et al. (2017).

Thus far, both the true experimental and quasi-experimental designs covered in this section have been group designs. In group designs, researchers report results for an average or typical member of a group (Cohen et al., 2018), as well as the spread of scores from low to high among group members. Although researchers occasionally might identify a member of a group who performed in an atypical way, usually the focus is on the collective performance of a group and not the performance of individual participants. Group designs are a dominant approach in many fields of study, including audiology and speech-language pathology. However, group designs might not be feasible for studying certain research questions. If the number of potential participants is relatively small, as in research focusing on treatment for a disorder with low prevalence, a group design often is not the best choice. A group design also is less suitable when researchers might expect participants to respond in distinctive ways to their treatment (Horner et al., 2005). When participant responses are highly individualistic, discussing findings in terms of the typical or average performance of a group is inappropriate. In the next section, we cover alternative, single-subject designs, which might be more appropriate in situations where the population of participants is small or participants' responses to the experimental manipulation are likely to be highly variable.

Single-Subject Designs

In research that employs a *single-subject design* (or single case) experimental design, researchers report the results for each individual participant separately. The term *single-subject design* refers to how researchers report their findings and does not mean that the study had only one participant in a literal sense. In fact, researchers often strengthen their findings by replicating their approach with two or more participants (Tate et al., 2013). Single-subject designs fit the category of quasi-experimental designs because such designs have one or more experimental manipulations but lack random assignment of participants to groups. As in repeated measures designs, participants in single-subject research experience both treatment and control conditions. The difference is that researchers report the combined results for all participants with repeated measures designs but report the results for individual participants with single-subject designs.

Often the notation system for single-subject designs employs the letters A, B, C, and so forth (e.g., Barlow et al., 2009; Byiers et al., 2012; Cohen et al., 2018; Tate et al., 2013). The letter A designates a baseline or no-treatment phase in a study, and the letter B designates the first treatment approach. If the study includes more than one treatment approach, the letter C designates the second treatment approach or sometimes designates a second element of treatment that combines with B (Byiers et al., 2012). To establish a functional relationship between a treatment and behavioral change, researchers measure the target behavior many times over a series of sessions. If the behavior remains relatively stable during the baseline, no-treatment phase and changes in a noticeable way during the treatment phase, the researchers have evidence for a relationship between the treatment and the change in behavior.

The simplest single-subject design is an A–B sequence, or a baseline-treatment design. Although an A–B sequence is the basis for all other single-subject designs, the design itself is rather weak and seldom found in reported research (Richards, 2019). Because the design includes only one A and one B phase, any changes that occur during the B phase could have alternative explanations, such as maturation or an extraneous environmental change. This simple single-subject design may have utility for audiologists and speech-language pathologists who need to document the effectiveness of their interventions for persons with speech, language, and hearing impairments.

A more sophisticated modification of an A–B design is an A_1–B–A_2 or *treatment withdrawal* design (Barlow et al., 2009), also sometimes called a reversal design (Leary, 2011). The subscripts on A_1 and A_2 indicate whether the baseline phase was the first or second in the series. In this design, researchers collect baseline data during a no-treatment phase first (A_1), implement an experimental intervention for several sessions, and then withdraw the intervention and collect data during a second no treatment phase (A_2). This design provides additional evidence for a functional (cause-and-effect) relationship between the experimental intervention and observed behavioral changes, if the behavior in the second baseline phase returns to levels observed during the first baseline phase. Consider the example of audiologists who want to test the effectiveness of an experimental amplification approach. They would collect baseline data by testing a participant without the experimental amplification for perhaps a minimum of five sessions; next they would implement the amplification phase for several sessions and then withdraw the amplification and test the participant for five additional baseline sessions. This hypothetical design is illustrated in Figure 8–1. In this figure, the vertical lines inserted between the A and B phases indicate the switch from no-treatment baseline to treatment phases. In this idealized experimental illustration, the behavior remained relatively stable during the initial five baseline sessions, the behavior immediately increased and stayed at a high level when treatment was implemented for 10 sessions, and finally the behavior returned to pretreatment levels during the second set of 5 baseline sessions. A treatment withdrawal design is appropriate when investigating experimental interventions that you expect to affect the target behavior only while the experimental intervention is occurring. With interventions that have a temporary effect, the participant's behavior should return to A_1 baseline levels once the intervention is no longer present. If the target

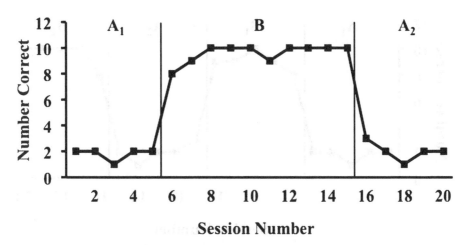

Figure 8–1. Illustration of an A_1–B_1–A_2 treatment withdrawal single-subject design.

behavior returns to levels present during the first baseline phase, you have evidence that the change in behavior resulted from the experimental intervention. If the target behavior remained at treatment levels after treatment withdrawal, the change in behavior could be attributed to some extraneous factor and the evidence for a treatment effect is weakened. For this reason, an A_1–B–A_2 design is not ideal for interventions that create lasting changes in the target behavior, because behaviors should remain at or near the levels present during the B or intervention phase.

Another modification of a simple baseline-treatment design is a *treatment replication* or A_1–B_1–A_2–B_2 design (Richards, 2019). In this design, illustrated in Figure 8–2, the researcher includes two A–B series to determine if effects that appear to be associated with treatment during the first phase can be repeated during a second treatment phase. After measuring behaviors during several baseline sessions, the investigator introduces an intervention and measures behaviors during a number of intervention sessions. Then, the investigator repeats the series by withdrawing intervention during a second baseline phase and reintroducing intervention during a second treatment series. If the behaviors return to baseline levels when intervention is withdrawn and change again when the intervention is reintroduced, the investigator has strong evidence that the intervention was the cause of the behavior change. If the behaviors do not return to baseline levels when intervention is withdrawn but change even more in a second intervention phase, as illustrated in Figure 8–3, the evidence for a cause-and-effect relationship between intervention and the behavior change is still relatively strong. On the other hand, if behaviors measured in the second baseline phase do not return to initial baseline levels, or the participant does not show any improvement in the second intervention, the evidence for a functional, cause-and-effect relationship is relatively weak.

Another variation on the treatment withdrawal design is a *multiple treatment* design. This design begins with an A_1–B_1–A_2

180 RESEARCH IN COMMUNICATION SCIENCES AND DISORDERS

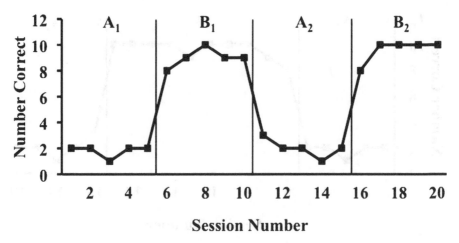

Figure 8–2. Illustration of an A_1–B_1–A_2–B_2 treatment replication single-subject design in which measured behaviors returned to initial baseline levels during the second baseline phase.

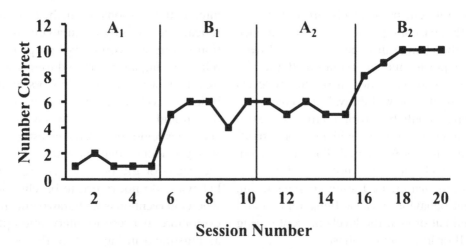

Figure 8–3. Illustration of an A_1–B_1–A_2–B_2 treatment replication single-subject design with incremental treatment effects in both B_1 and B_2 treatment phases.

series, but instead of following this with a second phase of the B intervention (B_2), the researchers implement a new intervention (e.g., C) (Leary, 2011; Richards, 2019). This notation for a multiple treatment design would be A_1–B_1–A_2–C_1, and often researchers follow C with a third baseline phase, A_1–B_1–A_2–C_1–A_3. Although this design allows the researchers to investigate the effects of a second treatment, the design does not provide evidence for the effectiveness of the C treatment by itself, only its effectiveness following prior administration of the B treatment. This is a serial order confound because the C treatment followed the B. Sometimes researchers employ this design with two or more participants and counterbalance the order. That is, one participant experiences the sequence A_1–B_1–A_2–C_1–A_3, whereas the other experiences the sequence A_1–C_1–A_2–B_1–A_3.

The basic single-subject baseline-treatment design can be extended in many ways and we have covered only a few of those options (Barlow et al., 2009; Richards, 2019). For example, researchers sometimes extend the treatment replication design for several A–B series or alternate treatment and baseline in a random manner. Sometimes, two treatment components are combined at the same time and designated as a BC phase.

Another alternative to strengthen the experimental control in a single-subject design is to use a *multiple baseline* design. Some of the common variations are multiple baseline across participants, behaviors, and settings (Barlow et al., 2009; Byiers et al., 2012; Richards, 2019). In a *multiple baseline across behaviors* design, researchers select two or more behaviors to observe and measure during the study. They determine baseline levels for both behaviors during the initial baseline phase and then initiate treatment for one of the behaviors. They continue to observe and measure the second behavior but do not immediately initiate treatment on that behavior. Sometimes the researchers continue to measure this behavior only, but often they begin treatment on this second behavior during a second treatment phase.

In the example illustrated in Figure 8–4, the researchers created two equivalent word lists. These could be lists of new vocabulary items, lists of words with speech sounds to discriminate, or other ideas you might generate. The researchers obtained baseline levels for both lists during the A_1 phase and then initiated treatment with the first word list. At the same time, they continued to observe the participant's performance with the second word list. You might think of this as an extended baseline phase for List 2. In this particular example, the improvements that occurred for List 1 words in the first treatment phase (B_1) were maintained during the second baseline or treatment withdrawal phase (A_2). Although maintenance of treatment gains during the treatment

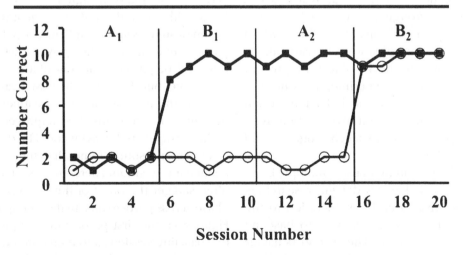

Figure 8–4. Illustration of an A_1–B_1–A_2–B_2 multiple baseline across behaviors single-subject design.

withdrawal phase weakens the evidence of a cause-and-effect relationship between the treatment and behavior change, this is often the kind of pattern audiologists and speech-language pathologists want to see. That is, clinicians try to identify treatment approaches that will produce lasting improvements in their clients. Fortunately, a multiple baseline across behaviors design provides an additional opportunity for researchers to demonstrate a functional relationship between the treatment and behavior changes. For the example in Figure 8–4, the number correct for the untreated words in List 2 remained at baseline levels during the first treatment phase (B_1) and second baseline phase (A_2). For the final treatment phase (B_2), the researchers started treatment on the words in List 2, and this is the point in the study when the participant's performance with these words improved. This multiple baseline design has several sources of experimental control to strengthen the evidence for a cause-and-effect relationship: (a) stable baselines for both word lists during the A_1 phase, (b) improved performance on the treated words in List 1 during the B_1 phase, (c) stable baseline levels for the untreated words in List 2 through phases A_1–B_1–A_2, and (d) improved performance on the words in List 2 with the initiation of treatment on those words in the B_2 phase. Because of these sources of experimental control, a multiple baseline across behaviors design is a good choice when investigating treatment approaches for speech, language, and hearing disorders.

When planning to use a multiple baseline across behaviors design, researchers need to give careful consideration to the choice of a second behavior to baseline and eventually treat. The second behavior should be generally equivalent to the first in difficulty and/or developmental level. For example, if researchers were constructing two word lists, it would be inappropriate to construct a treatment list with common, high-frequency words and to construct a probe list with less common, low-frequency words. Researchers also need to avoid behaviors that might change through treatment of the first behavior. One area in which this is an issue is in studies that address production and perception of speech sounds. If researchers selected a second speech sound to observe and measure in the A_1–B_1–A_2 phases of treatment, they need to avoid sounds that might improve because they share phonetic features with the trained phoneme. For example, if the first trained sound was /k/, /g/ would be a poor choice as a control phoneme. Because the /k/ and /g/ share phonetic features (velar, stop), training one of these sounds could lead to improvement in the other through feature generalization (Bernthal et al., 2013).

A final option covered here is a *multiple baseline across participants* (subjects) design (Barlow et al., 2009; Richards, 2019). In this kind of study, researchers replicate their intervention with one or more additional participants. A multiple baseline across participants design is often combined with an A_1–B_1–A_2–B_2 treatment replication design, as shown in Figure 8–5. Each participant could start the study at the same time and begin the treatment phase at the same time, but this is not the best arrangement. If the participants start treatment at the same time, any observed improvement in the participants' behavior could be due to an extraneous source rather than the experimental intervention. Therefore, researchers often stagger the onset of the intervention phase across participants. In the example in Figure 8–5, the first participant completed five baseline sessions and then entered the intervention phase, but the second participant completed two additional baseline ses-

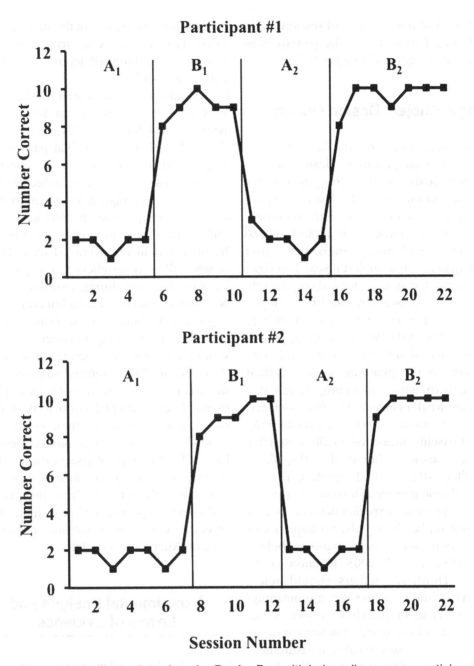

Figure 8–5. Illustration of an A_1–B_1–A_2–B_2 multiple baseline across participants single-subject design.

sions before beginning intervention. If the intervention is the cause of the observed change in the target skill, then the first participant should begin improving in sessions six and seven, but the second participant should continue exhibiting baseline levels and not start improving until sessions eight and nine. This in fact is the pattern illustrated in the graphs in Figure 8–5.

Single-Subject Design Quality

In the previous section, the descriptions of the various single-subject design options covered features that strengthened the design and enhanced the level of experimental control. Beginning with an influential article by Horner et al. (2005), several authors have discussed criteria that reflect high-quality single-subject research designs and presented systems for judging the reliability of evidence generated from single-subject designs (Reichow et al., 2008; Tate et al., 2008, 2013; Wendt & Miller, 2012). Researchers should take these criteria into account in the planning stages of their research to avoid conducting studies that provide weak evidence. The first consideration is a plan to collect an adequate number of baseline measures, ideally across five or more sessions (Tate et al., 2013; Wendt & Miller, 2012). Second, the design of the study should provide at least three opportunities to judge the experimental effect either through replications of the AB sequence or replications across participants or behaviors (Horner et al., 2005; Reichow et al., 2008). Third, researchers should select behaviors and measures that are meaningful in everyday life, that is, have social validity, and develop a working definition of the behaviors to ensure reliable measurement (Horner et al., 2005; Wendt & Miller, 2012). Fourth, researchers need a detailed description of the treatment or independent variable so that it can be administered consistently and replicated across experimenters. Finally, researchers should arrange for independent measurement of relevant behaviors by individuals who are unfamiliar with the participants and phases of the study, that is, blinded to the baseline versus experimental treatment conditions (Reichow et al., 2008; Tate et al., 2013).

Single-subject research designs are well suited to studying an individual's response to intervention (Leary, 2011; Lillie et al., 2011). If individual participants respond in unique ways to the intervention, the research is still valuable because findings are not aggregated across participants. In group research, individual variability in response to intervention tends to be obscured in the averaged data. These designs allow researchers to compare behaviors observed during baseline phases with those observed during intervention to determine if there is a functional, cause-and-effect relationship between an intervention and observed changes in behavior (Byiers et al., 2012). Because single-subject designs provide a researcher with ways to establish experimental control, they provide stronger evidence than nonexperimental case studies. Single-subject designs have a long history of use in the field of communication sciences and disorders in research with both children and adults, and Table 8–6 provides a brief summary of several recent studies that employed single-subject experimental designs.

Experimental Designs and Levels of Evidence

Previously we learned that the term *evidence-based practice* (EBP) refers to an approach in which clinicians use the best available research to guide their decisions about how to evaluate and treat persons with communication disorders. Some of the steps in EBP include identifying a clinical question, searching the professional literature, and

Table 8–6. A Sample of Studies in the Field of Communication Sciences and Disorders with Single-Subject Experimental Designs

Author(s)	Participants	Treatment
DeLong et al. (2015)	Three women and two men, ages 30 to 65, with chronic aphasia	Used a multiple-baseline design to investigate treatment outcomes for semantic feature analysis using probes of treated and untreated stimuli
Maas et al. (2012)	Four children, ages 5 years to 8 years, with a diagnosis of childhood apraxia of speech	Used a multiple-baseline, alternating treatments design to test the effects of high frequency vs. low frequency feedback in motor speech treatment
McDaniel et al. (2018)	Four preschoolers with hearing loss	Used an alternating treatment approach to assess word learning with auditory-only instruction compared to auditory-visual instruction
Palmer et al. (1999)	Eight individuals with Alzheimer's disease (AD) and their caregivers completed the study	Used a multiple-baseline design across participants to determine if receiving a hearing aid led to a reduction in reports of "problem behaviors" in persons with AD
Rudolph & Wendt (2014)	Three children, ages 4 years to 5 years, with speech sound disorders	Used a multiple-baseline design across participants and behaviors to investigate generalization and maintenance following treatment with the cycles approach
Tönsing et al. (2014)	Four children with limited speech who used graphic symbols	Used a multiple-baseline design for participants and behaviors to investigate the use of shared story-book reading to teach word combinations with semantic relations
Trussel et al. (2018)	Six preschoolers who were deaf/hard-of-hearing	Used a multiple probe across behaviors approach to assess interactive storybook reading as an intervention for word labeling and meaning
Wambaugh et al. (2013)	Three males and one female with chronic acquired apraxia of speech and Broca's aphasia	Used a multiple-baseline design across participants and behaviors to investigate the effects of different levels of treatment intensity and blocked vs. random practice

reading and evaluating research reports. In Chapters 3 and 4, we covered developing a clinical question and conducting a literature search as the initial steps in completing evidence-based practice research. The next step after completing the literature search is to select the most relevant articles to read and evaluate. An important consideration in evaluating research is to determine the *level of evidence* a study provides, and knowledge about research design is a key factor in making this judgment. As noted previously in this chapter, the strongest designs for establishing cause-and-effect relationships are true experimental designs: those with random assignment of participants to at least two groups, a treatment and a control group. True experimental designs, sometimes called randomized clinical trials, provide the strongest kind of evidence for intervention effectiveness and include studies that compare treatment and no-treatment conditions, as well as those that compare two or more different treatment approaches. Other experimental designs provide useful information, but the strength of evidence for a cause-and-effect relationship is weaker.

In addition to level of evidence, audiologists and speech-language pathologists consider the depth of evidence that supports the effectiveness of a particular intervention approach. For example, a well-designed, randomized clinical trial is considered a strong type of evidence, and several well-designed, randomized clinical trials that yielded similar results would be even stronger. If the studies yielded conflicting results, then the evidence in support of a particular intervention approach is undermined.

Sometimes your literature search might yield a systematic review or meta-analysis. From your reading, you might be familiar with a narrative review of literature in the introduction section of research reports. A *systematic review* is a special kind of review of existing research that employs a rigorous method of evaluation. The authors of a systematic review use a specific procedure to search the research literature, select the studies to include in their review, and critically evaluate the studies they find. In addition, authors of systematic reviews usually have identified a particular clinical question to answer when they begin their literature search (Trochim et al., 2016). A *meta-analysis* adds an additional component, a statistical analysis of the aggregated findings from several studies, and provides an estimate of the overall effectiveness of an intervention (Schlosser, 2006; Trochim et al., 2016). This combined estimate of effect should be less affected by random or systematic sources of bias in the individual studies and thus should be more stable.

Many organizations have published levels of evidence models to guide professionals in their evaluation of the strength of evidence obtained from different studies (e.g., American Speech-Language-Hearing Association [ASHA], 2004; Center for Knowledge Translation for Disability and Rehabilitation Research [KTDRR], 2020; OCEBM Levels of Evidence Working Group, 2011). The various models have more similarities than differences. For example, nearly all models place randomized clinical trials and meta-analyses at the highest level. A randomized clinical trial represents the highest level for individual studies: Several studies combined in a meta-analysis demonstrate the depth of evidence for a particular intervention. Similarly, nearly all models place expert opinion at the lowest level. One might, however, consider the convergent opinions of several experts (a panel of experts) to be stronger than the opinion of a single expert. Thus, judging the evidence in support of a particular intervention means considering the strength of the individual studies as well as the number of studies. At any level of evidence, having multiple sources that report similar findings is stronger than having a single source at that level. The strength of the evidence carries more weight than the amount of evidence. A single well-designed randomized clinical trial would generally outweigh the opinion of several experts. Figure 8–6 illustrates the concepts of strength of evidence and depth of evidence for intervention research.[3]

Finally, let's consider how the various nonexperimental and experimental research designs go with the common levels of evidence cited in the literature (ASHA, 2004; OCEBM Levels of Evidence Working Group, 2011). As noted previously, randomized clinical trials are at the highest level of evidence. Examples of designs that could be employed in such trials include pretest-posttest randomized treatment and control group designs, the Solomon four-group design, randomized switching replications designs, and randomized factorial designs. At the next lower level are various quasi-experimental designs with nonrandomized treatment and control groups such as a pretest-posttest nonequivalent treatment and control group design or a double pretest-posttest nonequivalent treatment and control group design. Toward the lowest level of evidence are quantitative and qualitative descriptive case studies and correlation/regression research. Single-subject designs like treatment replication design or multiple baseline across behaviors design usually fall in the middle of most evidence models. However, the Oxford Centre for Evidence-Based Medicine elevated some, particularly well-designed single-subject experimental designs to the highest level of evidence. Only single-subject designs with randomized baseline and treatment conditions (n of 1 trials) that meet other quality criteria are at this highest level. Table 8–7 gives examples of levels of evidence and the corresponding research designs.

When using levels of evidence, such as those in Table 8–7, we should keep in mind that many of the published models are for evaluating intervention research; the levels of evidence for other clinical questions, such as those related to diagnosis and prognosis, would be different. Phillips et al. (2009) provided a table with a side-by-side comparison of levels of evidence

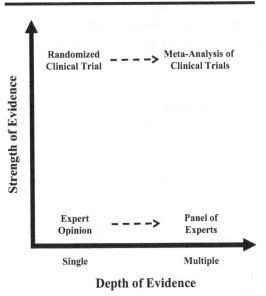

Figure 8–6. Illustration of contributions of strength and depth of research findings to decisions about levels of evidence.

---

[3]Those who are interested in the levels of evidence used in medicine and procedures for critical evaluation of research might consult Ebell et al. (2004) and Howick et al. (2011a, 2011b).

Table 8–7. Levels of Evidence for Intervention Research Commonly Cited in the Literature on Evidence-Based Practice and the Related Research Designs

Levels of Evidence	Research Designs
Meta-Analysis	• Combined analysis of several randomized clinical trials
Randomized Clinical Trial	• Posttest-only randomized groups designs • Pretest-posttest randomized groups designs • Solomon randomized four-group design • Randomized switching replications design • Randomized factorial designs
Nonrandomized Control Study	• Pretest-posttest nonequivalent groups designs • Switching replications design with nonequivalent groups • Double pretest-posttest nonequivalent groups designs
Other Quasi-Experimental Study	• Repeated measures experimental designs (with or without counterbalancing) • A_1–B_1–A_2 treatment withdrawal single-subject design • A_1–B_1–A_2–B_2 treatment replication single-subject design • A_1–B_1–A_2–C_1–A_3 multiple treatment single-subject design • Single-subject multiple baseline across behaviors design • Single-subject multiple baseline across participants design
Nonexperimental Studies	• Case-control studies • Correlation and regression research • Quantitative and qualitative descriptive case studies • Qualitative research approaches including ethnography, grounded theory, and phenomenology
Expert Opinion	• In the absence of previous empirical research

for several types of clinical studies: therapy, prognosis, diagnosis, differential diagnosis, and economic analysis. Qualitative research approaches, even though they fall at a lower level of evidence in levels of evidence models, would be considered a good choice for investigating some clinical questions, such as those related to how a disability or health condition affects an individual and how that individual perceives their care (Miller, 2010).

Summary

Experimental research designs are nearly always the best approach when the goal of a study is to establish a cause-and-effect relationship, such as between an intervention and improvement in the participants' behavior. All experimental designs share the feature of an experimental manipulation; the strongest experimental designs, called true experimental designs, also have the feature of random assignment of participants to at least one treatment and one control group. True experimental designs include variations with random assignment of participants to groups, such as posttest-only designs, pretest-posttest designs, switching replications designs, and factorial designs. When random assignment of participants to groups is impractical, researchers sometimes use a quasi-experimental design and compare preexisting groups. Quasi-experimental designs include variations that parallel the true experimental designs, except with nonrandom assignment of participants to groups. Some examples include a pretest-posttest nonequivalent control group design, switching replications design with nonequivalent control group, and a double pretest design with nonequivalent control group. Quasi-experimental designs also include time-series or single-participant designs with experimental manipulation of a treatment variable. Examples include treatment withdrawal, treatment replication, and multiple baseline designs.

In evidence-based practice investigations, research design is one of the key factors in determining the level of evidence a study provides. At the highest levels of evidence are true experimental designs, which are sometimes called randomized clinical trials, and meta-analyses. A meta-analysis is a study that involves a statistical analysis of the combined results of several experimental clinical trials. Quasi-experimental designs fall in the middle range of most levels of evidence models. Both quasi-experimental designs with nonequivalent treatment and control groups and single-participant research designs use experimental manipulation of at least one independent variable, but neither has the feature of random assignment of participants to groups. When judging the level of evidence for intervention studies, nonexperimental designs like descriptive case studies, correlation research, and qualitative designs fall at a relatively low level of evidence, and suggestions based on expert opinion with little or no supporting evidence are at the lowest level.

Review Questions

1. The purpose of _____ is to explore cause-and-effect relationships.

2. What are two important characteristics of a true experimental design?

3. Explain the following design notation:
   R   O   X   O
   R   O   O

4. What is the primary distinction between a true experimental design and a quasi-experimental design?

5. What is the design notation for a switching replications design?

6. Why is a switching replications design a good choice for intervention research?

7. Explain the concept of pretest sensitization (reactive effect of testing).

8. Identify each of the following statements as most likely to apply to single-subject or group research designs.
   a. Participants experience both the treatment and control conditions.

b. A good approach is when participants respond in unique ways to the experimental intervention.
c. Provide the best level of evidence when researchers use random assignment of subjects to treatment and control conditions.
d. Data are usually presented in graphs or tables for individual subjects and often no statistical analysis is completed.
e. Researchers usually report the combined results for all participants.

9. Explain how maturation is a threat to the internal validity of a study and how including both randomized treatment and control groups addresses this threat.

10. Explain how a repeated measures design would be different from a pretest-posttest randomized control group design.

11. A researcher wished to use a factorial design to study the length/scheduling of treatment sessions (30-minute sessions four times per week and 1-hour sessions two times per week) as well as two different approaches to providing feedback (immediate feedback following every response versus delayed feedback following each set of five responses). The researcher recruited 36 subjects with communication disorders for the study. Illustrate how the subjects would be randomly assigned to groups in this factorial design.

12. What is the meaning of the term *statistical regression* and how could this phenomenon affect the results of an intervention study?

13. What is the best way to control for most threats to internal validity?

14. Explain the difference between a multiple baseline across behaviors single-subject design and a multiple baseline across subjects single-subject design.

15. In most levels of evidence models, what kind of evidence is at the highest level and what kind is at the lowest level?

16. How are a systematic review and meta-analysis different from the narrative review of literature that usually begins a research report?

Learning Activities

1. Read one or more of the following published reports on research that employ a true experimental design. Identify the experimental manipulation and describe how participants were randomly assigned to groups.

Arnott, S., Onslow, M., O'Brian, S., Packman, A., Jones, M., & Block, S. (2014). Group Lidcombe program treatment for early stuttering: A randomized controlled trial. *Journal of Speech, Language, and Hearing Research, 57*, 1606–1618. https://doi.org/10.1044/2014_JSLHR-S-13-0090

Beukes, E. W., Baguley, D. M., Allen, P. M., Manchaiah, V., & Andersson, G. (2018). Audiologist-guided internet-based cognitive behavior therapy for adults with tinnitus in the United Kingdom: A randomized controlled trial. *Ear and Hearing*,

39(3), 423–433. https://doi.org/10.1097/AUD.0000000000000505

Capin, P., Vaughn, S., Gillam, S. L., Fall, A.-M., Roberts, G., Israelsen-Augenstein, M., Holbrook, S., Wada, R., Dille, J., Hall, C., & Gillam, R. B. (2023). Evaluating the efficacy of a narrative language intervention for bilingual students. *American Journal of Speech-Language Pathology*, *32*(6), 2999–3020. https://doi.org/10.1044/2023_AJSLP-21-00185

Cohen, W., Hodson, A., O'Hare, A., Boyle, J., Durrani, T., McCartney, E., Mattey, M., Naftalin, L., & Watson, J. (2005). Effects of computer-based intervention through acoustically modified speech (Fast ForWord) in severe mixed receptive-expressive language impairment: Outcomes from a randomized controlled trial. *Journal of Speech, Language, and Hearing Research*, *48*, 715–729. https://doi.org/10.1044/1092-4388(2005/049)

Doesborgh, S. J., van de Sandt-Koenderman, M. W., Dippel, D. W., van Harskamp, F., Koudstaal, P. J., & Visch-Brink, E. G. (2003). Effects of semantic treatment on verbal communication and linguistic processing in aphasia after stroke: A randomized controlled trial. *Stroke*, *35*(1), 141–146.

Humes, L. E., Rogers, S. E., Quigley, T. M., Main, A. K., Kinney, D. L., & Herring, C. (2017). The effects of service-delivery model and purchase price on hearing-aid outcomes in older adults: A randomized double-blind placebo-controlled clinical trial. *American Journal of Audiology*, *26*, 53–79. https://doi.org/10.1044/2017_AJA-16-0111

Murray, E., McCabe, P., & Ballard, K. J. (2015). A randomized controlled trial for children with childhood apraxia of speech comparing rapid syllable transition treatment and the Nuffield Dyspraxia Programme—Third Edition. *Journal of Speech, Language, and Hearing Research*, *58*, 669–686. https://doi.org/10.1044/2015_JSLHR-S-13-0179

Sapir, S., Spielman, J. L., Ramig, L. O., Story, B. H., & Fox, C. (2007). Effects of intensive voice treatment (the Lee Silverman Voice Treatment [LSVT]) on vowel articulation in dysarthric individuals with idiopathic Parkinson disease: Acoustic and perceptual findings. *Journal of Speech, Language, Hearing Research*, *50*, 899–912.

Spencer, R. D., Petersen, D. B., & Adams, J. L. (2015). Tier 2 language intervention for diverse preschoolers: An early-stage randomized control group study following an analysis of response to intervention. *American Journal of Speech-Language Pathology*, *24*, 619–636. https://doi.org/10.1044/2015_AJSLP-14-0101

van Kleeck, A., Vander Woude, J., & Hammett, L. (2006). Fostering literal and inferential language skills in Head Start preschoolers with language impairment using scripted book-sharing discussions. *American Journal of Speech-Language Pathology*, *15*, 85–95.

2. Think of an independent variable you would like to investigate. Perhaps focus on an intervention from the field of audiology or speech-language pathology. Think about whether you would investigate this variable with a treatment and control group or with two or more levels of treatment. Which of the true experimental designs discussed in this chapter would be appropriate for investigating the variable you chose? What measures will you use for your pretest and/or posttest? How many participants will you need to recruit and how will you assign them to the different groups?

3. Read the research scenario, "Participation in a Clinical Trial," provided in Appendix 8–1. Consider

how you would answer each of the discussion questions and compare your answers with those of your peers.

References

American Speech-Language-Hearing Association. (2004). *Evidence-based practice in communication disorders: An introduction* [Technical report]. https://www.asha.org/policy/tr2004-00001/

Antonucci, S. M., & MacWilliam, C. (2015). Verbal description of concrete objects: A method for assessing semantic circumlocution in persons with aphasia. *American Journal of Speech-Language Pathology, 24*, S828–S837. https://doi.org/10.1044/2015_AJSLP-14-0154

Arnott, S., Onslow, M., O'Brian, S., Packman, A., Jones, M., & Block, S. (2014). Group Lidcombe program treatment for early stuttering: A randomized controlled trial. *Journal of Speech, Language, and Hearing Research, 57*, 1606–1618. https://doi.org/10.1044/2014_JSLHR-S-13-0090

Baker, M., Buss, E., Jacks, A., Taylor, C., & Leibold, L. J. (2014). Children's perception of speech produced in a two-talker background. *Journal of Speech, Language, and Hearing Research, 57*, 327–337. https://doi.org/10.1044/1092-4388(2013/12-0287)

Barlow, D. H., Nock, M. K., & Hersen, M. (2009). *Single case experimental designs: Strategies for studying behavior change* (3rd ed.). Pearson.

Bernthal, J. E., Bankson, N. W., & Flipsen, P., Jr. (2013). *Articulation and phonological disorders* (7th ed.). Pearson.

Beukes, E. W., Baguley, D. M., Allen, P. M., Manchaiah, V., & Andersson, G. (2018). Audiologist-guided internet-based cognitive behavior therapy for adults with tinnitus in the United Kingdom: A randomized controlled trial. *Ear and Hearing, 39*(3), 423–433. https://doi.org/10.1097/AUD.0000000000000505

Byiers, B. J., Reichle, J., & Symons, F. J. (2012). Single-subject experimental design for evidence-based practice. *American Journal of Speech-Language Pathology, 21*, 397–414. https://doi.org/10.1044/1058-0360(2012/11-0036)

Capin, P., Vaughn, S., Gillam, S. L., Fall, A.-M., Roberts, G., Israelsen-Augenstein, M., Holbrook, S., Wada, R., Dille, J., Hall, C., & Gillam, R. B. (2023). Evaluating the efficacy of a narrative language intervention for bilingual students. *American Journal of Speech-Language Pathology, 32*(6), 2999–3020. https://doi.org/10.1044/2023_AJSLP-21-00185

Center for Knowledge Translation for Disability and Rehabilitation Research. (2020, March 20). *Strength of evidence* (KT strategies database). https://ktdrr.org/ktstrategies/evidence.html

Chapman, R. S., Sindberg, H., Bridge, C., Gigstead, K., & Hesketh, L. (2006). Effect of memory support and elicited production on fast mapping of new words by adolescents with Down syndrome. *Journal of Speech, Language, and Hearing Research, 49*, 3–15. https://doi.org/10.1044/1092-4388(2006/001)

Cohen, L., Manion, L., & Morrison, K. (2018). *Research methods in education* (8th ed.). Routledge.

DeLong, C., Nessler, C., Wright, S., & Wambaugh, J. (2015). Semantic feature analysis: Further examination of outcomes. *American Journal of Speech-Language Pathology, 24*, S864–S879. https://doi.org/10.1044/2015_AJSLP-14-0155

Doesborgh, S. J., van de Sandt-Koenderman, M. W., Dippel, D. W., van Harskamp, F., Koudstaal, P. J., & Visch-Brink, E. G. (2003). Effects of semantic treatment on verbal communication and linguistic processing in aphasia after stroke: A randomized controlled trial. *Stroke, 35*(1), 141–146.

Ebell, M. H., Siwek, J., Weiss, B. D., Woolf, S. H., Susman, J. Ewigman, B., & Bowman, M. (2004). Strength of recommendation taxonomy (SORT): A patient-centered approach to grading evidence in the medical literature. *American Family Physician, 69*, 548–556. https://www.aafp.org/afp/2004/0201/p548.html

Gordon-Salant, S., Fitzgibbons, P. J., & Friedman, S. A. (2007). Recognition of time-compressed and natural speech with selective temporal enhancements by young and elderly listeners. *Journal of Speech, Language, and Hearing Research, 50*, 1181–1193. https://doi.org/10.1044/1092-4388(2007/082)

Hesketh, A., Dima, E., & Nelson, V. (2007). Teaching phoneme awareness to pre-literate children with speech disorder: A randomized controlled trial. *International Journal of Language and Communication Disorders, 42*, 251–271.

Horner, R. H., Carr, E. G., Halle, J., McGee, G., Odom, S., & Wolery, M. (2005). The use of single-subject research to identify evidence-based practice in special education. *Exceptional Children, 71*, 165–179. https://doi.org/10.1177/001440290507100203

Howick, J., Chalmers, I., Glasziou, P., Greenhalgh, T., Heneghan, C., Liberati, A., Moschetti, I., Phillips, B., & Thornton, H. (2011a). *The 2011 Oxford CEBM evidence levels of evidence (introductory document)*. https://www.cebm.net/2016/05/ocebm-levels-of-evidence/

Howick, J., Chalmers, I., Glasziou, P., Greenhalgh, T., Heneghan, C., Liberati, A., Moschetti, I., Phillips, B., & Thornton, H. (2011b). *Explanation of the 2011 Oxford Centre for Evidence-Based Medicine (OCEBM) levels of evidence (background document)*. https://www.cebm.ox.ac.uk/resources/levels-of-evidence/explanation-of-the-2011-ocebm-levels-of-evidence

Humes, L. E., Rogers, S. E., Quigley, T. M., Main, A. K., Kinney, D. L., & Herring, C. (2017). The effects of service-delivery model and purchase price on hearing-aid outcomes in older adults: A randomized double-blind placebo-controlled clinical trial. *American Journal of Audiology, 26*, 53–79. https://doi.org/10.1044/2017_AJA-16-0111

Leary, M. R. (2011). *Introduction to behavioral research methods* (6th ed.). Pearson.

Lillie, E. O., Patay, B., Diamant, J., Issell, B., Topol, E. J., & Schork, N. J. (2011). The n-of-1 clinical trial: The ultimate strategy for individualizing medicine? *Personalized Medicine, 8*(2), 161–173. https://doi.org/10.2217/pme.11.7

Lundberg, M., Andersson, G., & Lunner, T. (2011). A randomized, controlled trial of the short-term effects of complementing an educational program for hearing aid users with telephone consultations. *Journal of the American Academy of Audiology, 22*, 654–662.

Maas, E., Butalla, C. E., & Farinella, K. A. (2012). Feedback frequency in treatment for childhood apraxia of speech. *American Journal of Speech-Language Pathology, 21*, 239–257. https://doi.org/10.1044/1058-0360(2012/110119)

Max, L., & Onghena, P. (1999). Randomized and repeated measures designs for speech, language, and hearing research. *Journal of Speech, Language, and Hearing Research, 42*, 261–270. https://doi.org/10.1044/jslhr.4202.261

McArdle, R. A., Killion, M., Mennite, M. A., & Chisolm, T. H. (2012). Are two ears not better than one? *Journal of the American Academy of Audiology, 23*, 171–181. https://doi.org/10.3766/jaaa.23.3.4

McDaniel, J., Camarata, S., & Yoder, P. (2018). Comparing auditory-only and audiovisual word learning for children with hearing loss. *Journal of Deaf Studies and Deaf Education, 23*(4), 382–398. https://doi.org/10.1093/deafed/eny016

Miller, W. R. (2010). Qualitative research findings as evidence: Utility in nursing practice. *Clinical Nurse Specialist: The International Journal for Advanced Nursing Practice, 24*(4), 191–193. https://doi.org/10.1097/NUR.0b013e3181e36087

Murray, E., McCabe, P., & Ballard, K. J. (2015). A randomized controlled trial for children with childhood apraxia of speech comparing rapid syllable transition treatment and the Nuffield Dyspraxia Programme–Third Edition. *Journal of Speech, Language, and Hearing Research, 58*, 669–686. https://doi.org/10.1044/2015_JSLHR-S-13-0179

Newhart, M., & Patten, M. L. (2023). *Understanding research methods: An overview of the essentials* (11th ed.). Routledge Taylor & Francis Group.

OCEBM Levels of Evidence Working Group. (2011). *The Oxford 2011 levels of evidence*. https://www.cebm.ox.ac.uk/resources/levels-of-evidence/ocebm-levels-of-evidence

Palmer, C. V., Adams, S. W., Bourgeois, M., Durrant, J., & Rossi, M. (1999). Reduction in caregiver-identified problem behaviors in patients with Alzheimer disease post-hearing-aid fitting. *Journal of Speech, Language, and Hearing Research, 42*, 312–328. https://doi.org/10.1044/jslhr.4202.312

Phillips, B., Ball, C., Sackett, D., Badenoch, D., Straus, S., Haynes, B., & Dawes, M. (2009, March). *Oxford Centre for Evidence-based Medicine levels of evidence* (Updated by J. Howick). https://www.cebm.net/2009/06/oxford-centre-evidence-based-medicine-levels-evidence-march-2009/

Reichow, B., Volkmar, F. R., & Cicchetti, D. V. (2008). Development of the evaluative method for evaluating and determining evidence-based practices in autism. *Journal of Autism and Developmental Disorders, 38*, 1311–1319. https://doi.org/10.1007/s10803-007-0517-7

Richards, S. B. (2019). *Single-subject research: Applications in educational and clinical settings* (3rd ed.). Cengage Learning.

Rosenthal, R., & Rosnow, R. L. (2008). *Essentials of behavioral research: Methods and data analysis* (3rd ed.). McGraw-Hill.

Rudolph, J. M., & Wendt, O. (2014). The efficacy of the cycles approach: A multiple baseline design. *Journal of Communication Disorders, 47*, 1–16. https://doi.org/10.1016/j.jcomdis.2013.12.003

Salkind, N. J. (2010). *Encyclopedia of research design: Volume 1*. Sage.

Salorio-Corbetto, M., Baer, T., & Moore, B. C. J. (2019). Comparison of frequency transposition and frequency compression for people with extensive dead regions in the cochlea. *Trends in Hearing, 23*, 1–23. https://doi.org/10.1177/2331216518822206

Sandage, M. J., Connor, N. P., & Pascoe, D. D. (2014). Vocal function and upper airway thermoregulation in five different environmental conditions. *Journal of Speech, Language, and Hearing Research, 57*, 16–25. https://doi.org/10.1044/1092-4388(2013/13-0015

Schlosser, R. W. (2006). *The role of systematic reviews in evidence-based practice, research, and development* (Technical Brief No. 15). https://ktdrr.org/ktlibrary/articles_pubs/ncddrwork/focus/focus15/Focus15.pdf

Shearer, W. M. (1997). Experimental design and statistics in speech. In W. J. Hardcastle & J. Laver (Eds.), *The handbook of phonetic sciences* (pp. 167–187). Blackwell Publishing.

Spencer, R. D., Petersen, D. B., & Adams, J. L. (2015). Tier 2 language intervention for diverse preschoolers: An early-stage randomized control group study following an analysis of response to intervention. *American Journal of Speech-Language Pathology, 24*, 619–636. https://doi.org/10.1044/2015_AJSLP-14-0101

Spratford, M., McLean, H. H., & McCreery, R. (2017). Relationship of grammatical context on children's recognition of s/z-inflected words. *Journal of the American Academy of Audiology, 28*(9), 799–809. https://doi.org/10.3766/jaaa.16151

Tate, R. L., McDonald, S., Perdices, M., Togher, L., Schultz, R., & Savage, S. (2008). Rating the methodological quality of single-subject designs and n-of-1 trials: Introducing the single-case experimental design (SCED) scale. *Neuropsychological Rehabilitation, 18*, 385–401. https://doi.org/10.1080/09602010802009201

Tate, R. L., Perdices, M., Rosenkoetter, U., Wakim, D., Godbee, K., Togher, L, & McDonald, S. (2013). Revision of a method quality rating scale for single-case experimental designs and n-of-1 trials: The 15-item Risk of Bias in N-of-1 Trials (RoBiNT) scale. *Neuropsychological Rehabilitation, 23*, 619–638. https://doi.org/10.1080/09602011.2013.824383

Tönsing, K. M., Dada, S., & Alant, E. (2014). Teaching graphic symbol combinations to children with limited speech during shared story reading. *Augmentative and Alternative Communication, 30*, 279–297. https://doi.org/10.3109/07434618.2014.965846

Trochim, W. M. K., Donnelly, J. P., & Arora, K. (2016). *Research methods: The essential knowledge base* (2nd ed.). Cengage Learning.

Trussell, J. W., Hasko, J., Kane, J, Amari, B., & Brusehaber, A. (2018). Interactive storybook reading instruction for preschoolers who are deaf and hard of hearing: A multiple probe across behaviors analysis. *Language, Speech and Hearing Services in Schools, 49,* 922–937. https://doi.org/10.1044/2018_LSHSS-17-0085

Wambaugh, J. L., Nessler, C., Cameron, R., & Mauszycki, S. C. (2013). Treatment for acquired apraxia of speech: Examination of treatment intensity and practice schedule. *American Journal of Speech-Language Pathology, 22,* 84–102. https://doi.org/10.1044/1058-0360(2012/12-0025)

Wendt, O., & Miller, B. (2012). Quality appraisal of single-subject experimental designs: An overview and comparison of different appraisal tools. *Education and Treatment of Children, 35,* 235–268. https://doi.org/10.1353/etc.2012.0010

APPENDIX 8-1

Research Scenario

Participation in a Clinical Trial

Please note that the following case description is a work of fiction. It is not intended to represent any actual individuals or events.

C. I. Jones is a speech-language pathologist (SLP) in an outpatient rehabilitation center affiliated with an acute care hospital. CI has worked in the facility for more than 5 years and had extensive training in the area of medical speech-language pathology from graduate coursework. CI has continued to acquire knowledge through personal reading, additional coursework, and continuing education activities. In the past 2 years, CI has been taking some courses toward a health care management degree at a nearby university. The university has a special distance learning program that allows students to complete their requirements on a part-time basis while continuing to be employed in the field. CI is highly regarded by the staff at the outpatient center and the director of rehabilitation services, Dr. V. Dedicated.

At a recent professional conference, CI attended a research seminar on a new approach for treating adult motor speech disorders, the Functional Speech Intelligibility Approach (FSIA). The presenters discussed the theory and principles underlying the approach, discussed the research that supported it, and presented some examples of its use in a clinical setting. What impressed CI was that the presenters described several research studies using the approach. Two of these were well-designed clinical trials that had a randomized pretest-posttest control group design, plus the researchers included procedures called "double blinding" to reduce the possibility of bias in their data collection. The researchers also had obtained long-term follow-up data, 6 months after treatment, to determine if the differences between experimental and control groups persisted. Both of the studies suggested FSIA was more effective than traditional therapy.

At the end of their presentation, the researchers described the next step in gathering data about the effectiveness of FSIA. They planned to conduct a multicenter clinical trial and asked SLPs in the audience to consider participating. SLPs in the multicenter trial would receive free training in how to administer FSIA treatment. They would need to treat five participants with FSIA and five with traditional treatment (determined randomly). SLPs would need to follow a protocol set up by the researchers for testing and treating the participants. As far as CI could tell, the protocol established appropriate pretest and posttest measures and adequate amounts of treatment. CI was interested in the study but wondered if participating in research would be feasible in the outpatient setting. CI knew that the hospital had an institutional review board and that other departments regularly participated in clinical trials. CI decided to talk to the director of rehabilitation services and maybe consult with the IRB members before making a decision.

Discussion Questions

1. Is the multicenter study described in this case a well-designed clinical trial? Explain your answer.

2. What do you think of the idea of conducting research in an actual clinical setting, such as an outpatient rehabilitation setting?

3. What are some of the issues CI would need to consider before making a decision about whether or not to participate in the clinical trial?

4. Do you think CI will be able to provide adequate speech and language services while gathering evidence about the approach? What are your reasons for answering yes or no?

9

Research Participants and Sampling

Main Points

- Researchers often make observations from a sample of a larger population. A population is all individuals who meet specific criteria; a sample is some of the individuals who meet specific criteria.
- A census is a summary of information from a population; an inference is a summary of information from a sample.
- A parameter is an observation of a population; a statistic is an observation of a sample.
- Participant recruitment procedures should attempt to minimize bias in the sample and be documented to help interpret inferential statistics. Recruitment procedures should also conform with the ethical principle of justice.
- The appropriate sample size depends on the population size, the study design, planned statistical analyses, degree of variability within the population, and ethical considerations. A large sample size is not necessarily a representative sample of the population.

When planning a study, researchers usually have a group of persons in mind who are the focal point of the study. These groups can be quite large, such as all persons in the United States who are age 65 and older or all children between the ages of 2 and 4, or the groups can be somewhat smaller, such as all persons between the ages of 45 and 65 with sensorineural hearing loss, 5-year-old children with specific language impairment, or adults between the ages of 18 and 25 with a traumatic brain injury. Even when a group is relatively small, studying everyone who is a member of the group is usually impractical. As an alternative, researchers try to identify a representative sample of individuals from the group to participate in their research. The strategies researchers use to select participants and criteria for obtaining a representative sample are topics covered in this chapter.

Populations and Samples

Ordinarily, researchers expect the findings from their studies to apply to a fairly large group of individuals and certainly to a larger group than actually participated in the study. Researchers use the term *population* to refer to all of the persons of interest for a particular study (Cohen et al., 2018; Newhart & Patten, 2023). This population is defined in the planning phase of the study, and all the members have one or more predetermined characteristics. For example, researchers might define the population of a study as all 4- and 5-year-old children who are bilingual Spanish-English speakers, all adults ages 45 to 65 who are native English speakers with no known medical conditions, or adults with a sensorineural hearing loss with an onset after age 50. Although the population of interest often is relatively large, this is not always the case. For example, audiologists and speech-language pathologists might conduct a study of the persons served in a particular speech-language-hearing center to determine how satisfied they were with the services provided. One of the criteria for establishing the population for a study is that all members have at least one characteristic in common (Newhart & Patten, 2023).

The persons who actually participate in a study usually are a *sample* from a larger population. Sometimes authors refer to research participants as the subjects of a study. Recent guidelines from the American Psychological Association (APA, 2020), however, suggest authors should refer to their participants in a way that either describes who they are (e.g., the first-grade children, the high school students, the parents, the teachers) or their role in the study (e.g., the participants, the listeners). One goal in identifying persons to participate in a study is to recruit a sample that represents the population well. This means all members of the population should have an equal chance of being recruited to participate (Newhart & Patten, 2023). Researchers particularly try to avoid systematically excluding some members of the intended population when they identify participants. Let's consider the example of a research team that wants to recruit preschool children for a study. The team members obtain the names and telephone numbers of potential volunteers by leaving a description of their study and a signup sheet at locations in their community frequented by parents and their children. They follow up by calling each of the families; however, because the researchers call between 9:00 a.m. and 5:00 p.m., they inadvertently exclude many families with working parents. This is an example in which some members of a population do not have an equal opportunity to take part in a study.

Trochim et al. (2016) make a distinction between the intended population for a study and the "accessible" population (p. 81). The intended population includes all persons to whom the researchers want to apply their results, and the accessible population represents the group from which the researchers actually recruit their participants. One reason for the difference between the intended and actual populations could be geographic proximity. The researchers might want to apply their findings to all persons in the United States with a particular speech, language, or hearing disorder, but the accessible population might only include those persons who live near the research facility. The accessible population might be a good representation of the intended population but, in some instances, could be systematically different. For example, researchers in a university setting could have more families with highly educated parents than would be the case in the general population. Sometimes researchers address issues such as geographic proximity by developing cooperative projects with researchers in other locations.

On occasion, researchers conduct a study in which they gather information from an entire population. When researchers attempt to gather data from all members of a population, the study is called a *census* (Newhart & Patten, 2023; Trochim et al., 2016). Perhaps the most familiar census is the U.S. Census that is conducted every decade by the United States Census Bureau (2020). Another example of a census would be research conducted on all members of a small population. Examples of these types of census studies would be research on persons served at a particular rehabilitation facility or on all first-grade children in a particular school district.

When researchers study a sample from a large population, they still want to draw conclusions about the population as a whole. Instead of knowing the characteristics of the population as they would if they conducted a census, however, researchers make *inferences* about the population based on the data they gather from their sample. An inference is a conclusion we draw in an indirect way. When researchers develop conclusions about a population based on data from a sample, their conclusions about the population are indirect and not based on actual observations of the entire population. Furthermore, the accuracy of these conclusions depends on how well the sample represents the population.

Usually, researchers want to study a population of persons, and the sample is a group of persons selected from that population. However, sometimes the population is defined in a different way, such as all first-grade classrooms in the United States or all utterances produced by a particular child (Woods et al., 1986), and the units sampled will be different as well (e.g., a sample of first-grade classrooms or a sample of utterances).

Often in group studies, researchers report their findings as numerical summaries (Pyrczak, 2010). If these numbers come from observations on the entire population, they are called *parameters*. If these numbers come from observations on a sample, they are called *statistics*. In other chapters, we discuss how researchers use statistics to describe their findings and to make accurate inferences about the populations of interest in their investigations.

Sample Characteristics

As noted earlier, the most common approach to group research is to study a sample and to infer characteristics of the population as a whole from the results of the sample. The value of this kind of research depends on how well the sample represents the population of interest. Thus, researchers want to know about sample characteristics, such as what population a sample represents and whether the sample is biased or unbiased.

A sample is representative if the characteristics of the sample are a good match for the characteristics of the population. One aspect of this is to understand the actual population from which you draw your sample. Sometimes it is difficult, if not impossible, to access the intended population. Perhaps researchers want to recruit 4-year-old children to participate in a study. They do not, however, have a readily available list of 4-year-olds and their parents. Instead, they have access to 4-year-olds who attend preschool programs in the community. If the researchers draw their sample from the preschool programs, this sample might not be an ideal match for the general population of preschoolers.

In addition to concerns about differences between the intended and accessible populations, researchers also need to avoid bias in selecting a sample. An unbiased sample is one in which all members of a population have an equal opportunity of being selected, whereas a biased sample is one in which some members of a population have an unequal opportunity, or perhaps no opportunity, of being selected (Newhart & Patten, 2023; Pyrczak, 2010). One source of bias in sampling *is failing to identify all members* of a population (Newhart & Patten, 2023), either because of differences in the accessible and intended populations or because the researchers used a sampling method that introduced a bias. For example, researchers might issue a call for participants in an ad in a newspaper and in flyers distributed throughout the community. If they select as their participants the first 50 persons who respond, it would be a biased way of selecting a sample. Persons who respond quickly to such an ad could be systematically different from those who take more time to respond.

Another source of bias is using a *sample of convenience*. This refers to using a group of participants who are easy to access (Pyrczak, 2010). A common example is research with college students and particularly research with students in introductory psychology courses. University professors often conduct research in their areas of professional interest, and if young adults are an appropriate population for the research, students in introductory courses are a readily available source of participants. Some professors might offer credit toward the course grade to students who volunteer for their research. From an ethical standpoint, however, professors should not require participation in research, nor should they offer such opportunities as the only way to earn extra credit.

Sometimes researchers recruit participants from existing community programs because contacting persons through these programs is less of an invasion of privacy. For example, researchers might make initial contact with a group of persons age 65 and older through a community activity center. The initial contact could be low key, perhaps through a flyer distributed at the community center, and potential participants could provide their contact information voluntarily without undue pressure. However, a sample recruited in this way might not be representative of the general population of persons age 65 and older. One might speculate that persons who attend the community programs might be more outgoing socially or in better general health than those who do not attend. If researchers wanted to apply their findings to all persons in this age group, they would need to develop ways to contact and sample from all members of the population of interest.

Another reason a sample could be biased is through *volunteerism*. This is a source of bias that cannot be avoided because the process of informed consent specifies that all persons who participate in research should do so on a voluntary basis. However, persons who volunteer to participate in research might differ from the general population in some systematic way. They might have a special interest in the topic of the research because of their own or a family member's experiences. They might have greater interest than usual in research because they have conducted studies of their own. These are just a few of the many ways research volunteers could differ from the overall population. To address this issue, researchers sometimes resort to incentives to increase the number who agree to participate, such as payments, extra credit points, and so forth.

Sampling Methods

Although certain types of problems in selecting a sample are difficult to avoid, particularly volunteerism, researchers prefer random sampling methods when they want to avoid systematic biases in choosing research participants. In this section, we cover some of the most common sampling methods.

Simple Random Sampling

The procedure researchers usually use to obtain an unbiased sample is *simple random sampling*. An important feature of this sampling approach is that every member of a population has an equal chance of being selected for the study (Cohen et al., 2018; Trochim et al., 2016). Theoretically, you could generate a random sample by writing participant identifiers on separate pieces of paper, placing them all in a hat, and drawing them out one at a time until you have the target number of participants. Researchers often use random numbers to choose participants, however. One approach is to assign all participants an identifying number. The researchers might start with a list of potential participants—for example, a list of 100 volunteers. Each person on the list is assigned a three-digit number from 101 to 200, and then the researchers could consult a table of random numbers and select participants in the order their numbers appear in the table. Example 1 is a series of random numbers representing the first 10 participants.

Example 1
154, 196, 191, 108, 157, 143, 188, 152, 183, 140

Another way to use random numbers to select a sample is to use the random number function in a spreadsheet program. First, you would list all possible participants in one column of a spreadsheet. Next, you would use the random number function to generate a random number for each participant in a second column, and then you would sort the participants using the random number column as the basis of your sort. Look at Table 9–1 for an example of this approach. The first column shows the potential participants listed by their participant identifier. The second column shows the random numbers generated for each participant. The last two columns show the participants and numbers after they were sorted. If the researchers in this example wanted a sample of 15 participants, they simply would take the first 15 persons in the sorted list (e.g., QQ through NN). This example only includes 26 possible participants, but the list often would be much longer.

Systematic Sampling

Another approach that generally yields a sample that is free from intentional bias is *systematic sampling*. In systematic sampling, you start with a list of potential participants, establish a sampling interval, and then select every so many participants according to the number representing your sampling interval (Cohen et al., 2018; Trochim et al., 2016). To illustrate, let's consider the case of a group of researchers who have a list of 2,500 potential participants. They want to select a sample of 125 actual participants from this list.

To determine the sampling interval, they divide 2,500 by 125, resulting in a sampling interval of 20. This means that the researchers will choose every 20th person from their list. Often, researchers using systematic sampling establish their starting point with a random number. For example,

Table 9–1. Illustration of the Use of a Spreadsheet to Generate a Randomized List of Research Participants

Participant Identifier	Random Numbers	Sorted Participants	Sorted Numbers
AA	87	QQ	10
BB	21	GG	11
CC	71	EE	14
DD	83	HH	18
EE	14	BB	21
FF	43	PP	23
GG	11	XX	26
HH	18	RR	29
II	40	JJ	32
JJ	32	UU	36
KK	52	YY	37
LL	99	II	40
MM	42	MM	42
NN	47	FF	43
OO	79	NN	47
PP	23	KK	52
QQ	10	ZZ	53
RR	29	VV	59
SS	60	SS	60
TT	61	TT	61
UU	36	CC	71
VV	59	OO	79
WW	97	DD	83
XX	26	AA	87
YY	37	WW	97
ZZ	53	LL	99

these researchers might have determined at random that Participant 110 would be the first selected. They would start at 110 and continue through their list choosing every 20th person until they have a sample of 125 persons (e.g., 110, 130, 150, 170, 190).

Stratified Random Sampling

When researchers want to increase the likelihood that their sample accurately represents the population of interest, they might use a strategy called stratified random sampling. In this approach, researchers identify one or more criteria or *strata* that characterize the population of interest. Examples include the percentage of men and women in the population, the distribution of persons by age group, family income levels, parent education levels, and whether the person lives in an urban, suburban, or rural area. Often the goal is to include a similar percentage of persons in the sample as was present in the population. For example, if the population percentages were 60% women and 40% men, and researchers want to match these percentages in a 125-person sample, they would include 75 women and 50 men. Speech-language pathology is an example of a field where including an equal number of men and women in a sample would not be representative of the population. Occasionally, the goal in stratified random sampling is to select an equal number of participants across the levels of a stratum. This is often true with sampling across age levels.

Variations on stratified random sampling are often employed in generating samples for test norms (e.g., Dunn & Dunn, 2007; Goldman & Fristoe, 2015; Newcomer & Hammill, 2008; Reynolds & Voress, 2008; Zimmerman et al., 2011) and less frequently in research reports (e.g., Phillips & Morse, 2011; Sharp & Shega, 2009; Smit et al., 1990; Trulove & Fitch, 1998). Usually the goal of stratified sampling is not to make comparisons across the subgroups but to generate a sample that represents the diversity present in the population of interest.

Cluster Sampling

One additional sampling approach that yields a random sample is *cluster sampling*. In this sampling approach, researchers begin by obtaining a random sample of predefined groups such as medical centers, classrooms, or communities. An example would be a random sample of all the kindergarten classrooms in a particular state. Sometimes cluster sampling is combined with simple random sampling in a procedure called *multistage sampling* (Newhart & Patten, 2023). In this procedure, researchers begin with a random sample from the previously identified clusters. They could start with a list such as a list of all communities in the United States with a population greater than 100,000 or a list of all universities that offer audiology and/or speech-language pathology graduate programs. Then, they would select a certain number of clusters at random from this list. Perhaps they could use random numbers to select 50 communities or 50 high schools. After selecting communities or high schools to investigate, the researchers could follow up by selecting actual participants from among those who volunteered in each high school or community using simple random sampling.

Newhart and Patten (2023) noted that predefined groups or clusters tend to be more similar to one another than the population as a whole. Therefore, researchers usually use cluster sampling in studies with relatively large numbers of participants. Such studies often include many clusters so that no single cluster will overly influence the research results. Tomblin et al. (1997) conducted a study in which they used a variation on cluster sampling, stratified cluster sampling. The clusters in this example were kindergarten children in previously identified elementary schools. The strata were schools classified as being in urban, suburban, and rural areas. These researchers sampled elementary schools or clusters from a group of urban, suburban, and rural schools, and then completed their research by testing the kindergarten children from each school who were eligible for the study.

The various options for random sampling are regarded as the best way to obtain a sample that is free from systematic bias. However, that does not mean that all random samples represent their populations well. On occasion, researchers obtain a sample that either overrepresents or underrepresents some aspect of the population. For example, the population might include fairly equal percentages of men and women, but after random sampling, researchers could end up with a sample that has 60% women and 40% men, or perhaps the researchers end up with a sample that includes a disproportionate percentage of children with college-educated parents compared with those whose parents have a high school education. When these kinds of variances occur by chance, and not through some bias in the sampling method, the errors that occur are less damaging than systematic errors such as failing to identify all members of a population or using a sample of convenience (Newhart & Patten, 2023).

Purposive Sampling

In some research, the goal is not to generalize findings to a larger population but rather to obtain an expert opinion or the perspectives of persons who have had a unique experience. Researchers use *purposive sampling* when they need to recruit participants they think will be the best source of information for a particular issue (Newhart & Patten, 2023). Professional expertise could encompass many areas of audiology, speech-language pathology, and speech, language, and hearing science. Perhaps researchers are interested in studying recommendations for feeding infants with a palatal cleft, services provided by speech-language pathologists in neonatal intensive care units, or industrial audiology services provided to a specific industry. The number of professionals who could provide meaningful information on topics such as these might be relatively small, and researchers would need to make a special effort to identify and recruit them as participants.

Qualitative researchers often are interested in studying persons or organizations that have had unique experiences and may employ purposive sampling to find appropriate participants. For example, they might be interested in how persons in a clinical or medical center react to an experience such as implementation of new regulations; how persons who faced a sudden-onset speech, language, or hearing impairment reacted and adjusted to the changes in their communication abilities; or how an adult who recently received a cochlear implant experienced the preparation for, and follow-up to, the surgery. When the answer to a research question requires input from special persons, researchers have to make a purposeful effort to identify those individuals.

Random Assignment

For some studies, researchers have to divide the participants into two or more groups. This is the case in any true experiment with treatment and no-treatment control groups or experimental and alternate treatment groups. The preferred method for generating groups is *random assignment* of participants to groups. Although both random assignment and random selection involve procedures such as a table of random numbers or the random number function of a spreadsheet, the two are different processes that serve different roles in research. The purpose of random selection is to identify a sample of individuals who will participate in the study from a larger population. The purpose of random assignment is to divide all the participants into different treatment groups. Sometimes in research, using random selection to choose participants is impractical (Cohen et al., 2018). This could be the case in audiology and speech-language pathology if the research involves persons with very specific diagnostic characteristics. For example, speech-language pathologists might want to conduct intervention research with 4-year-old children who have a moderate-to-severe phonological disorder and age-appropriate expressive and receptive language, or audiologists might want to conduct research with persons with bilateral sensorineural hearing loss with an onset after age 40 with certain audiogram characteristics. The number of individuals who fit these descriptions might be relatively small, particularly if the researchers are limited to working with individuals who live relatively close to their research site. In situations like this, you could begin with purposive sampling to identify as many individuals as possible that fit your criteria and were willing to participate in your study. After identifying your sample, you could use random assignment to divide the participants into different groups.

In the example in Table 9–2, the researchers identified 30 participants using purposive sampling. Each participant received a random number using the random number function in a spreadsheet program. The researchers sorted the list using the random numbers and then assigned the first 15 participants in the random list to treatment Group A and the next 15 to treatment Group B. This procedure would yield two treatment groups created at random that should be free of any systematic bias in the assignment of participants.

Sample Size

One additional thing to consider about the sample is the number of participants to include. In some types of research, such as single-subject designs or qualitative case studies, a single participant might be adequate. Having a sample that is too small, however, could affect the validity of the conclusions obtained from group studies. Even with random sampling methods, researchers might end up with a sample that does not represent their population well; this problem is more likely if the sample is very small. Pyrczak (2010) noted that increasing sample size should increase how well a sample represents a population, sometimes referred to as *sample precision*. On the other hand, increasing sample size does not decrease systematic bias. If researchers use a sample of convenience or fail to identify all members of a population, increasing sample size does not reduce the bias associated with these sampling problems. Thus, researchers recruiting 4-year-old children from local preschool programs will fail to include children who do not attend preschool in their sample: Even doubling the size of the sample does not reduce this source of bias.

Several factors affect decisions about sample size. When conducting a study to estimate characteristics of a population, such as a typical level of performance on some skill or the percentage of persons exhibiting a certain trait, these factors include the size of the population of interest, how variable the levels of performance are, and how frequent the trait is in the overall population (Newhart & Patten, 2023; Pyrczak, 2010). If a population is small (e.g., 50 members), the best strategy is to recruit all or nearly all members as participants. For moderately sized populations (such as

Table 9–2. Illustration of the Use of a Spreadsheet to Generate Two Treatment Groups Using Random Assignment

Participant Identifier	Random Numbers	Sorted Participants	Sorted Numbers	Treatment Group
P01	271	P26	006	A
P02	231	P20	058	A
P03	489	P07	068	A
P04	420	P14	079	A
P05	091	P05	091	A
P06	289	P19	095	A
P07	068	P15	098	A
P08	329	P17	107	A
P09	311	P10	114	A
P10	114	P18	125	A
P11	421	P23	151	A
P12	373	P24	181	A
P13	188	P13	188	A
P14	079	P28	194	A
P15	098	P30	198	A
P16	434	P02	231	B
P17	107	P21	245	B
P18	125	P22	251	B
P19	095	P01	271	B
P20	058	P06	289	B
P21	245	P09	311	B
P22	251	P29	317	B
P23	151	P08	329	B
P24	181	P12	373	B
P25	454	P27	386	B
P26	006	P04	420	B
P27	386	P11	421	B
P28	194	P16	434	B
P29	317	P25	454	B
P30	198	P03	489	B

1,000 members), the recommended sample is approximately 28% or about 280 participants, and for larger populations (100,000 members), the recommended sample size is approximately 0.4% or about 400 participants (Newhart & Patten, 2023). These sample size recommendations are not absolute and need to be modified to accommodate other factors such as population variability and high or low prevalence of the trait under study. Generally, the more variable a population is for a behavior, the larger the sample should be, and the rarer a particular trait, the larger the sample should be (Newhart & Patten, 2023; Pyrczak, 2010).

When conducting a study to investigate the difference between groups, such as between treatment and control groups, the factors that affect decisions about sample size include how large the group differences might be, variability of scores on the outcome measures, and how certain researchers want to be about detecting group differences (Bland, 2000; Trochim et al., 2016). If a sample is too small, a study has a low probability of detecting a difference that actually occurs in the population. Although failing to find a statistically significant difference would be disappointing for researchers, conducting a study with too few participants might have even more noteworthy consequences. If the treatment under investigation might expose participants to even a small level of risk, then conducting the study with little chance of finding a treatment effect violates standards for research integrity (Gardenier & Resnik, 2002).

Let's compare two hypothetical intervention studies. In this example, a group of researchers investigated two different language intervention approaches. Previous experience with the approaches suggested that Intervention A was slightly superior to Intervention B at the end of 3 weeks of treatment. The researchers expect participants receiving Intervention A to score on average about 2 points higher than those receiving Intervention B. Variability in performance would also be a factor and, in this example, the researchers expect 95% of the participants' scores to fall within ±12 points. The researchers found they would need to recruit approximately 400 participants for each intervention group to be reasonably sure of detecting this small difference. The researchers realized that recruiting 800 participants who fit their criteria was impractical.[1]

One solution the researchers considered was to extend the treatment time to 15 weeks. Their previous experience suggested that participants receiving Intervention A would score on average about 5 points higher than those receiving Intervention B after 15 weeks of treatment. Assuming the same amount of variability in participant scores, the researchers would only need to recruit approximately 25 to 30 participants for each intervention group to be reasonably sure of detecting this larger difference.

Let's also consider how differences in variability would affect sample size requirements. In the example above, the researchers needed 25 to 30 participants for each intervention group if the expected difference was approximately 5 points and variability was such that 95% of the participants' scores fell within ±12 points. How many participants would be needed if variability is greater and 95% of the participants' scores fall within ±18 points? The answer is that sample size requirements would increase

---

[1] These sample size estimates are based on Table 12–4 in Rosenthal and Rosnow (2008). The initial assumptions were that the outcome measure had a standard deviation (SD) of 6 and that this SD was the same for both intervention groups.

and the researchers might need to recruit as many as 65 participants for each group. Rosenthal and Rosnow (2008) noted that researchers need to attend to sample size requirements or run the risk of reaching conclusions that are inaccurate or invalid.

When researchers have too few participants, they are less likely to detect differences that would actually exist if they could study the entire population. Using a sample that is too small might lead researchers to discard a new intervention that actually could have improved professional practice.

A challenge in planning research is finding the information you need to make decisions about appropriate sample sizes. Conducting a pilot study is one of the best ways to determine how much difference to expect between groups or how variable participants will be on outcome measures. In a pilot study, researchers recruit a small number of participants and employ their research design with those participants. Through this procedure, they have an opportunity to identify any problems with their experimental procedures, determine how much change participants might make, and determine the amount of variability that occurs on their outcome measures. Although having data from a pilot study is extremely valuable in planning research, conducting one is not always feasible. As an alternative, Trochim et al. (2016) suggest careful review of published research that employed procedures and/or outcome measures similar to the ones you plan to use. The previous research should provide some guidance regarding how much variability to expect in performance on outcome measures and how much change to expect after a certain amount of treatment.

In an ideal world, researchers would always be able to conduct studies with an adequate number of participants. With many of the populations served by audiologists and speech-language pathologists, however, recruiting a large sample for a study is very challenging. Rather than settle for only a small chance of detecting differences that actually exist in a population, researchers in communication sciences and disorders might consider other ways to improve their research. As we saw in our first example above, even a relatively small sample would be adequate if the effect of a treatment is large. One way to increase the effectiveness of a treatment is to ensure that it is executed in a precise and accurate way, such as through extensive training of the person(s) who will provide the treatment (Trochim et al., 2016). The second example above illustrated how variability in performance affected sample size requirements. Thus, another way to improve the likelihood that you will be able to detect important differences is to reduce the variability associated with your outcome measures (Trochim et al., 2016). If you have a choice of outcome measures, using the one with a high degree of reliability or measurement consistency is important. If you are using a self-constructed measure, ways to increase reliability include increasing the number of items or trials and, possibly, improving the instruction for those who administer and score the measure. More reliable outcome measures could reduce the amount of variability researchers sometimes consider noise in their data relative to the systematic differences associated with the experimental manipulations.

Summary

One aspect of planning research is to define the population or group of persons who are potential participants. If this population is relatively large, a second aspect of planning is to consider how to obtain a representative, unbiased sample from this population. An unbiased sample is one in which all members of a population have an equal chance of being selected. A biased sample comes about when some members of a population are systematically excluded, such as when researchers fail to recruit some segment of a population or when they rely on a sample of convenience. Generating a sample in a random way—using methods such as simple random sampling, systematic sampling, or stratified random sampling—generally is the best way to obtain samples that are free of systematic bias.

In the field of communication sciences and disorders, researchers often engage in extensive, purposeful recruiting just to generate a sample of sufficient size. Samples generated in this way are not random samples, but researchers still could use random assignment to divide the participants into groups. Participants might receive their group assignment based on a series of random numbers, and thus each participant has an equal opportunity of being included in the various experimental and control groups.

Determining an adequate sample size is an issue that sometimes receives too little emphasis in research planning. A sample that is sufficiently large generally represents the characteristics of a population better than a sample that is too small. Furthermore, in intervention research, larger samples are more likely to reveal differences associated with treatment and control groups than samples that are relatively small. The appropriate sample size for research is not an absolute number but rather a variable number determined by factors such as how large the population is, how variable the population is for the characteristics under study, how frequent the trait is in the overall population, how large group differences might be, and how certain researchers want to be about detecting differences (Bland, 2000; Trochim et al., 2016). If researchers use samples that are too small, their findings are less likely to provide a true picture of the population as a whole and less likely to reveal differences that actually occur in the population.

Review Questions

1. What term refers to all persons of interest to researchers when they conduct a study? What term refers to the group of persons who actually participate in a study?

2. If all members of a population have an equal chance of being selected to participate in a study, is the sample biased or unbiased?

3. What is one reason that the intended population for a study and the accessible population could be different?

4. How could each of the following sources of bias affect the findings from a study?
   a. Failing to identify all members of a population
   b. Sample of convenience
   c. Volunteerism

5. Explain the procedures a researcher would use for each of the following approaches to random sampling.
   a. Systematic sampling
   b. Simple random sampling
   c. Stratified random sampling
   d. Cluster sampling

6. Which of the sampling approaches in Question 5 is often used in obtaining normative data for our clinical tests?

7. Explain the difference between random sampling and random assignment of subjects to groups.

8. Identify each of the following statements as true or false.
   a. You can reduce the potential errors from using a biased sample by selecting a very large sample.
   b. Generally speaking, a larger sample yields more precise results because the sample is more likely to be representative.

9. The following example illustrates the use of random numbers to select participants for a study. The potential participants, listed by identification letter in column 1, each received a random number, as shown in column 2. If a researcher selected participants by random number from lowest to highest, who would be the first five participants selected?

Column 1	Column 2
AB	105
CD	170
EF	129
GH	141
IJ	187
KL	158
MN	177
OP	121
QR	106
ST	131

10. Assuming all other factors are equal, which of the follow would require a larger sample?
    a. A behavior with high variability or a behavior with low variability
    b. A group difference of 10 points or a group difference of 20 points
    c. A trait that occurs frequently in a population or a trait that occurs rarely

Learning Activities

1. Use random assignment to divide your classmates into small discussion groups. You might use a spreadsheet application for this task. Start by listing all students in one column, and then assign each student a random number in a second column using the random number function. Finally, sort the students using the random numbers as your sort key. Once you have a randomized list, you can divide the class by grouping every three or every four students.

2. Read a published report on some form of group research. What was the intended population for the research and what was the accessible population? How did the researchers generate their sample?

References

American Psychological Association. (2020). *Publication manual of the American Psychological Association* (7th ed.).

Bland, J. M. (2000). Sample size in guidelines trials. *Family Practice, 17,* S17–S20.

Cohen, L., Manion, L., & Morrison, K. (2018). *Research methods in education* (8th ed.). Routledge.

Dunn, L. M., & Dunn, D. M. (2007). *Peabody Picture Vocabulary Test: Manual* (4th ed.). NCS Pearson.

Gardenier, J. S., & Resnik, D. B. (2002). The misuse of statistics: Concepts, tools, and a research agenda. *Accountability in Research, 9*, 65–74. https://doi.org/10.1080/08989620290009521

Goldman, R., & Fristoe, M. (2015). *Goldman-Fristoe Test of Articulation 3: Manual* (3rd ed.). Pearson Clinical.

Newcomer, P. L., & Hammill, D. D. (2008). *Examiner's manual: Test of Language Development–Primary* (4th ed.). Pro-Ed.

Newhart, M., & Patten, M. L. (2023). *Understanding research methods: An overview of the essentials* (11th ed.). Routledge Taylor & Francis Group.

Phillips, B. M., & Morse, E. E. (2011). Family child care learning environments: Caregiver knowledge and practices related to early literacy and mathematics. *Early Childhood Education Journal, 39*(3), 213–222. https://doi.org/10.1007/s10643-011-0456-y

Pyrczak, F. (2010). *Making sense of statistics: A conceptual overview* (5th ed.). Pyrczak Publishing.

Reynolds, C. R., & Voress, J. K. (2008). *Test of Memory and Learning: Examiner's manual* (2nd ed.). Pearson Clinical.

Rosenthal, R., & Rosnow, R. L. (2008). *Essentials of behavioral research: Methods and data analysis* (3rd ed.). McGraw-Hill.

Sharp, H. M., & Shega, J. W. (2009). Feeding tube placement in patients with advanced dementia: The beliefs and practice patterns of speech-language pathologists. *American Journal of Speech-Language Pathology, 18*, 222–230. https://doi.org/10.1044/1058-0360 (2008/08-0013)

Smit, A. B., Hand, L., Freilinger, J. J., Bernthal, J. E., & Bird, A. (1990). The Iowa articulation norms project and its Nebraska replication. *Journal of Speech and Hearing Disorders, 55*, 779–798. https://doi.org/10.1044/jshd.5504.779

Tomblin, J. B., Records, N. L., Buckwalter, P., Zhang, X., Smith, E., & O'Brien, M. (1997). Prevalence of specific language impairment in kindergarten children. *Journal of Speech, Language, and Hearing Research, 40*, 1245–1260. https://doi.org/10.1044/jslhr.4006.1245

Trochim, W. M. K., Donnelly, J. P., & Arora, K. (2016). *Research methods: The essential knowledge base* (2nd ed.). Cengage Learning.

Trulove, B. B., & Fitch, J. L. (1998). Accountability measures employed by speech-language pathologists in private practice. *American Journal of Speech-Language Pathology, 7*, 75–80. https://doi.org/10.1044/1058-0360.0701.75

United States Census Bureau. (2020). *About the decennial census.* https://www.census.gov/programs-surveys/decennial-census/about.html

Woods, A., Fletcher, P., & Hughes, A. (1986). *Statistics in language studies.* Cambridge University Press.

Zimmerman, I. L., Steiner, V. G., & Pond, R. E. (2011). *Preschool Language Scale: Examiner's manual* (5th ed.). Pearson Clinical.

10

Data Analysis: Tools for Describing Data

Main Points

- Often the first step in data analysis is summarizing the many data points obtained from the research.
- How you describe data depends on the level of measurement: *nominal*, *ordinal*, *interval*, or *ratio*.
- Visual representations such as tables, charts, and graphs are helpful when first beginning to interpret data.
- Basic descriptions of data include measures of central tendency, how much measures vary from the central tendency, and shape of the distribution.

Once researchers have the information they planned to gather from their participants, the next phase of scientific inquiry is to organize and analyze that information. The information or data obtained from research takes many forms.[1] In previous chapters, we discussed the basic distinction between qualitative or verbal forms of data, and quantitative or numerical forms. Even for quantitative data, the numerical information could represent one of several levels of measurement; these different levels of measurement go with various procedures for describing and analyzing data. Thus, before beginning an analysis, researchers need to consider the nature of their measures and what analysis tools are the best match for those measures.

Levels of Measurement

Level of measurement refers to the nature of the numbers associated with a particular set of observations. Any phenomenon could be measured in several different ways. Let's consider the example of a speech sound. Researchers could record several forms of information about a speech sound, including phonetically transcribing the sound;

---

[1] The word *data* refers to a collection of facts or information. The singular form is the word *datum*. In writing, you might see *data* used as either a singular or plural form.

judging the degree of nasality present during production of the sound; counting the number of correct productions of the sound in a list of spoken words; obtaining an ultrasound image during production of the sound; measuring electrical activity in selected muscles using electromyography (EMG); obtaining duration, intensity, and frequency measurements from a spectrogram; or measuring oral and nasal airflow during production of the sound. These procedures could yield various types of numbers, including frequency counts, ratings on a scale from 1 to 5, accuracy scores, or even proportions that reflect direct comparisons such as between oral and nasal airflow. These different types of data correspond to the different levels of measurement usually identified in most introductory statistics books. The field of statistics usually distinguishes four levels of measurement, nominal, ordinal, interval, and ratio, each with its own defining characteristics (Newhart & Patten, 2023; Oh & Pyrczak, 2023; Trochim et al., 2016).

The *nominal* level of measurement is sometimes referred to as the naming level (Trochim et al., 2016). When using a nominal level of measurement, researchers assign participants and their responses to categories such as male or female, type of utterance, type of hearing loss, type of aphasia, dialect of American English, and so forth. Nominal-level measures are not ordered, and being assigned to a particular category is not necessarily better or worse than being assigned to some other category. In analyzing nominal data, researchers could count the number of participants or behaviors that fit into a particular category, compare participants or behaviors by discussing whether they are members of the same or different categories, and discuss which categories have the most or fewest members. They would not compare categories directly, however, by suggesting a particular label is greater or less than or better or worse than another label.

Well-constructed nominal measures have categories that are exhaustive and mutually exclusive (Trochim et al., 2016). Categories are exhaustive if every participant or every behavior under observation fits into a category. Categories are mutually exclusive if each participant or instance of a behavior fits into only one category. Researchers might use strategies such as adding an "other" category and combining characteristics such as expressive and receptive language impairment to ensure having a set of categories that are both exhaustive and mutually exclusive.

The *ordinal* level of measurement corresponds to rank-ordered data (Trochim et al., 2016). Either researchers rank participants and observations from high to low relative to one another or researchers use a rating scale to assign an ordinal measurement to a series of observations (e.g., ratings from 1 to 5). With ordinal-level measurement, you know the relative positions of an observation or participant relative to others, but ordinal-level measurement does not provide information about the amount of difference (Oh & Pyrczak, 2023). In comparing ordinal measures, you can discuss who ranked higher or lower on a particular trait, but you cannot equate differences in ranks. Thus, the difference between a rank of 3 versus 4 is not necessarily the same degree of difference as a rank of 5 versus 6. Let's say a researcher ranked a group of 10 preschool children on talkativeness during a 30-minute play session. The degree of difference between the child ranked 3 and the one ranked 4 could be unlike the degree of difference between the child ranked 5 and the one ranked 6. In one case, the difference could be quite small, but in the other case fairly large.

Although ordinal measures often involve assigning numbers, using labels that represent relative traits is another possibility (e.g., mild, moderate, severe; poor, fair, good, very good, excellent; strongly disagree, moderately disagree, undecided, moderately agree, strongly agree). Furthermore, having a low rank might be desirable or undesirable. For some attributes or events, it might be better to be ranked lower; for other attributes, it might be better to be ranked higher. For example, a rank of 2 would be more desirable than a rank of 5 if the scale of measurement was a severity rating scale where a 1 corresponded to a mild impairment and 5 corresponded to a severe impairment. However, the reverse would be true if the scale of measurement was an intelligibility rating scale where a 1 corresponded to always unintelligible and 5 corresponded to always intelligible.

The *interval* level of measurement provides information about which participants have higher or lower scores, as well as by *how much* participants differ (Trochim et al., 2016). To interpret "how much," you need a measure that yields equal intervals. This means that the difference between scores of 25 and 35 is the same amount as the difference between scores of 50 and 60. Let's revisit the example of the researcher who studied the talkativeness of 10 preschool children. Instead of ranking the children on talkativeness, the researcher might have used a more direct measure such as the number of words produced during 30 minutes of play. If the child ranked 3 produced 25 words and the child ranked 4 produced 35 words, whereas the child ranked 5 produced 50 words and the one ranked 6 produced 60 words, then we would know the amount of difference was the same (10 words).

The numbers on an interval scale can be added, subtracted, multiplied, and divided in a meaningful way without affecting the comparable intervals between numbers. For example, if we had a series of numbers that differed by 5 points, such as 20, 25, 30, 35, 40, 45, and 50, we could add 10 points to each number and the difference would still be 5 points: 30, 35, 40, 45, 50, 55, and 60. If we multiplied each number by 2 (40, 50, 60, 70, 80, 90, and 100), the interval between numbers would also double but would still be comparable. One characteristic that is lacking in interval-level measurement is the ability to compare numbers directly. In comparing two interval level scores, such as 25 and 50, you could say the scores differ by 25 points, but not that a score of 50 is twice as good as a score of 25. This type of direct comparison, expressed in a proportion or quotient, requires a level of measurement with a true zero, a characteristic that is absent in interval-level measures.

Many behavioral measures, such as achievement tests, aptitude tests, expressive and receptive language tests, and perceptual tests, are interval-level measures. Even when a participant receives a score of zero on such a test, it is difficult to claim that the participant has absolutely no ability on the skills assessed (a true zero). The participant might be able to score a few points if tested with other items and words that sample the same behaviors.

The *ratio* level of measurement has all of the features of interval-level measurement, plus a true zero (Trochim et al., 2016). Ratio-level measurements have three characteristics: (a) the ability to arrange numbers on a continuum, (b) the ability to specify amount and differences between amounts, and (c) the ability to identify an absolute zero relative to a characteristic. Thus, the difference between 20 and 30 is the same as the difference between 55 and 65. Furthermore, a score of 60 would represent twice as much of the characteristic as a score of 30. Often, ratio-level measures are assessments of physical attributes such as intensity, duration, or frequency measurements; electrophysiological measurements like EMG and auditory brainstem response (ABR) testing; or airflow measurements.

With knowledge of the level of measurement, researchers can make decisions about the most appropriate ways to represent and analyze their data. Some of these options include visual representations and descriptive statistics and are covered in the following sections.

Visual Representation of Data

One way to visually represent numerical information is to arrange it in a *table*. Research reports often include tables to convey information about participants, as well as the statistical findings of the study. The example in Table 10–1 illustrates a common way of representing participant information in a table. Publication manuals, such as the one from the American Psychological Association (APA, 2020), provide guidelines for how to organize and format tables.

Charts and graphs are ways to visually represent numerical information. These come in several forms and are useful either as supplements to information presented in tabular or text form or as the primary means of presenting data. Charts and graphs are particularly useful for live presentations and posters where numbers in a table could be difficult to read. Often graphs are the primary means of presenting and interpreting data in single-subject design research (Barlow et al., 2009; Byiers et al., 2012; Parsonson & Baer, 2016; Richards, 2019).

A type of chart that is appropriate for nominal, categorical measures is a *pie chart*. Pie charts are useful for illustrating the percentages or proportions of observations that fit particular categories. You can use a pie chart if you have percentages or proportions that total to 100% or 1.0. An example of a pie chart is shown in Figure 10–1. This example figure shows hypothetical data from graduate students in communication sciences and disorders regarding where they plan to seek employment in the future. The size of a "slice of pie" corresponds to the percentage value. In the example, the smallest slice corresponds to private practice (10%), and the largest slice corresponds to school setting (37%).

A *scatterplot* is another type of graph that is useful for illustrating the relationship between two, and even three, continuous measures. An XY scatterplot is a special graph that illustrates the relationship between two sets of scores, usually from the same participants. Scatterplots are useful for

Table 10–1. Illustration of the Use of a Table to Present Participant Information Including Participant Identifier, Age in Months, and Test Scores

		Test Scores	
Identifier	Age	Percentile Rank	Standard Score
AB	48	9	80
CD	52	2	70
EF	46	2	68
GH	54	5	75
IJ	50	8	79
KL	46	5	76
MN	51	7	78
OP	45	6	77
QR	47	5	75
ST	53	10	81

depicting relationships between measures, as in correlation research. The example in Figure 10–2 illustrates a hypothetical study with 20 participants. This plot depicts a situation in which low scores on Test 1 correspond to low scores on Test 2, midrange scores on Test 1 correspond to midrange scores on Test 2, and high scores on Test 1 correspond to high scores on Test 2. The relationship depicted in Figure 10–2 also would be described as a linear relationship because the plot corresponds roughly to a

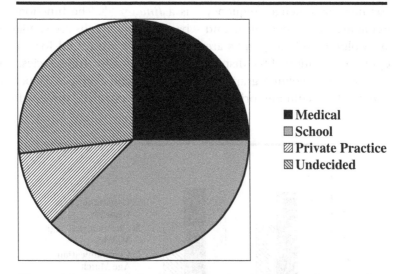

Figure 10–1. Illustration of the use of a pie chart to show nominal data by percentage.

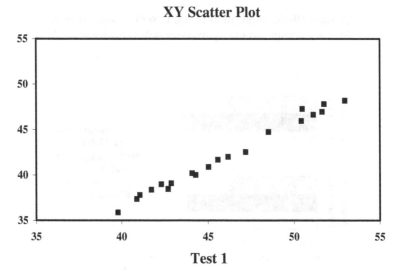

Figure 10–2. Illustration of the use of an XY scatterplot to show the relationship between two continuous variables.

straight line; however, scatterplots are not always linear, and some relationships might be nonlinear, such as those shown by a U shape.

Column and bar graphs are useful for illustrating the magnitude or frequency of one or more variables. Researchers often use these types of graphs to depict group differences on measures such as frequency counts, percentages of occurrence, and group means. Column and bar graphs are similar except for orientation of the display relative to the axes. In a column graph, as shown in Figure 10–3, columns originate from the horizontal axis, and the height of the columns corresponds to the values for frequencies, means, and so forth. In a bar graph, as shown in Figure 10–4, bars originate from the vertical axis and the length of the bars corresponds to the different values.

One final type of graph that is common in research presentations and reports is a *line graph*. The functions of column, bar, and line graphs are similar because all three types are useful for illustrating different values for frequencies, counts, percentages, and averages. Depending on the nature of your data, these values could be

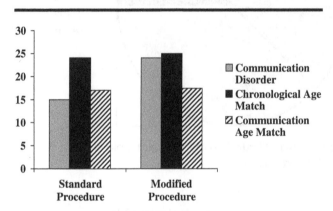

Figure 10–3. Illustration of the use of a column graph to show group means by experimental condition.

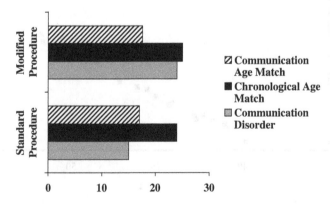

Figure 10–4. Illustration of the use of a bar graph to show group means by experimental condition.

associated with different groups, different tasks, different behaviors, changes over time, and so forth. Line graphs might be particularly suitable for depicting several values in a series or for depicting a special kind of nonlinear relationship called an interaction. An interaction occurs when two or more groups respond in unique ways to the experimental manipulations. The example line graph in Figure 10–5 illustrates an interaction in a simple 2 × 2 design, that is, a design with two different groups (e.g., persons with a hearing impairment or those with normal hearing) and two levels of the experimental manipulation (e.g., standard or modified test procedure). This example shows the use of a line graph to depict group means as well as variability within each group, as shown by the vertical lines extending from each mean.[2] By examining such a graph, you can readily see differences between the groups as well as differences associated with the experimental manipulation. Another characteristic to note in Figure 10–5 is that the lines representing each group are not parallel. The scores of persons with a hearing impairment improved more with the modified test (5 points higher) than the scores of the persons with normal hearing (1 point higher). This is what is meant by an interaction: The two groups responded to the change in test procedures in different ways, and these unique responses perhaps are easier to visualize with a line graph than with any other type of chart or graph.

Due to the greater cost of publishing graphic material as compared to textual information, researchers traditionally were fairly conservative about including charts and graphs in research reports. Visual representation of data has a role in the initial stages of data analysis even if the graphs and charts produced are not part of the final, published report; with greater reliance on electronic distribution of journals via websites, authors currently have greater flexibility in choosing how to display their

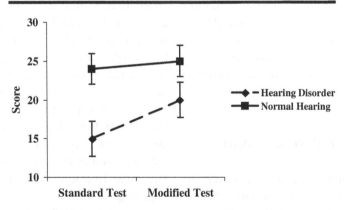

Figure 10–5. Illustration of the use of a line graph to show group means and standard deviations by experimental condition.

---

[2]These vertical lines are sometimes referred to as error bars. One use of error bars is to depict group variability by showing the mean ± 1 standard deviation as shown in Figure 10–5. Another use of error bars is to show confidence intervals as illustrated later in the chapter.

data. Furthermore, visual representations are an essential part of live presentations and poster sessions, such as the ones you would see at local, state, national, and international conferences. The tools for generating charts and graphs are readily available in computer software you might already be using, such as spreadsheet and presentation programs.

Descriptive Statistics

Although charts and graphs provide an attractive way to display information, reporting quantitative data in numerical form is more common. Often, the starting point in reporting results is to provide descriptive information about your data (Oh & Pyrczak, 2023; Trochim et al., 2016). *Descriptive statistics* might be thought of as a way of summarizing data to convey the main information. Rather than presenting raw scores, researchers present a few summary measures that capture the key characteristics of their data. Some of these key characteristics might include how often and how consistently particular behaviors occurred, what was typical or average among the participants or observations, and how variable behaviors were among participants.

Frequencies and Percentages

A frequency count or percentage could be the preferred descriptive measure when researchers want to convey how often particular phenomena occurred in a set of data. Frequencies and percentages are the primary descriptive statistics for nominal-level measures. You might obtain a frequency count of the number of participants who fit a particular nominal category or the number of behaviors that fit a particular classification. For example, a university with a graduate program in audiology might survey its recent graduates to determine their primary work setting. This example is shown in Table 10–2. The frequencies in this case represent the number of survey participants who reported working in each setting. The most frequently reported settings were hospital, health clinic or other nonresidential facility, and physician's office. The least frequently reported settings were school, university, and other.

Although research often involves classification of individual participants, sometimes frequency counts are based on a series of observations from the same participant. The data in Table 10–3 illustrate this possibility. In this example, a speech-language pathologist (SLP) was concerned about the behavior of a child who participated in small group treatment. The child exhibited frequent off-task behaviors and the SLP decided to document these behaviors before implementing an intervention to reduce their occurrence. The SLP videotaped two 30-minute group sessions and analyzed the middle 20 minutes of each session by classifying the child's behavior every minute. Thus, the SLP made 40 behavioral observations and classified these behaviors into seven categories, as shown in Table 10–3. The hypothetical data show that on-task behaviors occurred in 10 of the observations, and various off-task behaviors occurred in the other 30 observations. The most frequent off-task behavior was fidgeting.

A *percentage* (%) of occurrence is calculated by dividing the number of participants or observations in a particular category (i.e., the smaller number) by the total number across all categories (the larger number), and then multiplying the result by 100. Allowing for some minor differences

Table 10–2. Hypothetical Results from a Survey of Audiologists Who Graduated from a University Program in the Last Five Years: Frequencies and Percentages by Work Setting

Work Setting	Frequency	Percentage
School	6	10%
University	5	8%
Hospital	16	27%
Physician's office	16	27%
Health clinic or other nonresidential	15	25%
Other	2	3%
Total	60	100%

Source: These data are hypothetical. Demographic information for employment settings of audiologists is available from the American Speech-Language Hearing Association (2021).

Table 10–3. Hypothetical Results from a Series of Observations of a Child's Behavior During Small Group Language Activities

Behavior	Frequency	Percentage
On-task behavior	10	25%
Fidget in chair	8	20%
Talk/act while receiving an instruction	6	15%
Talk/act during another child's turn	4	10%
Prolonged look away from activity	6	15%
Leave seat at inappropriate time	4	10%
Other off-task	2	5%
Total	40	100%

associated with rounding, the percentages for each category should add to 100%. When reporting percentages, researchers usually include the raw numbers as well to clearly convey the nature of their data. Sample size is important for determining how well a set of observations might represent the population as a whole. A behavior that occurs 2 times out of 10 and one that occurs 10 times out of 50 both occur 20% of the time, but a sample of 50 should be more representative than a sample of 10.

An alternative to a percentage is to calculate a *proportion*. Proportions and percentages yield related numbers. A proportion is calculated by dividing the number for a particular category by the total number, yielding a number between 0 and 1.0 because the number for a particular category could range from none to all. If you went one step further and multiplied by 100, you obtain a percentage, a number between 0 and 100. When using percentages, you think of the construct under study as having multiple instances, such as 60 graduates of the audiology program (see Table 10–2) or 40 behavioral observations (see Table 10–3). When using proportions, you think of the construct as a unitary phenomenon, such as one sample of recent graduates or one sample of behaviors. Thus, you could pose a question like, "What percentage of graduates work in a hospital setting?" or "What proportion of the sample works in a hospital setting?" Based on the data in Table 10–2, the answer to the first question would be 27%, and the answer to the second question would be .27.

When data involve information from participants or observations of a series of behaviors, researchers typically report frequencies and percentages. Conceptually, the notion of a proportion associated with persons, such as .27 audiologists, is awkward. Some entities are easy to think of in proportions, on the other hand. For example, we might ask for a slice of pie that is one-sixth or one-eighth the size of the whole pie, corresponding to proportions of .167 and .125, respectively. As another example, we could think of a consonant sound, such as /z/, as a unitary construct. One could measure the duration of such a sound, perhaps finding that one such production in the word *buzz* had a duration of 250 milliseconds. Another characteristic of /z/ is that speakers tend to devoice this sound at the end of words (Small, 2020). Thus, we could ask a question like, "What proportion of /z/ is devoiced when produced at the end of words?" If we analyzed a production and found the first 150 milliseconds were voiced and the final 100 milliseconds were devoiced, we could state that a proportion of .40 was devoiced (i.e., 100 divided by 250). Frequencies, percentages, and proportions are important ways of reporting nominal-level data. Frequency counts are useful in reporting other measures as well, such as the number of participants receiving a particular rating on an ordinal-level scale or the number of participants receiving a certain score on an interval/ratio-level measure.

Measures of Central Tendency

Measures of central tendency convey information about typical and usual responses of participants, or the score that falls toward the middle of a set of scores (Oh & Pyrczak, 2023; Trochim et al., 2016). In everyday life, we use the word *average* to refer to a typical response. Researchers identify specific ways to measure central tendency, and the three common ways are the mode, median, and mean. The *mode* is based on frequency information and is the category, response, or score that occurs most often. The mode is the primary measure of central tendency for nominal measures; however, you can compute a mode for all levels of data, nominal, ordinal, interval, or ratio. First, let's consider the data in Table 10–3. In this example, the mode, or most frequently occurring category, was "on-task behavior." For the data in Table 10–2, two categories were most frequent. Both "hospital" and "physician's office" had frequencies of 16, and this was the highest number in the set, so these data could be called *bimodal*. You can determine the mode for a set of interval/ratio-level measures too, as illustrated in Example 1. In this set of numbers, a score of 75 occurs most often and is the mode.

Example 1

50, 55, 60, 65, 75, 75, 75, 80, 80, 85, 90

The mode is not always in the center of a set of scores, as illustrated in Example 2. In this series of numbers, a score of 55 occurs most often. Thus, the mode in Example 2 is 55, a number in the low end of the series.

Example 2

50, 55, 55, 55, 60, 65, 70, 70, 75, 80, 85

The *median* is a number that occurs at the midpoint in a series of scores. In publications, the abbreviation for median is *Mdn* (APA, 2020). To compute a median, you need numbers that can be ordered from low to high (or from high to low). Because of this, a median is appropriate for ordinal-, interval-, and ratio-level measures but not appropriate for nominal-level measures. If a series of scores represents an odd number of observations, calculating the median is straightforward. The median will be the middle score with an equal number of scores falling above it and below it. Example 2 above has a series of 11 scores. The middle score and median is 65, which has 5 scores above it and 5 scores below it. If a series of scores represents an even number of observations, determining the median is slightly more complex. First, you identify the two middle scores that divide the series in half. Then, you use a process of interpolation to determine the number that falls halfway between the two middle scores. If a series of numbers has 10 scores, for example, the lower half will have 5 scores and the upper half will have 5 scores. The median will be the value that falls halfway between the fifth and sixth scores. Let's add a score to the series in Example 2 and create a series with 12 scores (see Example 3). In this example, the middle two scores are 65 and 70, and the number that falls halfway between them is 67.5.

Example 3

50, 55, 55, 55, 60, 65, 70, 70, 75, 80, 85, 90

Identifying the median in a small set of scores is relatively easy. However, with a large set of scores, you might consider entering the data in a spreadsheet and using a statistical function for calculating medians or even using software designed specifically for statistical computations. If you have ever administered a test and determined the percentile rank for a client's raw score, you have used numbers that share a relationship with the median. If a client's score fell at a percentile rank of 50, that score would be at the midpoint in the distribution, half of the scores falling above it and half falling below it.

The *mean* is a common measure of central tendency, and when persons use the term *average*, they usually are referring to a mean. The recommended publication abbreviation for mean is *M* (APA, 2020), although some statistical textbooks might still use an X-bar symbol. You compute a mean by summing all of the scores in a series and dividing by the total number of scores. The mean is most appropriate for data at the interval or ratio level of measurement. In general, the mean is most reflective of data when the distribution of scores fits a normal distribution or close to it. If your data seriously violate a normal distribution, such as with extreme outliers, then you might consider a median rather than mean as your measure of central tendency. Example 4 includes two sets of data.

In the first series, the mean and median are both 75. In the second series, one number was replaced with an outlier, an extremely low score. This extreme score impacted the value of the mean by lowering it to 70.9 but had no effect on the median.

Example 4

55, 60, 65, 70, 75, 75, 75, 80, 85, 90, 95
(M = 75.0 and Mdn = 75.0)

30, 55, 60, 65, 70, 75, 75, 80, 85, 90, 95
(M = 70.9 and Mdn = 75.0)

Calculating a mean may yield a number that never occurred in your data set. In the example above, all of the scores are whole numbers, but the mean is a decimal number. Similarly, one often reads statements such as, "The average number of students in graduate classes is 24.5," even though you cannot literally have half a person.

Measures of Variability

Usually, descriptions of a series of scores include measures of variability as well as measures of central tendency. Variability refers to the distribution or spread of scores around the midpoint of the scores (Oh & Pyrczak, 2023). As with measures of central tendency, researchers have many options for conveying the amount of variability in their data. The simplest way to convey variability is to report the *minimum and maximum* scores in a series. The scores in Example 4 illustrate one of the weaknesses of using this simple approach. In the first set of scores, the minimum value is 55 and the maximum is 95. The midpoint between these two scores is 75, which does correspond to the mean and median. In the second series, the minimum is 30 and the maximum is 95. The midpoint between these scores is 60, which is much lower than the actual mean and median.

Another relatively simple measure of variability is the *range*. The calculation of a range utilizes the minimum and maximum scores in a series; however, we need to distinguish between reporting a true range and the actual minimum and maximum scores. An actual range, as defined by statisticians, is the *difference* between the highest and lowest scores. If the minimum value is 55 and the maximum is 95, the range is 40 (95 minus 55). In the field of communication sciences and disorders, researchers often report minimum and maximum scores using statements such as, "The scores ranged from 75 to 125." We need to keep in mind that the phrase "ranged from" is associated with reporting the lowest and highest scores and not the difference between these scores (125 − 75 = 50). Like minimum and maximum scores, a major disadvantage of the range is that a single extremely low or extremely high score could make a set of numbers appear more variable than they actually are.

When a set of scores has an extremely high or low value, an alternative to the range is an *interquartile range*. The interquartile range is similar to the range, except it represents the difference between the score that falls at the 75th percentile and the score that falls at the 25th percentile. Interquartile range characterizes the spread of scores in the middle 50% of your data. If 60 was the score that fell at the 75th percentile and 40 was the score that fell at the 25th percentile, then the interquartile range would be 20 (60 − 40 = 20). An interquartile range is a more stable measure of variability than the range because extreme scores have less impact on its value. Computation and interpretation of an interquartile range are less straightforward than calculation of a range. For this reason, researchers are less likely to report interquartile ranges than other measures of variability.

When the level of measurement is interval or ratio, the most commonly used measure of variability is a *standard deviation*. The recommended publication abbreviation for standard deviation is *SD* (APA, 2020). The standard deviation reflects the dispersion of scores around the mean. Unlike the range, the calculation of a standard deviation uses all scores in the set; therefore, extreme scores have less influence on a standard deviation than a range (Oh & Pyrczak, 2023; Trochim et al., 2016). A larger standard deviation means you have a larger spread of scores around the mean. Thus, a set of scores that clusters close to the mean will have a relatively small standard deviation, and a set of scores that disperses widely from the mean will have a relatively large standard deviation.

Calculation of a standard deviation is fairly easy to understand. Usually, all scores are listed in a column as shown in Table 10–4. First, you need to compute the mean for the set of scores. Then, you obtain the difference between each score and the mean, as shown in the second column. If you simply summed these differences, however, the numbers would sum to zero with the differences above the mean canceling the differences below the mean. Therefore, the next step involves squaring the differences to eliminate the negative numbers, as shown in the third column. At this point, you sum the squared differences, yielding a value called the *sum of squares*. When you are working with a sample from a larger population, the next step is to divide the sum of squares by the number of participants minus 1 ($n - 1$). This value is referred to as the *variance*, and the standard deviation is the square root of the variance. Although calculation of a standard deviation is relatively clear-cut, the easiest way to obtain this value is to use the standard deviation statistical function that is available in most spreadsheet programs. Using a spreadsheet or statistical software for this calculation is particularly valuable when you are working with a large set of numbers.

Means as Estimates

One of the concepts discussed in Chapter 9 (Research Participants and Sampling) was the difference between a sample and a population. As noted in that chapter, researchers usually study a sample of participants from a larger population with the goal of generalizing what they learn from the sample to the larger population. Any statistic calculated for a sample is just an estimate of the population parameter and might or might not be an accurate estimate. Hypothetically, if the researcher conducted a study many times with different random samples from the larger population, the calculated statistics could be somewhat different for each sample. The possibility that a random sample might yield an estimate of a population characteristic that is not perfectly accurate is referred to as *sampling error*. Professional societies and other publishers recently began encouraging researchers to acknowledge the possibility of sampling error in the way they report statistics (Cumming, 2012; Kline, 2004). For example, rather than report just a single mean score for a sample, researchers might calculate a *margin of error* and use the margin of error to establish a *confidence interval* for the estimate of the population mean. Margin of error reflects the potential distribution of means, the *sampling distribution*, that would emerge if you took many samples from a population and calculated a mean

Table 10–4. An Example of the Calculation of a Standard Deviation Using a Sample from a Hypothetical Set of Data

Raw Score	Minus the Mean	Difference Squared
20	−31.2	973.44
30	−21.2	449.44
70	18.8	353.44
60	8.8	77.44
45	−6.2	38.44
60	8.8	77.44
60	8.8	77.44
35	−16.2	262.44
35	−16.2	262.44
45	−6.2	38.44
35	−16.2	262.44
45	−6.2	38.44
35	−16.2	262.44
70	18.8	353.44
30	−21.2	449.44
65	13.8	190.44
65	13.8	190.44
45	−6.2	38.44
50	−1.2	1.44
55	3.8	14.44
55	3.8	14.44
60	8.8	77.44
70	18.8	353.44
75	23.8	566.44
65	13.8	190.44
Mean = 51.2	Sum = 0.0	Sum of Squares = 5614.00
		Divided by $n - 1$ = 233.92 (Variance)
		Square Root = 15.29 (Standard Deviation)

for each of those samples (Trochim et al., 2016). To determine the margin of error and establish a confidence interval, researchers first calculate a standard error of the sampling distribution. This measure is similar to a standard deviation but reflects the distribution of mean scores in the hypothetical sampling distribution rather than in the actual sample. If we knew the population standard deviation, we could use that in calculating the standard error, but that is seldom available to researchers. Therefore, researchers use the standard deviation calculated for their sample as an estimate of the population standard deviation (Cumming, 2012; Kline, 2004). That is the procedure used in the example that follows.

To illustrate the concept of margin of error, we will use the mean and standard deviation from the hypothetical sample in Table 10–4. The first step is to calculate a standard error, and this measure is based on the standard deviation (*SD*). The formula below uses the sample *SD* as an estimate of the *SD* in the population.

Standard error (*SE*) = *SD* divided by the square root of *N* (i.e., number of samples)

SE = 15.29/square root of 25 or 15.29/5

Thus, *SE* = 3.058

To complete the calculation of margin of error, you need a number to reflect your level of confidence, usually the 95% confidence level. If we were working with population parameters, we could use a known distribution of scores based on the normal curve, *z* scores, for the 95% confidence level. Because we are working with an estimate, however, we are going to use a different distribution for the 95% confidence level (i.e., *t* score for a sample with 25 participants, which would be 2.064). Using this number, we can calculate the margin of error for our example as follows:

Margin of error (MOE) = $t_{.95}$ * *SE* or 2.065 * 3.058

Thus, MOE = 6.315

The confidence interval for our example is the mean of 51.2 ± the MOE of 6.315, which yields a confidence interval of 44.885 to 57.515. Rather than reporting just the static estimate of the mean, reporting that the mean for the population most likely falls somewhere between 44.885 and 57.515 highlights the fact that our calculation of the mean is an estimate of the population mean and that estimate has a margin of error (Cumming, 2012; Kline, 2004).

Shapes of Distributions

Now that we have information about measures of central tendency and variability, we will consider one additional topic related to description of data. Certain measures such as the mean and standard deviation are easiest to interpret when scores disperse in a certain way, called a normal distribution. Figure 10–6 illustrates a set of data that are roughly normally distributed. In a normal distribution, the dispersion of scores around the mean is symmetrical, and half of the scores fall above the mean and half fall below the mean. Furthermore, the mean and median reflect the same value (50 in the example in Figure 10–6). Another characteristic of a normal distribution is that about 34% of the scores fall within 1 standard deviation below the mean and another 34% fall within 1 standard deviation above the mean. Thus, approximately 68% of the scores fall within ±1 standard deviation from the mean. If you consider 2 standard deviations above and below the mean, you would find approximately 95% of the scores fall within ±2 standard deviations from the mean.

Knowing how your data distribute from low to high around the mean is important because it helps you select appropriate descriptive and inferential statistics. Usually, selection of procedures for statistical analysis depends on the distribution of data in a population. However, researchers seldom have access to actual population parameters; the best alternative is to examine the distribution of scores in your sample (Coladarci & Cobb, 2014). A special type

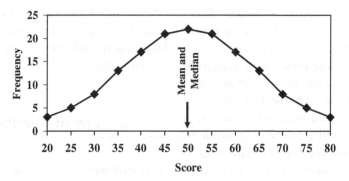

Figure 10–6. A frequency polygon illustrating a set of scores that are roughly normally distributed.

of graph, a *frequency polygon*, is a way to examine the shape of your distribution. The graph in Figure 10–6 is a frequency polygon, as are the examples in the figures that follow. To construct a frequency polygon, first determine how many persons achieved a certain score (e.g., how many had a score of 50, a score of 45, and so forth). Sometimes researchers group scores to construct the polygon by counting how many scores fell in a certain interval (e.g., how many fell from 46 to 50, from 41 to 45, and so forth). Once you determine the frequency of each score, you simply plot frequency on the vertical axis and scores on the horizontal axis using a graph such as a scatterplot with lines. After making your plot, you visually inspect the plot and decide whether or not the shape approximates that of a normal curve. Keep in mind that a distribution will not be very smooth unless you have a large sample. Figure 10–6 illustrates a distribution that is roughly normally distributed with a relatively wide spread of scores from 20 to 80. In contrast, Figure 10–7 illustrates a distribution that also is roughly normally distributed but with a relatively narrow spread of scores from 35 to 65.

Another way to think about generating a frequency polygon and inspecting the plot is that you are looking for the presence of scores that separate quite a bit from the other scores. These are sometimes called *outliers*. When a set of scores has outliers, the shape of the frequency polygon changes and the distribution no longer approximates a normal curve. Researchers often describe sets of scores with outliers as having a positive or negative skew. In a frequency polygon with a positive skew, the distribution has an abnormally long tail that stretches in the positive direction, as shown in Figure 10–8. The lengthened tail occurs when the set of scores includes a few that are higher than would be expected in a normal distribution. Another consequence, as we noted when discussing the computation of the mean and median, is that extreme positive scores pull the mean higher, producing a set of data in which the mean is higher than the median.

Outliers could occur in the opposite direction as well. In a frequency polygon with a *negative skew*, the distribution has an abnormally long tail that stretches in the negative direction, as shown in Figure 10–9. In this case, the lengthened tail occurs when the set of scores includes a few that are lower than would be expected in a normal distribution. These extreme negative

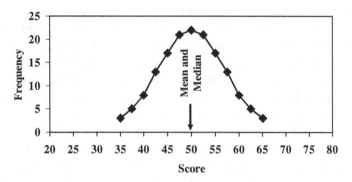

Figure 10–7. A frequency polygon illustrating a set of scores that are roughly normally distributed but have a relatively narrower spread and smaller standard deviation than the scores in Figure 10–6.

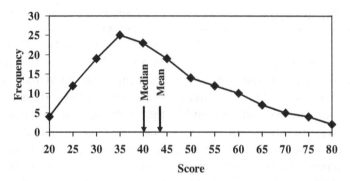

Figure 10–8. A frequency polygon illustrating a set of scores with a positive skew.

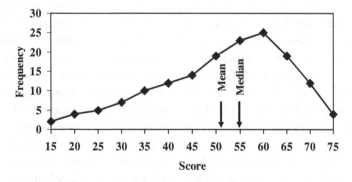

Figure 10–9. A frequency polygon illustrating a set of scores with a negative skew.

scores pull the mean lower, producing a set of data in which the mean is lower than the median, as shown in Figure 10–9.

When data are skewed, measures of central tendency and variability are more difficult to interpret (Oh & Pyrczak, 2023). A few extreme scores might create the illusion of a difference that does not really exist or even mask a true difference. Departures from a normal distribution are most likely with small sample sizes; when working with small groups of participants, researchers need to be careful about their choice of statistical analysis procedures (Cohen et al., 2018; Gibbons & Chakraborti, 2003).

Summary

One of the first steps in reporting research findings is to describe and summarize your findings. For quantitative data, researchers typically use descriptive statistics and/or visual displays; the choice of appropriate procedures depends in part on the level of measurement for the outcome or dependent variables. The field of statistics usually distinguishes four levels of measurement: nominal, ordinal, interval, and ratio. The nominal level of measurement encompasses naming or categorizing observations, the ordinal level of measurement relates to placing observations in order or ranking them, and the interval-level measures enable you to specify how much scores differ and not just which scores are higher or lower. Ratio-level measures have all the characteristics of interval-level measures and also have a true zero. Because of this, ratio-level measures allow researchers to directly compare scores in proportional relationships.

Researchers have many options for the visual representation of data, ranging from numerical tables to various types of charts and graphs. The choice of visual display depends in part on your level of measurement and also on the nature of your research design. For example, a pie chart is a visual display that is appropriate for nominal measures that can be summarized with percentages or proportions. A scatterplot is useful in showing the relationship between two continuous measures, as in correlation studies. Other options for visual displays include column, bar, and line graphs. These types of graphs are often used to display data from group comparison research. Descriptive statistics are summary measures that convey the key characteristics of a data set. The options for describing data include frequency counts and percentages; measures of central tendency, including the mode, median, and mean; and measures of variability such as the range and standard deviation. Each of these options fits certain types of data, and the challenge for researchers is to select descriptive statistics that are a good match to their outcome measures and research design. When reporting descriptive statistics like means, researchers need to keep in mind that these statistics are estimates of population characteristics and might or might not be accurate estimates.

One final consideration in describing your data is to determine how the scores distribute or spread around the center. Often, data fit a special kind of distribution called a normal distribution. Data that approximate a normal curve have a symmetrical distribution with roughly equal numbers of scores above and below the mean. However, data sometimes include extreme or outlying scores that alter the shape of the distribution. When a set of scores includes extreme outliers, the shape of the distribution is asymmetrical with an abnormally long tail in either the positive or negative direction. Outliers have a greater impact on certain descriptive statistics such as the mean and range, whereas other measures such as the median and standard deviation are more stable. Thus, the shape of the distribution, whether it is symmetrical or asymmetrical, has an impact on the researchers' decisions regarding what descriptive statistics to report.

Review Questions

1. Match the level of measurement with its brief description

    _____ Nominal
    _____ Ordinal
    _____ Interval
    _____ Ratio

    a. Rank order from highest to lowest
    b. Shows how much participants differ but no true 0
    c. Measures with a true 0
    d. Naming or mutually exclusive categories

2. Subjects in a study indicated where they live, which the researcher classified by geographic regions (e.g., Northeast, Midwest, Southeast, West). What scale of measurement would this be?

3. Researchers classified preschool children's history of middle ear infections as frequent/moderate/infrequent based on the number of reported episodes. What scale of measurement would this be?

4. The scores obtained from articulation/phonology or language tests most likely measure at what level?

5. What level of measurement would allow you to say that a score of 30 was three times as much as a score of 10?

6. What kind of chart or graph could you use if your level of measurement was nominal and you had percentages that totaled to 100%?

7. Explain when a researcher would use each of the following:
    a. Scatterplot
    b. Column graph
    c. Line graph

8. What descriptive statistics are used most often with nominal-level measures?

9. Three measures of central tendency are the mode, median, and mean. What measure of central tendency provides information about the most frequently occurring category or score? What measure of central tendency is calculated by summing all the scores in a set and dividing that sum by the number of scores? What measure of central tendency provides information about the score that falls at the midpoint of a distribution?

10. What measure of variability is calculated by determining the difference between the minimum and maximum scores?

11. What is the relationship between the standard deviation and variance?

12. Will an extreme, outlying score have a greater impact on the range or the standard deviation of a set of scores?

13. What is the relationship between the mean and median in (a) a normal curve, (b) a curve with a positive skew, and (c) a curve with a negative skew?

14. Draw a distribution that illustrates data that approximate a normal curve, one that illustrates data with a positive skew, and one that illustrates data with a negative skew.

15. Draw the following:
    a. A roughly normal distribution with a mean of 50 and an *SD* of 5
    b. A roughly normal distribution with a mean of 50 and an *SD* of 10

    Try to use a similar scale of measurement in your drawings. Which distribution has the most variability?

Learning Activities

1. You have video recorded a conversation between an adult with expressive aphasia and her spouse. Think of two examples of quantitative measures you could obtain from the speech sample and two qualitative descriptors you could use for the conversation. For your qualitative descriptors, try to use a precise level of description with minimal inference.

2. If you have access to a spreadsheet program, enter the sets of scores below into two columns. After entering the numbers, select the cell immediately below the first column, find the menu item for functions, and select the statistical function for average or mean. This should enable you to calculate the mean for the first set of data. Repeat this procedure for the second column of data. You can add the computation for standard deviation by selecting the menu item for functions and finding the standard deviation function. If your spreadsheet has a graphing function, you might try selecting both columns and generating a scatterplot for the two sets of scores. You also might try generating a column or bar graph for the two means.

Set A	Set B
48	51
54	55
48	51
61	61
44	47
62	65
39	41
63	66
48	49
57	58
53	56
45	47
44	45
48	50
55	56
64	66
44	46
43	46
49	51
36	39

References

American Psychological Association. (2020). *Publication manual of the American Psychological Association* (7th ed.).

American Speech-Language-Hearing Association. (2021). *2021 audiology survey*. https://www.asha.org/research/memberdata/audiology-survey/

Barlow, D. H., Nock, M. K., & Hersen, M. (2009). *Single case experimental designs: Strategies for studying behavior change* (3rd ed.). Pearson.

Byiers, B. J., Reichle, J., & Symons, F. J. (2012). Single-subject experimental design for evidence-based practice. *American Journal of Speech-Language Pathology, 21*, 397–414. https://doi.org/10.1044/1058-0360(2012/110036)

Cohen, L., Manion, L., & Morrison, K. (2018). *Research methods in education* (8th ed.). Routledge.

Coladarci, T., & Cobb, C. D. (2014). *Fundamentals of statistical reasoning in education* (4th ed.). John Wiley & Sons.

Cumming, G. (2012). *Understanding the new statistics: Effect sizes, confidence intervals, and meta-analysis*. Routledge.

Gibbons, J. D., & Chakraborti, S. (2003). *Nonparametric statistical inference* (4th ed.). CRC Press-Taylor & Francis Group.

Kline, R. B. (2004). *Beyond significance testing: Reforming data analysis methods in behavioral research*. American Psychological Association.

Newhart, M., & Patten, M. L. (2023). *Understanding research methods: An overview of the essentials* (11th ed.). Routledge Taylor & Francis Group.

Oh, D. M., & Pyrczak, F. (2023). *Making sense of statistics: A conceptual overview* (7th ed.). Routledge Taylor & Francis Group.

Parsonson, B. S., & Baer, D. B. (2016). The visual analysis of data, and current research into the stimuli controlling it. In T. R. Kratochwill & J. R. Level (Eds.), *Single-case research design and analysis: New directions for psychology and education* (Re-issue ed., pp. 15–40). Routledge Taylor & Francis Group.

Richards, S. B. (2019). *Single subject research: Applications in educational and clinical settings* (3rd ed.). Cengage Learning.

Small, L. H. (2020). *Fundamentals of phonetics: A practical guide for students* (5th ed.). Pearson Education.

Trochim, W. M. K., Donnelly, J. P., & Arora, K. (2016). *Research methods: The essential knowledge base* (2nd ed.). Cengage Learning.

11

Data Analysis: Measures of Association and Difference

Main Points

- To identify an appropriate statistical test, first determine if the goal of your data is to describe, relate, or compare.
- To identify an appropriate statistical test, also determine the number of samples you will be comparing/relating, the level of measurement, whether samples are independent or paired, and if parametric or nonparametric.
- For interval- or ratio-level data where the goal is to compare, use *t*-tests to compare two samples and ANOVAs to compare three or more samples.
- Measures of association are generally correlation or regression, with regression adding the element of a predictive value.
- Correlation will describe both the strength and the direction of the relationship between samples.

In Chapter 10, we read about ways in which researchers might describe and summarize their data. A few summary measures that capture the key characteristics of the data frequently are more meaningful than the raw scores themselves. Researchers often want to go beyond describing just the actual observations and want to develop answers that apply to a larger population. When researchers obtain information from a sample, one question they need to ask is whether their findings reflect the situation in the population in general or whether the findings occurred because of some idiosyncrasy in the sample. Another way of phrasing this question is to ask if the findings from a sample represent the "true" situation in the population. Fortunately, the field of statistics provides researchers with tools for quantitative data analysis that allow them to draw meaningful conclusions about a population, even when they were only able to study a sample from that population.

Inferential Statistics

Once researchers have completed their observations and obtained a set of scores from their participants, they usually use some type of inferential statistical analysis to determine the likelihood that the findings from their sample represent the situation in the population as a whole. If the researchers, hypothetically, could study the population as a whole, would they obtain the same results? *Inferential statistics* are a tool that helps researchers test their findings to establish how representative these findings are. In a sense, one might think of inferential statistics as a tool for bridging the gap between the actual observations of research participants to hypothetical observations of the population they represent. In generalizing from observations on a sample to the entire population the sample represents, researchers do not draw absolute conclusions. They do not make statements such as, "Our findings are or are not representative of the population in general." Rather, they make statements about how much *confidence* they have in their findings or about the *probability of error* associated with the results they reported. When you read a statement in a research report such as, "This difference was statistically significant," it means the researchers tested their data using some kind of inferential statistic(s).

The need to submit research findings to a statistical test arises from the possibility of a sampling error or the possibility that a sample does not represent the entire population (Newhart & Patten, 2023; Oh & Pyrczak, 2023). Sampling errors occur inadvertently and can be present even in random samples from a population. Imagine that a researcher could draw 100 different random samples from a population. With that many samples, there is a possibility that at least a few samples have some peculiar characteristics and do not reflect the true nature of the population. If a researcher studied one of these unique samples, then the findings could reflect the unique characteristics of the sample rather than the effects of an experimental manipulation. The role of inferential statistics is to provide information about the probability that the findings of a study were due to a sampling error rather than a true experimental difference (Oh & Pyrczak, 2023; Trochim et al., 2016).

Authors are guided to use careful language when discussing probability and the outcomes of a statistical analysis (Wasserstein & Lazar, 2016). In one sense, inferential statistics indicate the probability of a calculated result given the assumption that the null hypothesis is true or accurately represents conditions in the population. Recall that a null hypothesis is a negative statement such as, "The experimental and control groups are not significantly different" or "Scores from the experimental test and traditional test are not correlated." If the statistical test is significant, the experimental findings would be unlikely if the null hypothesis were true. Researchers sometimes specify a predetermined probability for statistical tests. Common levels for statistical tests are .05 or 5 in 100, .01 or 1 in 100, or the very conservative .001 or 1 in 1,000. Most statistics applications calculate an exact probability, and reporting the actual probability associated with a statistical test, for example, a probability of .04 or .003, is the preferred practice (American Psychological Association [APA], 2020). As we stated in the chapter on research questions (Chapter 3), research reports do not always include an actual statement of a null hypothesis or research hypothesis. Rather, researchers often formulate questions or a statement of purpose to provide information about the intent of their study. Therefore, you seldom read a formal statement about testing the findings against the null hypothesis. Researchers are more likely to conclude that the results were *statistically significant* or were *not significant*.

You might think of inferential statistics as providing information about the probability that the findings of a study accurately portray the entire population. What many statistical procedures test is the probability or likelihood of obtaining a calculated result given the assumption that the null hypothesis is true. Thus, if a statistic is significant at the .05 level, it means that the probability of obtaining those results would be less than 5 in 100 given a true null hypothesis. Similarly, a statistic that is significant at the .01 level means that the probability of obtaining those results if the null hypothesis were true would be less than 1 in 100. When researchers conclude that a difference is *not significant*, they have concluded that the probability of obtaining that statistic is unacceptably high assuming a true null hypothesis.

Examples of things you might test with a significance test are associations or correlations, in which the null hypothesis would be that there is "no relationship between the two variables," or differences, in which the null hypothesis would be "no difference between the two groups." When researchers complete an inferential statistical analysis, they might report their findings with statements such as the examples below:

1. The difference between means was statistically significant ($p = .003$).[1]
2. The difference between groups was significant at the .01 level.
3. The correlation between the two scores was significant at the .05 level.
4. The difference between groups was not significant at the .05 level ($p = .38$).

One final concept to discuss is what researchers and statisticians mean when they talk about the possibility of making an error. Actually, researchers could make two types of errors when drawing conclusions about their data. The first kind of error is a *Type I error*. This error occurs when a researcher concludes that findings are significant when, in fact, the difference or correlation was not significant (i.e., the null hypothesis was actually true). The goal of researchers is to keep the likelihood of making a Type I error very low. Type I errors could occur because of sampling issues, when the participants in a study did not represent the general population very well.

The second kind of error is a *Type II error*. This error occurs when a researcher finds that a result is not significant when it is, in fact, a significant difference or correlation. In other words, the researchers concluded that the difference between two treatment groups was not significant when the treatments actually were different, or the researchers concluded that the correlation between two measures was not significant, when a correlation between the variables actually existed. One reason that researchers might make a Type II error is that the study lacked sufficient power. As we discussed in the chapter on sampling (Chapter 9), the best way to increase statistical power is to recruit an appropriate number of participants. Other ways to reduce the likelihood of making a Type II error are to provide the experimental treatment with appropriate intensity and precision and to measure your outcomes as accurately and consistently as possible.

In the sections that follow, we discuss two broad categories of inferential statistics, measures of association and difference tests. The intention is to provide information that will contribute to your understanding of the role of statistics in research but not at the

---

[1] A lowercase *p* is the statistical symbol for probability.

depth needed to actually complete a statistical analysis. For additional information on calculation and use of statistics, readers might check out a book on statistics for education or the behavioral and clinical sciences, such as Coladarci and Cobb (2014), Cumming (2012), Pagano (2013), and Satake (2015). Those looking for more advanced information on statistics might refer to recent articles related to the fields of audiology and speech-language pathology that covered some common statistical errors that occur in research publications (Oleson et al., 2019a) and new approaches for analyzing data (Gordon, 2019; Oleson et al., 2019b). Another possibility is to identify a professional statistician and obtain assistance on your statistical analysis prior to starting your study. Many universities offer statistical consulting services for their students and faculty.

Measures of Association

Researchers use measures of association when they are interested in investigating the relationship between two or more sets of scores. For measures of association, each participant in a sample receives all of the tests or other observation procedures. If the researcher is comparing two different tests, then each participant completes both tests. Measures of association usually yield information about the strength of the relationship as well as the direction of the relationship (positive or negative) between measures. Some commonly used measures of association are correlation coefficients, such as the Pearson product-moment correlation coefficient and Spearman rank-ordered correlation coefficient. Other examples include chi-square analysis and contingency coefficients as well as simple regression and multiple regression.

Pearson Product-Moment Correlation Coefficient

If a researcher is investigating the relationship between two measures and the level of measurement is interval or ratio, the most widely used measure of association is the *Pearson product-moment correlation coefficient*. The recommended symbol for the Pearson correlation coefficient is r (American Psychological Association [APA], 2020), and this measure of association is often called the Pearson r. The potential values of the Pearson r range from 0 to ±1.00 (plus or minus 1.00). A value of .00 would indicate that two sets of measures have no relationship, whereas a value of ±1.00 would indicate that two sets of measures have a perfect relationship (Oh & Pyrczak, 2023). The closer the correlation coefficient is to ±1.00, the stronger the relationship. The plus or minus indicates the direction of the relationship, but a *negative* correlation (e.g., −.90) is just as strong as a *positive* correlation (e.g., +.90). In some statistics textbooks, the term *direct relationship* is used as a synonym for a positive relationship, and *inverse relationship* is used as a synonym for a negative relationship (Newhart & Patten, 2023; Oh & Pyrczak, 2023).

Perhaps the best way to understand the nature of the relationship expressed in a correlation coefficient is to produce a scatterplot of two measures and then compute the correlation coefficient. Figure 11–1 depicts the relationship between two variables that have a strong, positive correlation of $r = .98$. A few points to note about Figure 11–1 are that each participant completed both Test 1 and Test 2. The participants' scores on Test 1 are plotted on the vertical axis and Test 2 on the horizontal axis, and each point corresponds to a participant. In this scatterplot, persons who obtain high scores on Test 1 also obtain high scores on Test 2, persons who obtain mid-range scores on Test 1 also obtain mid-range scores on Test 2, and persons who obtain low scores on Test 1 also obtain low scores on Test 2.

Thus, the direction of the relationship is positive or direct. Furthermore, the relationship between the two tests is a strong one. The Pearson r is .98 and the scores tend to plot along a straight line with only small deviations away from the line.

Figure 11–2 illustrates a strong negative or inverse relationship between two variables. In this example, persons who score high on Test 1 score low on Test 2, whereas persons who score low on Test 1 score high on Test 2. Finally, Figure 11–3 illustrates a weak positive relationship between two variables ($r(23) = .25, p = .228$).[2] Note how

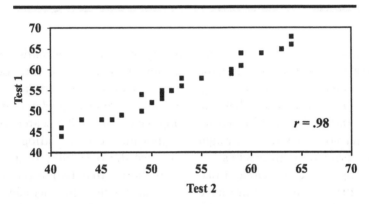

Figure 11–1. An XY scatterplot depicting the relationship between two variables with a strong, positive correlation.

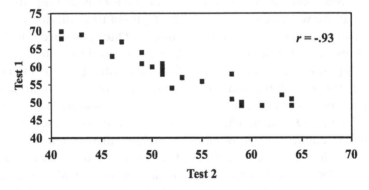

Figure 11–2. An XY scatterplot depicting the relationship between two variables with a strong, negative correlation.

---

[2]We used the website "Free Statistics Calculators" to generate the p value for the Pearson r correlations (Soper, 2006–2020).

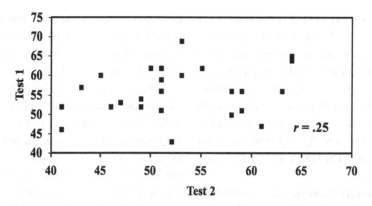

Figure 11–3. An XY scatterplot depicting the relationship between two variables with a weak, positive correlation.

the scores in this example scatter widely, approximating a wide oval shape. When the correlation between two variables is strong, the scatterplot approximates the shape of a straight line, and with a perfect correlation, the scatterplot looks like a straight line. When the correlation approaches .00, the scatterplot approximates a circle (Coladarci & Cobb, 2014). Some authors have suggested verbal descriptors to use with different correlation values. For example, Newhart and Patten (2023) suggested that a correlation of .25 was *weak*, .50 was *moderate*, and .75 and above was *strong*.

When interpreting a correlation coefficient, researchers consider the direction of the relationship, the magnitude of the correlation, and the possibility that the observed relationship between the variables occurred because of random chance. That is, researchers conduct a test of significance to determine if the correlation between two variables is statistically significant. If researchers found that a correlation was significant at the .05 level, they determined that the probability of obtaining this result given a true null hypothesis was low and less than 5 out of 100. Typically, researchers are comfortable that a probability of .05 provides sufficient protection against a Type I error (i.e., deciding that two variables were correlated, when they actually were not correlated in the general population). Plus, if researchers made their significance tests too stringent, they might increase the possibility of a Type II error (concluding that two variables were not correlated when they actually were in the population as a whole).

Because the Pearson r is commonly used, most spreadsheet programs provide a function for calculating this statistic, as do most programs dedicated to statistical calculation. Once you have calculated a correlation, you need to evaluate the probability that the resulting r value might represent a spurious result rather than a true correlation. If the application did not report a p value for the correlation, you might find an online calculator to obtain that value. Alternately, to determine if an r value is significant, you could consult a correlation table for the Pearson r and these are generally included in most introductory statistics textbooks (e.g., Coladarci & Cobb, 2014). To use a correlation table you need to know the number of participants in a study and a related concept referred to as *degrees of freedom*.[3] The degrees of freedom for a statistic relate to the number of participants but reflect the number of data points that are independent or free to vary, or the number of observations that have no restrictions on their values (Cohen et al., 2018; Coladarci & Cobb, 2014). Degrees of freedom for a statistic are always the number of participants minus some number and, for a Pearson *r* correlation statistic, the degrees of freedom are the number of pairs minus 2.

Let's consider the examples in Figures 11–2 and 11–3. The figures illustrate two different associations; however, both hypothetical studies included 25 participants. The measures plotted along the vertical and horizontal axes might be two different ways to measure some aspect of speech, language, or hearing. The researchers selected a random sample of 25 participants and administered both measures to each person. In these examples, the samples included 25 participants; thus, the degrees of freedom for evaluating the significance of the correlation and probability would be 23 (25 − 2 or the number of participants/paired scores minus 2). When the researchers consulted a statistical table for the Pearson *r*, they found that the critical value of *r* was .396 with 23 degrees of freedom and a probability of .05. If the computed value of *r* is greater than or equal to the critical value, .396 in our example, the correlation would be significant. If the computed value of *r* is less than the critical value in the table, the probability would be greater than .05 and the correlation would be nonsignificant. Therefore, the correlation associated with Figure 11–2 was significant at the .05 level, but the one associated with Figure 11–3 was not.

Guidelines in the publication manual of the American Psychological Association (APA, 2020) suggest including the statistical symbol, degrees of freedom, computed value, and probability when reporting statistics. The results in Figure 11–2 would be reported as $r(23) = -.93, p < .001$, and the results in Figure 11–3 would be reported as $r(23) = .25, p > .228$.

Sample size and degrees of freedom have a strong influence on the likelihood that a computed correlation would be significant. Even a weak correlation could be significant in a statistical sense if the sample size is large enough. For example, if our researchers had a larger sample of 102 participants and 100 degrees of freedom, the critical value for *r* would be only .195 at the .05 level. On the other hand, if they had a small sample, perhaps 12 participants and 10 degrees of freedom, the critical value for *r* would be .576. In research, obtaining a result that is statistically significant is not the same as obtaining an important result. If a weak correlation (e.g., $r = .25$) is significant, it means that the probability that it would occur given a true null hypothesis is low. It does not mean this correlation would be particularly useful to a researcher who wanted to show that two tests measured a skill in highly similar ways.

When conducting a significance test, researchers need to keep in mind one caution. The probability associated with a level of significance, such as .05, usually is for a single test of significance. If a research team conducted a study and computed the correlations among several measures, they need to be cautious about the probability of a Type I error. Although the significance level for an individual correlation might be set at .05, the probability of a Type I error for the entire study could be much higher. The example in Table 11–1 shows a problem with computing several correlation coefficients

---

[3] The abbreviation for degrees of freedom is *df* (APA, 2020).

Table 11–1. Illustration of a Table with Several Correlation Coefficients and the Possibility of an Inflated Error Rate

	Speech Discrimination	Phonological Awareness	Consonant Composite	Digit Span	Picture Vocabulary
Speech Discrimination					
Phonological Awareness	0.48*				
Consonant Composite	0.36	0.40			
Digit Span	0.22	0.10	0.35		
Picture Vocabulary	0.30	0.30	0.20	0.15	

$n = 20$.
*$p < .05$.

and making multiple comparisons. In this example, the researcher obtained scores from five different measures and wished to determine if these scores were intercorrelated. In this example study, the researchers calculated 10 correlation coefficients and tested each for significance at the .05 level. The researcher found a single correlation (.48) with a probability of less than .05. A careful researcher would ask if the probability was still .05 after running 10 different statistical tests, however, and the answer to that question would be "no." The actual probability is much higher and is based on the number of individual correlations. For the example in Table 11–1, you could determine the actual error rate by using the following formula: $p = 1 - (1 - .05)^{10}$ (Ottenbacher, 1986). In this formula, the value of $(1 - .05)$ is .95 and when .95 is multiplied by itself 10 times, the resulting value is .60. Thus, the actual probability in a series of 10 separate correlation computations is $1 - .60$ or .40 (Jacobs, 1976). This suggests the chance of a Type I error is much higher than the chance of error that most statistical textbooks recommend. When calculating multiple correlation coefficients, one recommendation is to adopt a more conservative error rate such as .01. Researchers should also be highly suspicious of their findings when only one correlation coefficient in a large table meets the test of significance (i.e., is significant at the .05 level).

Another caution in interpreting a significant correlation coefficient is to consider whether a tested relationship makes logical sense. Sometimes you can obtain a significant correlation between two variables that are not directly related. Rather, the two variables both relate to a third variable you did not measure. Consider the hypothetical example of a researcher who measured height in inches and also gave the same children a language test that yielded an age-equivalent score. The researcher might obtain a significant correlation between height in inches and language age, but logically these two variables should not be directly related. Children who are relatively tall can have language delays and children who are relatively shorter can be quite expressive. If the sample included children across a wide age range, such as from ages 3 to 7, however, then one would expect to see both growth in height and language age with increases in chronological age. The two variables would appear to be correlated because both height and language age correlated to a third variable, chronological age, which was not evaluated.

Coefficient of Determination

The coefficient of determination is a measure that is closely related to the Pearson r. Its symbol is r^2 (Coladarci & Cobb, 2014; Oh & Pyrczak, 2023). Calculation of the coefficient of determination is straightforward; you simply square the Pearson r. Some examples are listed below:

Pearson r	r^2
.20	.04
.50	.25
.80	.64

The coefficient of determination provides information that is helpful in interpreting the magnitude or importance of a correlation. By multiplying a coefficient of determination by 100, a researcher obtains a percentage that reflects the degree of association between two variables. Literally, an r^2 tells you what percentage of variation in one measure can be accounted for by variation in the other measure (Oh & Pyrczak, 2023). Consider the correlation depicted in Figure 11–1. If you knew a participant's score on Test 1, you could guess the score on Test 2 and come very close. An r of .98 corresponds to an r^2 of .96, and knowing one of the scores lets you account for 96% of the variation in the other score. On the other hand, the correlation depicted in Figure 11–3 was weak. An r of .25 only lets you account for 6% of the variation in the other measure.

Spearman Rank-Order Correlation

If the level of measurement is ordinal, researchers often use the Spearman *rank-order correlation* coefficient (*Rho* or r_s) rather than a Pearson r. The Spearman correlation coefficient is a nonparametric statistic and also might be useful when your data do not meet the assumptions associated with use of the Pearson r. For example, researchers might prefer the Spearman *Rho* if the data have a substantial positive or negative skew. Calculation of a Spearman *Rho* involves comparing two sets of rank-ordered measures (Coladarci & Cobb, 2014; Gibbons & Chakraborti, 2011). The range of values for a Spearman *Rho* is similar to a Pearson r: from 0 to ±1.0. The closer the value is to ±1.0, the stronger the correlation, and the closer the value is to 0.0, the weaker the correlation. A value of −1.0 indicates a perfect negative relationship, a +1.0 indicates a perfect positive relationship, and a zero indicates no relationship.

The example in Table 11–2 illustrates two sets of rank-ordered scores and the procedures for calculating a Spearman *Rho*. To compute *Rho*, you determine the difference in ranks, square the difference to remove negative values, and then sum the squared ranks. This information is entered into the formula as shown in Table 11–2. Most commercially available statistical applications include a function for computing a Spearman correlation coefficient, but this function might not be available in a

Table 11–2. Example of Using Rank–Ordered Scores in the Calculation of a Spearman Rank-Order Correlation Coefficient

Participant Identifier	Participant Ranks on Measure 1	Participant Ranks on Measure 2	Difference in Ranks	Difference Squared
A	10	9	1	1
B	2	1	1	1
C	1	2	−1	1
D	6	7	−1	1
E	3	8	−5	25
F	9	10	−1	1
G	7	5	2	4
H	8	4	4	16
I	4	3	1	1
J	5	6	−1	1

Sum of squared differences = 52

Rho = 0.685

Formula for calculating *Rho* is $1 - (6*52/(10*(10^2 - 1)))$

basic spreadsheet program. If the application you use to calculate a Spearman correlation does not provide the *p* value, you can look up the critical value in a statistical table to determine if the statistical value is significant at an appropriate error rate such as .05, as you would for the Pearson *r*.

Chi-Square and Contingency Coefficient

Researchers also have tools for investigating associations among sets of observations when their level of measurement is nominal. One procedure for investigating the degree of association between two categorical variables is a chi-square analysis and contingency table (Coladarci & Cobb, 2014; Gibbons & Chakraborti, 2011). The hypothetical example in Table 11–3 illustrates a 2-by-3 contingency table with two variables: area of specialization in communication sciences and disorders and primary factor in employment decisions. The specialization variable has two levels, and the employment factors variable has three levels. The numbers in the table are frequencies and represent the number of persons in a particular category (e.g., audiologists, speech-language pathologists) who chose each reason for making an employment decision. The logic underlying a chi-square is that an association between the two variables would appear as a difference in the observed frequency compared to the *expected* frequency. The expected frequency is similar to a null hypothesis and represents the situation that would occur if the two variables had no association. In our example, the number of audiologists and speech-language pathologists is equal,

Table 11–3. Example of a 2-by-3 Contingency Table and Chi Square Computation

	Most Important Factor in Employment Decisions			Row Subtotal
	Annual Salary	Work Setting	Other	
Audiologists	80 (Observed) 100 (Expected)	80 60 (Expected)	40 40 (Expected)	200
Speech-language pathologists	120 100 (Expected)	40 60 (Expected)	40 40 (Expected)	200
Column subtotal	200	120	80	Total = 400

Note: The numbers in this table are entirely hypothetical.
Chi square = $((80 - 100)^2 \div 100) + ((80 - 60)^2 \div 60) + ((40 - 40)^2 \div 40) + ((120 - 100)^2 \div 100) + ((40 - 60)^2 \div 60) + ((40 - 40)^2 \div 40)$.
Chi square = $4 + 6.67 + 0 + 4 + 6.67 + 0$.
Chi Square = 21.33.
Contingency coefficient = square root of $(21.33/(400 + 21.33))$ or .225.

so the expected frequencies reflect equal distribution of the professions under each decision factor. The actual computation uses the value of the following for each cell: (Observed − Expected)² ÷ Expected. As with other statistical values, you determine if the probability is greater than .05 by consulting a chi-square table. The degrees of freedom for a chi-square are based on the number of rows and columns [(rows − 1) * (columns − 1)]. For the example in Table 11–3, the degrees of freedom would be (2 − 1) * (3 − 1) or 2. Contingency tables with two rows and two columns are also common, but the table could have different numbers of rows and columns (e.g., 3 by 3, 4 by 3).

Sometimes researchers need to estimate the magnitude of the association between two categorical variables. One way to make such an estimate is to compute a *contingency coefficient* (abbreviated as *C*) (Oh & Pyrczak, 2023). Because contingency coefficients are computed from a chi-square, you complete the chi-square analysis first and then compute a contingency coefficient from the chi-square, in which *C* is equal to the square root of (chi-square/(N + chi-square)). This value is shown in Table 11–3 along with the chi-square computation. Contingency coefficients may range from 0 to 1.0 but are distributed differently depending on the size of the contingency table. Thus, 0 to 1.0 reflects the maximum range; meanwhile, the actual upper limit could be less. For this reason, contingency coefficients cannot be compared directly unless they are yielded by tables of the same size (Oh & Pyrczak, 2023). Due to the computational procedures, contingency coefficients are always positive and do not convey information about the direction of a relationship.

Simple Regression and Multiple Regression

Sometimes researchers want to investigate the predictive value of an association. In these instances, they might conduct a regression analysis rather than a correlation analysis. A simple regression with two variables is similar to a correlation, except that one variable is the independent or predictor variable and the other is the dependent variable. A regression analysis allows you to predict or estimate the value of a dependent variable if you know the value of the independent variable. One thing that researchers might do is generate a regression line to show where predicted scores would fall. This possibility is illustrated in Figure 11–4. These are the same data portrayed in Figure 11–1, but in this case, we added a regression line to the display and designated the variable along the x-axis as the independent variable (predictor) and the variable along the y-axis as the dependent variable (predicted). The slope of the line represents the amount of change in Y that corresponds to a change of one unit in X. The regression line is the line of "best fit" or the line about which the scores would deviate the least.

In the case of a simple regression with two variables, the regression statistic (r^2) and the Pearson r relate to one another in a direct way. The regression statistic is the square of the Pearson r. You might recall this value from our discussion of the coefficient of determination. In the case of a regression, you might think of the r^2 as reflecting the extent to which changes in the Y variable are predictable if you know the person's score on the X variable. One common use of regression analysis is to determine the value of the independent (X) variable for predicting future performance on the dependent (Y) variable. An example of this would be research in the area of reading where researchers have investigated the predictive value of various measures of phonemic awareness to determine if they would provide early identification of children who would be at risk for reading problems in the future. In this example, measures of phonemic awareness would be the independent variables, and measures of reading skills would be the dependent variables.

Sometimes questions about the relationships among variables are too complex to analyze with a simple regression model. For example, a researcher might be interested in investigating the simultaneous pre-

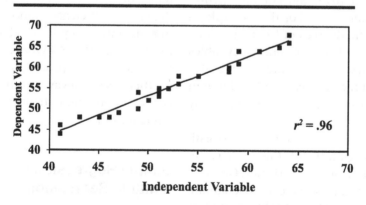

Figure 11–4. An illustration of a simple regression model with one dependent variable, one independent variable, and a linear regression line representing the predicted relationship between the two variables.

dictive value of two or more independent variables, or perhaps a researcher discovered that the independent and dependent variables in a study are related in a nonlinear manner. Simple regression works well for investigating the predictive relationship between two variables whose relationship roughly approximates a straight line but, for the more complex examples, a researcher might consider using a *multiple regression* analysis and/or a *nonlinear regression* analysis (Cohen et al., 2018).

Multiple regression techniques allow you to determine the strongest combination of variables for predicting outcomes on a dependent variable. Often with regression analysis, researchers are interested in predicting a future outcome. Our simple regression example involved predicting future reading skills from a measure of phonemic awareness. Another example might be predicting future speech sound production abilities of preschool children with hearing impairment. Perhaps researchers have developed a new way to test speech discrimination abilities of young children at ages 3 and 4. They also know the children's average pure-tone thresholds. The researchers want to determine if one or both of these measures would enable them to accurately predict speech production abilities at age 6 as measured by the percentage of intelligible words in conversational speech. Such a study would require a longitudinal research design because the researchers need to measure the *independent* variables at ages 3 and 4, and then reassess the children at age 6 to determine their speech intelligibility. Once they have collected these measures, the researchers can complete a multiple regression analysis with speech intelligibility as the dependent variable and speech discrimination and average pure-tone threshold as independent variables. The results of the regression analysis will provide information to determine the strength of the predictive relationship, expressed as an r^2; the probability associated with the analysis; and the extent to which each of the independent variables made a significant contribution to the prediction. The computation and interpretation for a multiple regression analysis are complex, and those who might need to use such an analysis need to consult more advanced data analysis textbooks (e.g., Rosenthal & Rosnow, 2008).

One final consideration in designing a regression analysis is whether or not the relationships among the dependent and independent variables are linear. Some variables might actually have a highly predictable relationship, but because the relationship is curvilinear rather than linear, a simple regression on the variables would yield disappointing findings. Figure 11–5 illustrates one example of a curvilinear relationship. This type of curve sometimes is called an inverted U shape, but more formally, it is a quadratic relationship (Velleman, 1997). If you completed a simple regression and obtained an r^2 for these two variables, the value would be very low, $r^2 = .006$. This would mean that only 0.6% of the variability in the dependent variable could be accounted for by its relationship with the independent or predictor variable. However, the two variables are actually more closely related than that. The problem is that both low scores and high scores on the independent variable are associated with low scores on the dependent variable, whereas mid-range scores on the independent variable are associated with high scores on the dependent variable. If the researcher used an appropriate type of nonlinear regression to analyze this relationship, the resulting r^2 would be much larger, $r^2 = .61$. This means

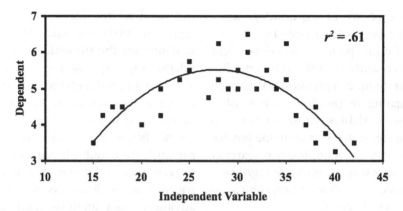

Figure 11–5. An illustration of a nonlinear relationship with one dependent variable, one independent variable, and a line of best fit representing the curvilinear relationship.

that the relationship between the independent and dependent variables, when treated as a nonlinear relationship, accounted for 61% of the variability. This example illustrates two important points about data analysis. First, examining a graphic display of your data is helpful for determining how to approach the analysis. This is one way to determine important characteristics such as the linearity of relationships and the shapes of distributions. Second, choosing an appropriate analysis procedure has a definite impact on the accuracy of your findings. An inappropriate analysis might mask a relationship that actually exists in the data.

Thus far, our discussion of data analysis has focused on procedures for investigating associations among variables. In this type of study, researchers look at a single group of participants and obtain two or more measures from each participant. Studies that employ correlation and regression analyses are usually nonexperimental designs in which the researchers examine preexisting relationships among variables. The next section focuses on data analysis procedures for examining differences between groups. Although difference tests are useful for analyzing group differences in nonexperimental designs, one of their main uses is in analyzing results from randomized experimental designs.

Testing for Differences Between Two Samples

Many statistical tests are available for analyzing differences between groups. In deciding which test is most appropriate, you need to consider how many groups you are going to compare, as well as what kind of differences you are analyzing. Additionally, some statistical tests are recommended for interval- and ratio-level measurements, observations that fit certain assumptions about the distribution of data around the mean, and larger sample sizes. These are called parametric statistics. Other statistical tests, called nonparametric statistics, are recommended for ordinal-level measurements, situations in which you are uncertain about the distribution of data or have smaller sample sizes (Gibbons & Chakraborti, 2011). Thus, researchers also need to consider whether a parametric or nonparametric statistic would be a better choice for analyzing their data.

Independent and Paired *t*-Tests

The *t*-test is the most common procedure used for analyzing the difference between two sets of data when you have interval- or ratio-level measures. A *t*-test specifically tests the difference between means to determine if two groups are significantly different. Figures 11–6 and 11–7 illustrate the types of group differences that could be analyzed with a *t*-test. Each figure contains a frequency polygon for two different groups. In each instance, the group means are 10 points apart, as shown by the arrows, and in each instance, the groups partially overlap. However, the two groups represented in Figure 11–6 overlap more than the two groups in Figure 11–7. This greater overlap occurs because the scores

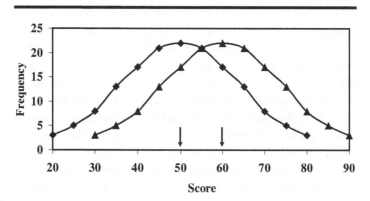

Figure 11–6. A frequency polygon illustrating the difference between means for two groups with relatively greater variability among scores.

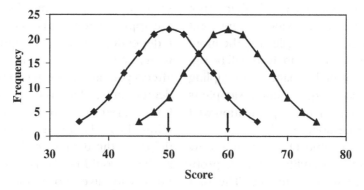

Figure 11–7. A frequency polygon illustrating the difference between means for two groups with relatively less variability among scores.

in Figure 11–6 are more widely dispersed around the mean. Whenever researchers analyze data with a *t*-test, they are trying to determine if an observed difference between groups means is a true difference. A significant result means that the observed difference is most likely a real difference with a low probability (e.g., less than .05 or less than .01).

Three factors influence whether or not you will find a significant difference when analyzing data with a *t*-test (Oh & Pyrczak, 2023). One of these factors is the magnitude of the difference between means. All other factors being equal, the larger the difference between means, the more likely the *t*-test analysis will come out significant. A second factor that influences the likelihood of obtaining a significant outcome is the amount of variability in your data. The less variable the scores, as measured by variance and standard deviation, the more likely a difference between means will come out significant. Figures 11–6 and 11–7 both illustrate situations in which the group means differ by 10 points. The groups illustrated in Figure 11–6 have greater variance, however, than the groups in Figure 11–7. When scores are more widely dispersed around the mean, you need a larger mean difference to obtain significance. Sample size is a final factor that influences whether or not a statistical analysis will yield a significant result. The larger the sample size, the more likely the outcome of an analysis will be significant. Recall from the chapter on sampling (Chapter 9) that a larger random sample is more likely to represent the population well than a smaller random sample.

The data in Table 11–4 illustrate how sample size and variability influence probability and significance testing. The first four columns present scores randomly selected from distributions similar to the ones depicted in Figure 11–6. Columns 1 and 2 are relatively larger samples ($n = 25$), whereas columns 3 and 4 are relatively smaller samples. The group means differ by approximately 10 points, and the data in columns 1 through 4 are relatively more variable with standard deviations of 10.8 and above. The last four columns present scores randomly selected from distributions similar to the ones depicted in Figure 11–7. Again, the group means differ by approximately 10 points; however, the data in columns 5 through 8 are less variable, as reflected by the smaller standard deviations. Although computing a *t*-test by hand is possible, it is safer to use a spreadsheet statistical function or dedicated statistical software for the task. The results reported in Table 11–4 are from a dedicated statistical software package, DataDesk® 6.3 (2011).

When using *t*-tests, you need to consider whether the two samples being compared are related or independent. Related samples are either two measures on the same participants, such as measures at two different times, or measures from samples of matched participants. Sometimes researchers create participant pairs by matching them on some pretest measure. After the matching, the researchers randomly assign the participants to one of two treatment groups. With either two measures on the same participants or matched participants, the appropriate *t*-test is a *paired t-test*. With independent samples, the appropriate *t*-test is an *independent t-test*. One way this choice affects your analysis is when you determine degrees of freedom. The degrees of freedom for a paired *t*-test are the number of pairs minus 1 ($n - 1$). If you had 25 matched participants, the degrees of freedom for your analysis would be 24. For an independent *t*-test, you have two options for determining degrees of freedom. The most common when you have equal numbers of participants in each group is called the *pooled*

Table 11-4. Example of Computation of *t*-Tests for More Variable and Less Variable Groups with Different Sample Sizes

	More Variable				Less Variable			
	n = 25		n = 10		n = 25		n = 10	
	1st	2nd	3rd	4th	5th	6th	7th	8th
	57	70	57	70	55	67	55	67
	33	49	33	49	55	65	55	65
	47	49	47	49	39	50	39	50
	40	50	40	50	40	51	40	51
	40	44	40	44	57	67	57	67
	51	58	51	58	60	70	60	70
	52	69	52	69	52	61	52	61
	38	51	38	51	45	54	45	54
	57	67	57	67	43	53	43	53
	73	73	73	73	59	69	59	69
	33	48			40	48		
	67	75			49	61		
	47	52			45	53		
	49	64			49	59		
	60	72			56	65		
	43	53			52	64		
	29	31			50	59		
	64	72			51	62		
	61	73			44	56		
	62	75			45	55		
	69	82			54	65		
	39	52			57	67		
	55	72			49	60		
	50	50			59	69		
	27	41			40	49		
M =	49.6	59.6	48.7	57.9	49.8	60.0	50.5	60.8
SD =	12.9	13.4	11.8	10.8	6.7	6.9	7.9	8.0

variance t-test. You add the number of participants in each group and subtract 2 ($n_1 + n_2 - 2$). If you had 25 participants in each group, the degrees of freedom would be 25 + 25 – 2 or 48. When you have two independent samples, and the variances of the two groups are different, using the pooled variance *t*-test is inappropriate. Determining the degrees of freedom for groups with different variances is beyond the scope of our discussion. You might consult other sources if confronted with this situation (Coladarci & Cobb, 2014).

Let's return to the data in Table 11–4. These data represent independent samples, so we are going to analyze the mean differences using an independent t-test. First, we are going to report the results for the larger samples (n = 25). Oh and Pyrczak (2023) recommended always reporting the values of your means and standard deviations before reporting the results of a t-test, so this information is included in Table 11–4. The results from the analysis of the more variable groups revealed a significant difference between the first and second groups, $t(48) = -2.69, p < .001$. Repeating the analysis for the data in columns 5 and 6 revealed a significant difference between the fifth and sixth groups as well, $t(48) = -5.33, p < .001$. Thus, with samples of 25 participants, the differences between groups were significant for both the more variable and less variable samples.

Let's repeat our analyses with the smaller samples, starting with the more variable groups in columns 3 and 4. In this case, our degrees of freedom will be 10 + 10 − 2 or 18. The results from this analysis revealed the mean difference between the third and fourth groups was not significant at the .05 level, $t(18) = -1.82$, $p = .09$. Finally, let's complete our example by analyzing the data in columns 7 and 8. The results from the analysis of the less variable groups revealed a significant difference between the seventh and eighth groups, $t(18) = -2.86, p = .01$.[4] The t-test results reported here follow the guidelines in the APA (2020) publication manual by including the statistical symbol, degrees of freedom, statistical value, and probability.

Confidence Intervals

Although difference tests, such as the t-test, are common in published articles, investigators have been encouraged to consider alternative procedures such as reporting confidence intervals (Cumming, 2012; Kline, 2004). In keeping with this suggestion, let's calculate and display the confidence intervals for the data in Table 11–4. A *confidence interval* is a way of estimating the margin of error associated with your sample. Remember that researchers study a sample in order to make inferences about the entire population from that sample. However, a sample may or may not represent the population well. If you could obtain 100 different samples from a population and calculate a mean from each sample, some of those samples would provide very close estimates of the population mean, but other samples would provide estimates that were somewhat distant from the population mean. This is the notion of margin of error. Researchers calculate a confidence interval to establish a range that has a high probability of capturing the true population mean.

To calculate a confidence interval, we need four numbers: the number of participants (N), mean (M), standard deviation (SD), and a critical value for the t statistic at a particular level of confidence, for example, .05 or .01. Researchers obtain the first three numbers from their data and look up the final number in a statistical table. The formula for calculating margin of error

---

[4]Many dedicated statistical software packages report the actual probability, and the p values reported by DataDesk® 6.3 are included here.

(MOE) and the 95% confidence interval was first described in Chapter 10. The calculation involved determining the standard error (*SE*) and then using that value to determine MOE and the 95% confidence interval.[5] Recall that the *SE* was the *SD* divided by the square root of *N* and that MOE was $t_{.95}$ * *SE*, where $t_{.95}$ was obtained from a table for the *t* statistic, and finally, the confidence interval was the mean ± the MOE (Cumming, 2012). Means and standard deviations for each of the groups are already included in Table 11–4. To complete our calculation, we need the *t* for the 95% confidence level, which is 2.065 for our larger groups (for $n - 1$ or 24 degrees of freedom) and 2.262 for our smaller groups (for $n - 1$ or 9 degrees of freedom). The confidence intervals (CIs) for each group are reported below and plotted in Figure 11–8.[6] Our population means would probably fall within these ranges 95% of the time (i.e., 95% confidence interval). In the following examples, the first number in brackets is the lower limit and the second number is the upper limit.

More variable n = 25, first group (A1)
95% *CI* [44.54, 54.66]

More variable n = 25, second group (A2)
95% *CI* [54.35, 64.85]

More variable n = 10, first group (B1)
95% *CI* [41.39, 56.01]

More variable n = 10, second group (B2)
95% *CI* [51.29, 64.59]

Less variable n = 25, first group (C1)
95% *CI* [47.17, 52.43]

Less variable n = 25, second group (C2)
95% *CI* [57.3, 62.7]

Less variable n = 10, first group (D1)
95% *CI* [45.6, 55.4]

Less variable n = 10, second group (D2)
95% CI [55.84, 65.76]

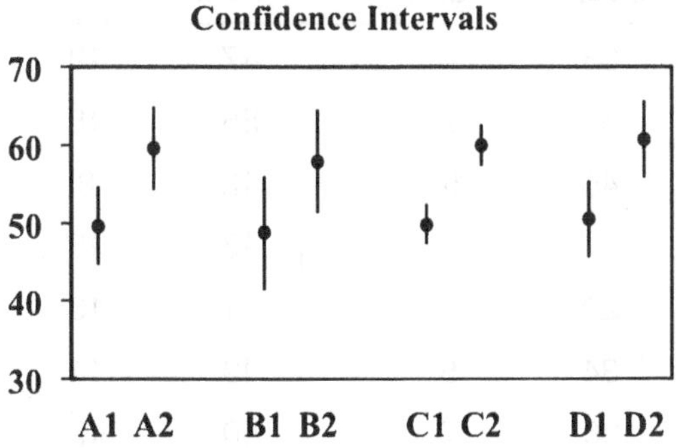

A couple of points to note about the confidence intervals calculated above and displayed in Figure 11–8 are, first, that the larger groups tended to have smaller confidence intervals, indicating that our estimates of the means are more precise with a larger sample size. Second, the more the confidence intervals for two groups in each comparison overlap, the less definitive are the group differences (Cumming, 2012; Kline, 2003). This was particularly true for the more variable, small groups (B1 and B2). Finally, the less variable groups yielded more definitive results, and this is

Figure 11–8. A plot showing the confidence intervals for the mean ± the margin of error for each of the groups compared in Table 11–4.

---

[5]As with effect size, tools for calculating a confidence interval are available via the Internet, for example, the EasyCalculation.com website (https://www.easycalculation.com/statistics/data-analysis.php).
[6]Although you could compute these confidence intervals manually with a calculator, these examples were generated using Exploratory Software for Confidence Intervals (ESCI), free software that accompanies the Cumming (2012) textbook.

most evident for the less variable, larger group comparison (C1 and C2). As shown in Figure 11–8, the confidence intervals for C1 and C2 were small and did not overlap. In some fields of study, confidence intervals replace difference tests such as the t-test. Even if researchers still calculate and report difference tests, confidence intervals are a useful way to more accurately depict the relationship between groups.

In Chapter 8, we covered different experimental designs. Each of those designs would correspond to one of the data analysis procedures we are covering in this chapter. An independent t-test might be used to analyze data from a randomized, posttest-only design. An independent t-test also might be appropriate for analyzing data from a nonexperimental design, such as when researchers compare random samples from two populations with preexisting differences. In the field of communication sciences and disorders, studies often focus on comparing persons with a communication disorder and those with typical communication skills. If only two groups are being compared, an independent t-test would be one way to analyze the data.

Sometimes researchers want to investigate the differences between two groups but find that using a t-test or confidence intervals would be inappropriate. One reason could be that the level of measurement was ordinal rather than interval or ratio. Otherwise, the researchers might be concerned that their data do not meet the assumptions associated with a parametric test such as a t-test. Perhaps their sample sizes are quite small or they are uncertain how their measures distribute about the mean. For example, they might have noted an obvious positive or negative skew in a plot of the scores. In these situations, alternative, nonparametric procedures such as the Mann-Whitney U test, sign test, or the Wilcoxon signed-ranks test might be better choices for analyzing the data.

Mann-Whitney U

The Mann-Whitney U test is a nonparametric test that is appropriate for testing the difference between two independent groups (Gibbons & Chakraborti, 2011). This test can be used with ordinal, ranked scores or you can convert a set of measures to ranks. An example of the setup and computation of a Mann-Whitney U is shown in Table 11–5. In this hypothetical study, some graduate students conducted a small study to test the

Table 11–5. Example Computation of a Mann Whitney U Test for Examining the Difference Between Two Independent Samples

Treatment Procedure			
Traditional		Experimental	
Score	Rank	Score	Rank
33	4	47	12
30	2	55	18
45	10	42	8
31	3	48	13
20	1	51	16
34	5	49	14
36	7	50	15
46	11	52	17
44	9		
35	6		
			$R_1 = 113$

$U = n_1 n_2 + n_1 (n_1 + 1)/2 - R_1$.
$U = 10*8 + 8(8 + 1)/2 - 113$.
$U = 3, p = .0003$.

effectiveness of a new treatment procedure. They were able to randomly assign their participants to groups, but the sample sizes were small and the groups had different numbers of participants. The students were advised by a statistical consultant at their university to use a Mann-Whitney U test to analyze their data. Computing this statistic is relatively easy, as shown in Table 11–5. The students used a statistics software program to complete their analysis in this case. To calculate a Mann-Whitney U, the scores of the two groups are ranked as if they were from a single group, and then the ranks for the smaller group are summed (e.g., R_1 in the table). If the two groups are different, the highest ranks should cluster in one group, whereas the lowest ranks should cluster in the other group. The sum of the ranks is entered into a special formula for computation of the U statistic (Gibbons & Chakraborti, 2011), as shown in Table 11–5. In our example study, the students found that the higher-ranking scores tended to occur in the experimental group and that this difference was significant: $U = 3$, $p = .0003$. The statistical analysis software reported the p value as well as the value of the U statistic. If the students had looked up the value in a statistical table, they would have used the number of participants in each of the two groups to determine the critical value of U. For $n_1 = 8$ and $n_2 = 10$, the critical value for U at the .05 level was 17. The computed value had to be less than or equal to the value in the table, so the U of 3 was significant.

Sign Test and Wilcoxon Matched-Pairs Signed-Ranks Test

If your scores are from related samples, such as two scores from the same participants, the sign test and the Wilcoxon matched-pairs signed-rank test are useful statistical tests. Like the Mann-Whitney U test, these two procedures would be appropriate for ordinal-level measures or in situations where the distribution of scores around the mean is irregular (Gibbons & Chakraborti, 2011). The sign test and the Wilcoxon test are nonparametric alternatives to a paired t-test. The sign test is the simplest to compute but only reflects the direction of a difference and not the magnitude of the difference. Consider the situation depicted in Table 11–6. In this example, participants listened to two computer-generated voices and chose the one they preferred. The + or – signs represent the direction of these differences. As long as you are consistent in making the comparisons, the value will be the same. For example, if A was designated as the – and B as the +, the value of x would be the same because you still would count

Table 11–6. Example Computation of a Sign Test for Examining the Difference Between Two Related Samples

Participant	Preferred Voice	Sign
#1	A	+
#2	A	+
#3	A	+
#4	A	+
#5	B	–
#6	A	+
#7	A	+
#8	A	+
#9	A	+
#10	A	+
$x = 1$*	(Count the number of the less frequent sign to obtain x.)	

*$p < 0.05$.

the less frequent sign. With 10 participants and an x of 1, the probability would be less than .05, indicating that the subjects preferred voice A over voice B significantly more often.

The Wilcoxon matched-pairs signed-rank test uses rank-ordered level measurement in its computation. An example of the use of this test is shown in Table 11–7. In this example, the researchers matched their participants on their pretest scores and then randomly assigned one participant from each pair to the computer activity and one to the paper-and-pencil activity. They found that scores were higher with the computer activity for 8 out of 10 participants. To compute the Wilcoxon matched-pairs signed-rank test (T) statistic, you determine the difference between the scores of the matched pairs, rank those differences with their sign, and then determine the sign (+/−) that occurred less frequently. The T statistic is the sum of the ranks with the less frequently occurring sign, $T = 3$ in our example. For some sample sizes, you simply look up the probability associated with T in a table. For example, Gibbons and Chakraborti (2011) include a table for sample sizes up to 15. For larger samples, the computation is complex, and the safest approach would be to complete the calculation using a statistics software program.

Testing for Differences Among Three or More Samples

If the design of a study involves three or more groups, usually the technique for data analysis will be an *analysis of variance* (ANOVA). In one sense, the analysis of vari-

Table 11–7. Example Computation of the Wilcoxon Matched-Pairs Signed-Rank Test for Examining the Difference Between Two Related Samples

Type of Activity				
Computer	Paper and Pencil	Difference	Rank of Difference	Less Frequent Sign
51	41	10	8	
65	61	4	4	
40	42	−2	−2	2
60	51	9	7	
38	39	−1	−1	1
63	51	12	10	
65	58	7	5	
57	54	3	3	
58	50	8	6	
50	39	11	9	
Sum the ranks of the less frequent sign, ignoring the sign.				$T = 3$*

*$p = 0.005$.
Source: Gibbons & Chakraborti (2011).

ance is an extension of the *t*-test because the outcome is affected by the same factors: mean differences among the groups, amount of variability within and across the groups, and sample size. Although researchers could use an ANOVA to analyze differences between two groups, this is seldom the practice. Usually, ANOVA analyses are reserved for designs with several groups or designs with more than one independent variable.

One of the simplest designs for a *one-way ANOVA* is illustrated in Figure 11–9. This shows three different frequency polygons, each representing a different group. The distributions are roughly normal, with scores spreading in a symmetrical way around the group means. An ANOVA computation involves a comparison of different sources of variance in the data. In the example in Figure 11–9, one source of variance is the dispersion of scores around the individual group means. A second source of variance is the overall dispersion of scores across all three groups. If the groups are different, then the overall spread of scores will be much larger than the spread of scores within the individual groups. When you examine Figure 11–9, the three groups stand out and are easy to identify. A different situation occurs in Figure 11–10. The

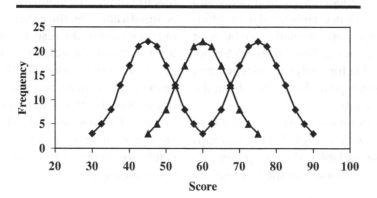

Figure 11–9. A frequency polygon illustrating differences among three groups associated with mean differences and amount of variability.

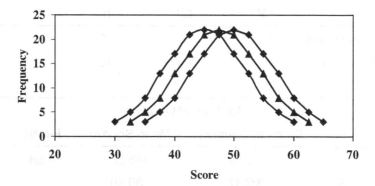

Figure 11–10. A frequency polygon illustrating three groups with relatively greater overlap associated with lesser mean differences relative to variability.

three groups overlap to a great extent and are not clearly separated. The overall variance across all three groups and the variance for each individual group are similar, and it is more difficult to identify the three separate groups. A researcher conducting an ANOVA on data similar to that shown in Figure 11–9 would be much more likely to identify a significant difference among the groups than a researcher with data similar to that shown in Figure 11–10.

Analyzing data using analysis of variance is appropriate if you have interval- or ratio-level measures. The statistic associated with an ANOVA is an F test (Oh & Pyrczak, 2023). This statistic is sometimes called an F ratio because its computation takes into account the variance associated with differences among groups in relation to the error variance. Like t-tests, different ANOVA models are available for analyzing independent groups versus repeated measures from the same participants.

Next, let's review an example of a one-way ANOVA with a single between-groups independent variable. The design in this example is an extension of the randomized posttest-only design we analyzed with a t-test. The difference is that we now have three independent groups: an experimental treatment group, a traditional treatment group, and a no-treatment control group. The means and standard deviations for each group, along with the results from a one-way ANOVA, are shown in Table 11–8. The computational procedures for an ANOVA are complex, so the results in Table 11–8 are from a statistical software package (DataDesk®, 2011). From the standpoint of the researchers, the most important number in the ANOVA table is the probability. With a p of .014, they know that probability value is low, less than 5 in 100, in concluding that the difference among the three groups is significant. For the purposes of reporting their results, the researchers also would want to know the value of the F ratio and the degrees of freedom for the groups and error sources. Note that the total degrees of freedom are the number of participants minus 1. The degrees of freedom for groups are the number of groups minus 1. What is left over represents the error degrees of freedom (e.g., 36 – 1 – 2 = 33). When report-

Table 11–8. Example of a One-Way Analysis of Variance (ANOVA) with Three Groups

	Descriptive Statistics		
	M	**SD**	**n**
Experimental Treatment	46.5	5.53	12
Traditional Treatment	40.1	5.50	12
No Treatment Control	39.8	5.51	12

		Analysis of Variance			
Source	**df**	**Sums of Squares**	**Mean Square**	**F-ratio**	**Probability**
Groups	2	296.72	148.36	4.88	0.014
Error	33	1003.17	30.40		
Total	35	1299.89			

ing the results of the analysis in Table 11–8, you would first report the means and standard deviations for each group (Oh & Pyrczak, 2023) and then the following: $F(2, 33) = 4.88, p = .014$. This format follows the APA (2020) guidelines.

If you obtain a significant result after conducting an ANOVA, you know that one or more of the group differences were significant. Meanwhile, you do not know exactly which group differences were the significant ones. Examining descriptive statistics, such as the group means and standard deviations, generally is not sufficient for identifying the specific differences. Rather, researchers follow up a significant ANOVA result with an additional post hoc statistical test (i.e., one conducted after the initial analysis). Several different procedures are available specifically for post hoc analysis and making multiple comparisons among means. Some examples include the Bonferroni correction, the Scheffé test, and Tukey's honest significant difference (HSD) test (Coladarci & Cobb, 2014). Examples that follow in a later section of this chapter include use of the Scheffé post hoc test.

A different version of the ANOVA test, a repeated measures ANOVA, is available for situations in which researchers obtained several measures from the same participants. Sometimes these kinds of designs involve participants being observed under three or more experimental conditions. Another application of this kind of design is to obtain repeated measures over time to document growth and/or change with treatment. In the chapter on experimental research design, we noted that a one-group pretest-posttest design was a weak experimental design. One of the major problems with this design is that participants could change over time due to maturation and/or recovery. Such changes would confound any treatment effects that you hoped to observe. Trochim et al. (2016) noted that adding a second pretest before initiating treatment was a way to address this issue, at least partially. Our example of a one-way repeated measures ANOVA, shown in Table 11–9,

Table 11–9. Example of a One-Way Repeated Measures Analysis of Variance (ANOVA) with Measures from the Same Participants at Three Different Times

	Descriptive Statistics				
	M	SD	n		
Pretest #1	46.0	5.89	12		
Pretest #2	45.3	5.79	12		
Posttest	52.2	5.81	12		
	Analysis of Variance				
Source	**df**	**Sums of Squares**	**Mean Square**	**F-ratio**	**Probability**
Participants	11	1023.00	93.00	20.60	≤0.0001
Times	2	340.67	170.33	37.73	≤0.0001
Error	22	99.33	4.52		
Total	35	1463.00			

is an analysis of this type of design. The researchers recruited 12 participants for an exploratory treatment study. Because they were not able to use random assignment to treatment and control groups, they decided to add a second pretest to their design. As with the example in Table 11–8, these data were analyzed using a statistics software package (DataDesk®, 2011). The means and standard deviations for each time, along with the results from a one-way repeated measures ANOVA, are included. The results of the analysis revealed a significant difference in the participants' performance over time, $F(2, 22) = 37.73, p < .001$. In this example, the researchers would want to use a post hoc test to verify that the participants did not make a significant change between Pretest 1 and Pretest 2 and that the only significant difference occurred on the posttest after treatment.

You might examine the ANOVA results in Tables 11–8 and 11–9 and identify some of the similarities and differences between the one-way ANOVA for independent groups and the repeated measures ANOVA. Both analyses include similar information: degrees of freedom, sum of squares, mean square, F ratio, and probability. The variance in the scores is divided among several sources. In the case of the repeated measures analysis of variance, however, an additional source associated with participants was added. This reduced the number of degrees of freedom associated with the error source (i.e., total of 35 − 11 − 2 for error degrees of freedom). The F ratio is still the mean square for times divided by the mean square for error.

If your level of measurement is ordinal or you have concerns that your data do not meet the assumptions associated with an ANOVA, you might consider one of the nonparametric alternatives to the one-way ANOVA. Nonparametric tests are available to analyze both related and unrelated samples. *Friedman's two-way analysis of variance* is appropriate if you have repeated measures from the same participants or related samples due to matching. Although this test is called a two-way analysis of variance, it is an alternative to a one-way repeated measures ANOVA. A second nonparametric test, the *Kruskal-Wallis test*, is equivalent to a one-way ANOVA for independent samples. Gibbons and Chakraborti (2011) provide a detailed discussion of the nature and computation of these nonparametric alternatives.

Statistical Analysis for Factorial Designs

A one-way analysis of variance is useful for studies with one independent variable or factor. Although the example in Table 11–8 had three levels of the independent variable, such an analysis could compare even more groups. However, sometimes researchers want to investigate two or more independent variables in the same study. We learned in Chapter 8 that designs with more than one independent variable are factorial designs. The analyses for these designs are called two-way ANOVAs, three-way ANOVAs, and so forth, depending on the number of factors or independent variables. Theoretically, researchers could design a study with many different independent variables. In practice, you seldom see more than four or five different factors, and even those designs are relatively rare. The interpretation of multiway ANOVAs is complex, and the more variables you add, the more challenging it becomes to explain your findings.

The example in Table 11–10 illustrates a 2-by-2 analysis of variance. This is one of

Table 11–10. Example of a Two-Way Analysis of Variance (ANOVA) with Two Independent Variables, Treatment Type and Intensity

	Descriptive Statistics	
	Two Sessions/Week	**Four Sessions/Week**
Experimental	M = 13.60 SD = 4.60 n = 10	M = 23.20 SD = 4.54 n = 10
Traditional	M = 13.40 SD = 4.62 n = 10	M = 13.30 SD = 4.55 n = 10

Analysis of Variance					
Source	**df**	**Sums of Squares**	**Mean Square**	**F-ratio**	**Probability**
Intensity	1	225.63	225.63	10.77	0.0023
Treatment	1	255.03	255.03	12.17	0.0013
Int. by Trt.	1	235.23	235.23	11.22	0.0019
Error	36	754.50	20.96		
Total	39	1470.37			

the simplest factorial designs. The notation 2 by 2 means you have two independent variables and each of those variables has two levels. In this example, the independent variables are intensity of treatment and type of treatment. The levels for the intensity variable are two sessions per week and four sessions per week, and the levels for type of treatment are experimental and traditional. The researchers randomly assigned 10 participants to each treatment/intensity combination. Although this study has two independent variables, the design is still a randomized posttest-only design because the researchers only tested their participants one time at the end of treatment.

The ANOVA results are shown at the bottom of Table 11–10, and much of the information is familiar from our discussion of one-way analysis of variance: degrees of freedom, sums of squares, mean square, F ratio, and probability. In the case of this two-way ANOVA, the sources of variance include the two independent variables, intensity and treatment, and an additional source called the intensity-by-treatment interaction. Any differences associated with the two independent variables often are called *main effects*, and differences associated with the intensity-by-treatment interaction are called *interaction effects*.

A two-way ANOVA would enable you to determine if there are differences associated with your main effects (the main levels), as well as any interactions between the levels. For the example in Table 11–10, the main effects for intensity of treatment, $F(1, 36) = 10.77$, $p = .0023$, and type of treatment, $F(1, 36) = 12.17$, $p = .0013$, were significant, as was the intensity-by-treatment interaction, $F(1, 36) = 11.22$, $p = .0010$. A significant interaction means that the outcome for one of the independent variables was different depending on the level of the other independent variable. In our example, the outcome for treatment was different depending on the level of intensity. When you have a significant interaction, it is good practice to examine this source first rather than focus on the main effects. A beginning step in analyzing an interaction is to plot the individual group or cell means; a line graph is a useful tool for generating this plot. Figure 11–11 shows the interaction of treatment and intensity. As shown in this graph, the mean for the experimental treatment was greater than the mean for traditional treatment when the treatment was intense (four times per week) but not when the treatment was less frequent. Researchers also use post hoc tests like the Scheffé test and Tukey's HSD test to further analyze significant interactions as well. These post hoc tests are designed to tell you which individual group comparisons were significant. The results for the Scheffé test as reported by DataDesk® (2011) revealed the following significant differences:

1. Difference between two sessions and four sessions per week for the experiment treatment was 9.60, $p < .0001$.
2. Difference between traditional treatment with two sessions per week and experimental treatment with four sessions per week was 9.80, $p < .0001$.
3. Difference between traditional treatment and experimental treatment with four sessions per week was 9.90, $p < .0001$.

Hypothetically, an interaction such as the one illustrated in Figure 11–11 could occur with persons with communication disorders. Perhaps a subgroup did not respond well to traditional treatment, so researchers decided to study an experimental treatment program. The experimental program was not effective either, unless it was presented more intensely. On the other hand, more intense treatment did not improve the effectiveness of the traditional treatment approach.

The final example, shown in Table 11–11, is an analysis of a randomized pretest-posttest design. The analysis procedure for

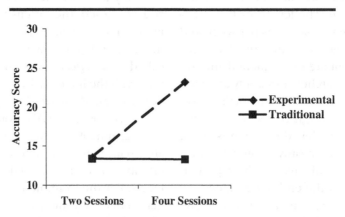

Figure 11–11. A line graph illustrating an interaction between type of treatment and intensity of treatment.

Table 11–11. Example of a Two-Way Mixed-Model Analysis of Variance (ANOVA) with One Between and One Repeated Measures Variable

	Descriptive Statistics	
	Pretest	**Posttest**
Experimental	$M = 6.80$	$M = 13.70$
	$SD = 2.30$	$SD = 2.31$
	$n = 10$	$n = 10$
Traditional	$M = 6.70$	$M = 13.20$
	$SD = 2.31$	$SD = 2.35$
	$n = 10$	$n = 10$

Analysis of Variance					
Source	**df**	**Sums of Squares**	**Mean Square**	**F-ratio**	**Probability**
Participants	18	116.70	6.48	1.52	0.1908
Treatments	1	0.90	0.90	0.14	0.7138
Time	1	448.90	448.90	105.35	≤0.0001
Trt. by Time	1	0.40	0.40	0.09	0.7628
Error	18	76.70	4.26		
Total	39	643.60			

a randomized pretest-posttest design is a *mixed-model ANOVA*. The procedure is called a mixed model because it has both a repeated measure factor, the pretest and posttest, and a between-group factor, experimental or traditional treatment. In a mixed-model ANOVA, one source of variance is associated with participants. The other sources are associated with the between-group factor (treatments), the repeated measures factors (time of test), the interactions (treatments by time), and the error term. In this analysis of a randomized pretest-posttest design, only the main effect for time of test was significant, $F(1, 18) = 105.35$, $p < .0001$. Examination of the means and standard deviations at the top of the table revealed that both the experimental and traditional treatment groups improved from the pretest to posttest, and the amount of improvement was approximately equal. This type of design and analysis is particularly important in the field of communication sciences and disorders because it often is employed in randomized clinical trials.

Additional Tools for Analyzing Clinical Data

Historically, researchers conducted data analyses to identify any statistically significant relationships or difference and reported these statistics along with a probability or p value. The standards for analysis of clinical data are changing, however, and many publications have policies that require additional analyses, such as effect size measures and/or confidence intervals (Cumming, 2012; Kline, 2004; Newhart & Patten, 2023; Trochim et al., 2016). Although detailed procedures for calculating these measures are beyond the scope of this chapter, clinician-investigators should have some familiarity with effect size measures to better understand the research articles they read.

For studies that involve comparisons of treatment/no-treatment conditions or alternate treatment options, current research reports frequently include one or more measures of effect size, such as *Cohen's d*, an *effect size r*, or *number needed to treat*. Cohen's *d* actually has several variations, and researchers should specify which one they used in reporting their results. Cumming (2012) provides a comprehensive explanation of the options for calculating Cohen's *d* with guidance for researchers to consider when choosing the best option for their research.

Cohen's *d* is one of the commonly reported effect size measures. To explain the calculation of this measure, we will use a basic treatment and no-treatment comparison. The calculation involves converting the mean difference between groups into a common unit of difference based on standard deviations (Newhart & Patten, 2023). To compute this measure, you need to know the means and standard deviations for each group. A basic Cohen's *d* is calculated as follows: $M_1 - M_2$/pooled standard deviation[7] (Cumming, 2012; Hargrove, 2002; Newhart & Patten, 2023). Let's consider the following example.

A group of audiologists and speech-language pathologists conducted a posttest-only study with randomized experimental treatment and control groups. The experimental group received an *M* of 59.6 with an *SD* of 13.4, whereas the control group had an *M* of 49.6 with an *SD* of 12.9. Each group had 25 participants. One way to calculate a pooled standard deviation for the two groups is as follows: take the square root of $((25 - 1)13.4^2 + (25 - 1)12.9^2)/(25 + 25 - 2)$ or 13.15. Then you would use this value to compute the effect size represented by Cohen's *d* as $(59.6 - 49.6)/13.15$ or 0.76. Cohen (as cited in Newhart & Patten, 2023) suggested that a *d* of 0.20 corresponded to a small treatment effect, a *d* of 0.50 corresponded to a medium treatment effect, and a *d* of 0.80 corresponded to a large treatment effect.

Another option for conveying effect size includes an effect size *r*, which is similar to a Pearson *r* (Meline & Paradiso, 2003; Newhart & Patten, 2023). Like the Pearson *r*, the values of an effect size *r* range from 0 to ± 1.00. Newhart and Patten (2023) noted that an effect size *r* could be estimated if you know Cohen's *d* using the formula: $r_{es} = d$ divided by the square root of $(d^2 + 4)$. Newhart and Patten also noted r_{es} is easier to interpret when you convert it to an r^2 and multiply r^2 by 100. This yields a number similar to a coefficient of determination, as discussed earlier in this chapter. Thus, for the example we calculated above, with a *d* of 0.76, the r_{es} = 0.76/square root of $(0.76^2 + 4)$ or r_{es} = .36 and r^2 = .13, for a percentage of 13%.[8]

---

[7]The formula for computing a pooled standard deviation is available from several sources (e.g., Hargrove, 2002; Newhart & Patten, 2023; Yampolsky & Matthies, 2002). The formula is as follows: square root of $((n_1 - 1) SD_2 + (n_2 - 1) SD_2)/(n_1 + n_2 - 2)$.

[8]Although these measures were relatively easy to calculate, several effect size calculators are available on the Internet, such as the one by Wilson (n.d.) at the Campbell Collaboration website (https://campbellcollaboration.org/research-resources/effect-size-calculator.html).

One additional effect size measure is *number needed to treat* (Trochim et al., 2016). This is an effect size measure often used in the field of medicine. It reflects how many patients' doctors would need to treat before they found someone who experienced a benefit from a treatment. For example, you might compare a new medication and a placebo and ask how many patients needed to take the new medicine before someone experienced an improvement. A lower number needed to treat is better; thus, a new medicine that is effective for 1 out of 3 patients is better than a new medicine that is effective for 1 out of 10 patients. Although effect size measures were seldom reported for older studies, new research reports should include this information because reporting effect sizes is one component in current standards for research publications (American Speech-Language-Hearing Association, 1997–2024; Enhancing the QUAlity and Transparency Of health Research [Equator], 2024).

The effect size measures for clinical research that address questions of diagnostic accuracy are different from those for studies of group differences. Two important concepts for diagnostic tests are *sensitivity* and *specificity*. Sensitivity refers to the extent to which a diagnostic test identifies all of the individuals who have a disorder (Centre for Evidence-Based Medicine, n.d.). Specificity refers to the extent to which a diagnostic test excludes all of the individuals who are free of a disorder. In order to determine sensitivity and specificity, a researcher needs to compare the experimental diagnostic test to a standard, typically an existing test that is highly regarded or the "gold standard" (Dollaghan, 2004). An accurate diagnostic measure will have both high sensitivity and high specificity.

Caution in the Use and Reporting of Statistics

Although editors and publishers of professional journals endeavor to provide information that is accurate, experts who have critiqued articles published in journals have found some issues with the use and reporting of statistics (Gardenier & Resnik, 2002; Horner & Minifie, 2011; Marco & Larkin, 2000; Max & Onghena, 1999; Oleson et al., 2019a). Usually, these issues are associated with inadvertent mistakes and insufficient knowledge of statistical analysis. In some rare instances, researchers have deliberately misrepresented their data and engaged in research misconduct. An ethical researcher will avoid any temptation to disguise problems with outcome data, such as failing to report that some data points are missing or omitting inconsistent or outlying data without justification or explanation (Gardenier & Resnik, 2002).

Although spotting deliberate misrepresentations would be difficult, clinician-investigators should be aware of some of the issues that appear relatively frequently in research reports across many disciplines. In a review of published research reports, Marco and Larkin (2000) identified a number of problems that occurred with some consistency. Several of these related to the reporting of statistical information, including inappropriate use of percentages, reporting differences that were not statistically significant, inadequate power, and performing multiple tests without correction. According to Marco and Larkin, it is inappropriate to report percentages without the actual numbers on which the percentages were based (e.g., the number of participants). If a difference test, such as a *t*-test, shows no significant differences between groups, researchers should not dismiss this finding by pointing out mean differences anyway, that is, by saying something similar to "Although the difference between means was not significant, the mean for Group A was higher than the mean for Group B." The issue of sample size and statistical power was covered in the chapter on sampling (Chapter 9). In brief, if the sample size for a study is too small, researchers run the risk of making a Type II error; that is, the researcher falsely concludes that there is no difference between groups. Finding that two groups were not significantly different based on a statistical test is not equivalent to finding that the two groups were the same. The final issue occurs in studies with many possible comparisons, such as computing correlations among several measures or difference tests for many different outcome measures. When researchers conduct multiple statistical tests, the accepted practice is to make some type of correction, either in the choice of statistic (e.g., a statistical test designed for multiple comparisons) or in the level of probability (e.g., conduct each individual test at the .01 level rather than the .05 level). The specific corrections researchers might use are beyond the scope of this chapter, but it is important to watch for these kinds of problems when reading research articles and to avoid them in your own analyses.

Summary

Inferential statistics are a valuable tool for helping researchers determine the likelihood that their observations, based on a small sample, represent the actual situation in a population. Statistical tests provide information about the probability that results reflect the true situation in a population or a spurious finding associated with some idiosyncrasy in the sample. Inferential statistics convey information about the probability of obtaining a calculated result given the assumption that the null hypothesis is true. Thus, if a statistic is significant at the .05 level, it means that the probability is less than 5 in 100.

Measures of association are statistical tools for investigating the relationship between two or more measures. These measures usually yield information about the strength of a relationship as well as whether it is a direct or inverse relationship. Some examples of measures of association are the Pearson product-moment correlation coefficient for interval- and ratio-level data, the Spearman rank-order correlation coefficient for ordinal-level data, and the chi-square analysis for nominal data.

Simple regression and multiple regression are ways of analyzing associations among variables for the purpose of making predictions. In a simple regression, one variable is the independent or predictor variable, and the other is the dependent variable. The simple regression statistic, an r^2, has a direct relationship to the Pearson r. Other types of regression analyses, such as multiple regression and nonlinear regression, are useful when researchers want to explore the predictive value of more than one independent variable or to analyze variables that have a curvilinear relationship.

Many statistical tests are designed to test the differences between groups. The t-test is one of the most common analysis procedures when the comparison involves two sets of scores. Different versions of the t-test are available for independent samples and matched or related samples. When the design of a study involves three or more groups, the most common data analysis procedure is an analysis of variance (ANOVA).

A one-way ANOVA is appropriate for analyzing experimental research with one independent variable that has three or more levels, such as a no-treatment control group, a traditional treatment group, and an experimental treatment group. As with a t-test, different versions of the one-way ANOVA are available for analyzing independent samples and repeated measures on the same participants. When researchers want to investigate two or more independent variables in the same study, the choice of analysis procedure usually is a multiway analysis of variance. If the study has two independent variables, the analysis is a two-way ANOVA; if the study has three independent variables, the analysis is a three-way ANOVA; and so forth. A special version of a multiway analysis of variance, called a mixed-model ANOVA, is particularly important for conducting clinical research. A two-way mixed-model ANOVA would have one between-group independent variable and one repeated measure variable. This type of analysis is appropriate for randomized pretest-posttest designs. In this kind of design, the pretest and posttest are repeated measures and the experimental treatment is the between-group variable.

Review Questions

1. What does it mean when a researcher reports that the probability for a statistic was $p < .01$?

2. What does it mean when a researcher reports that the probability for a statistic was $p = .089$?

3. When the relationship between two variables is perfect and inverse, what is the value of r?

4. Is an r of $-.90$ stronger than an r of $.50$? Explain.

5. For a Pearson r of $.50$, what is the value of the coefficient of determination? What does this coefficient mean?

6. If you read that the value of a Pearson r is $.45, p = .09$, should you have confidence that this correlation represents the actual situation in the population? Why or why not?

7. If you make an error of rejecting the null hypothesis when it is true, what type of error have you made?

8. Which is the stronger level of significance, $.01$ or $.001$?

9. Would you say that the following is statistically significant or not statistically significant?

    $(r = .40, df = 18, p = .26)$

10. What is the difference between a simple regression and a multiple regression?

11. What difference is tested for significance using a t-test?

12. Identify three factors that affect whether or not the results of a t-test will be significant.

13. If you are conducting a t-test on two scores from the same subjects or scores from a matched sample, what kind of t-test will you use?

14. What nonparametric statistic can be used to test the difference

between two groups when you have independent samples?

15. If you have two random samples with 12 subjects in each, how many degrees of freedom do you have for the *t*-test?

16. If you read the following, $t(18) = 1.38$, $p > .05$, what conclusion would you make?

17. What are two reasons that you might select a nonparametric alternative to a *t*-test, such as the Wilcoxon signed-ranks test or the Mann-Whitney *U* test?

18. You had a sample with six matched pairs of participants. One participant from each pair was randomly assigned to Treatment A and the other to Treatment B. The participants' scores are listed below. Show how you would compute the sign test for these data.

Score for Subject Receiving Treatment A	Score for Subject Receiving Treatment B
56	62
50	52
53	49
48	54
57	61
51	59

19. Interpret the parts of the following one-way ANOVA statistic: $F(2, 43) = 6.45, p < .05$.

20. Explain what it means when you have a significant interaction in an ANOVA analysis.

Learning Activities

1. The analysis in Table 11–12 is from a hypothetical study comparing performance of children with communication disorders, their chronological age-matched peers, and their communication age-matched peers. The study had two independent variables: a group variable that was nonexperimental and a method variable that was experimental. The information reported includes descriptive statistics for the three groups of children across the two methods. The inferential data analysis was a two-way analysis of variance (ANOVA) with group and method as the independent variables. First, examine the descriptive statistics. What do you think might have happened in this study? You might consider entering the means in a spreadsheet and generating a bar graph or line graph. Second, examine the ANOVA table. What information in this table is important? Write out the statistical results in the style recommended by the American Psychological Association (2020). Would you need to complete post hoc testing with these results? Explain.

2. Select an article that includes quantitative data analysis in the results section. You might select one of the articles from Appendix 11–1 or something on a topic of interest. Make a point to read the results section carefully. What statistical information did the authors report? Descriptive statistics? Inferential statistics? Did the authors use an analysis of variance?

Table 11–12. Hypothetical Study Comparing Performance of Children with Communication Disorders (CD), Their Chronological Aged-Matched Peers (Chron-matched), and Their Communication-Age Matched Peers (Comm-matched)

	Descriptive Statistics		
	Children with CD	**Chron-Matched**	**Comm-Matched**
New Method	$M = 54.00$	$M = 49.33$	$M = 51.33$
	$SD = 2.28$	$SD = 2.16$	$SD = 2.28$
	$n = 6$	$n = 6$	$n = 6$
Old Method	$M = 45.92$	$M = 51.17$	$M = 47.41$
	$SD = 2.20$	$SD = 2.14$	$SD = 2.24$
	$n = 6$	$n = 6$	$n = 6$

Analysis of Variance					
Source	**df**	**Sums of Squares**	**Mean Square**	**F-ratio**	**Probability**
Group	2	6.51	3.26	0.52	0.60
Method	1	88.67	88.67	14.07	0.0008
Group by Method	2	140.51	70.26	11.15	0.0002
Error	30	189.04	6.30		
Total	35	424.74			

If yes, what were the results? How did they present the information from their statistical analysis?

References

American Psychological Association. (2020). *Publication manual of the American Psychological Association* (7th ed.).

American Speech-Language-Hearing Association. (1997–2024). *ASHA journals author resource center: A step-by-step guide to publishing your research*. https://academy.pubs.asha.org/asha-journals-author-resource-center/

Centre for Evidence-Based Medicine. (n.d.). *Diagnostic study appraisal worksheet*. https://www.cebm.net/wp-content/uploads/2018/11/Diagnostic-Accuracy-Studies.pdf

Cohen, L., Manion, L., & Morrison, K. (2018). *Research methods in education* (8th ed.). Routledge.

Coladarci, T., & Cobb, C. D. (2014). *Fundamentals of statistical reasoning in education* (4th ed.). John Wiley & Sons.

Cumming, G. (2012). *Understanding the new statistics: Effect sizes, confidence intervals, and meta-analysis*. Routledge.

DataDesk® (Version 6.3) [Computer software]. (2011). Data Description.

Dollaghan, C. A. (2004). Evidence-based practice in communication disorders: What do we know and when do we know it? *Journal of Communication Disorders, 37*, 391–400. https://doi.org/10.1016/j.jcomdis.2004.04.002

Enhancing the QUAlity and Transparency Of health Research. (2024, January). *CONSORT 2010 statement: Updated guidelines for reporting parallel group randomised trials.* Equator network. https://www.equator-network.org/reporting-guidelines/consort/

Gardenier, J. S., & Resnik, D. B. (2002). The misuse of statistics: Concepts, tools, and a research agenda. *Accountability in Research, 9,* 65–74. https://doi.org/10.1080/08989620290009521

Gibbons, J. D., & Chakraborti, S. (2011). *Nonparametric statistical inference* (5th ed.). CRC Press, Taylor & Francis Group.

Gordon, K. R. (2019). How mixed-effects modeling can advance our understanding of learning and memory and improve clinical and educational practice. *Journal of Speech, Language, and Hearing Research, 62,* 507–524. https://doi.org/10.1044/2018_JSLHR-LASTM-18-0240

Hargrove, P. (2002, October). Evidence-based practice tutorial #3: Identifying the magnitude of the effect. *Perspectives on Language Learning and Education, 9*(3), 34–36.

Horner, J., & Minifie, F. (2011). Research ethics II: Research ethics II: Mentoring, collaboration, peer review, and data management and ownership. *Journal of Speech-Language-Hearing Research, 54,* S330–S345. https://doi.org/10.1044/10924388(2010/09-0264)

Jacobs, K. W. (1976). A table for the determination of experiment wise error rate (alpha) from independent comparisons. *Educational and Psychological Measurement, 36,* 899–903.

Kline, R. B. (2004). *Beyond significant testing: Reforming data analysis methods in behavioral research.* American Psychological Association.

Marco, C. A., & Larkin, G. L. (2000). Research ethics: Ethical issues of data reporting and the quest for authenticity. *Academic Emergency Medicine, 7,* 691–694. https://doi.org/10.1111/j.1553-2712.2000.tb02049.x

Max, L., & Ohghena, P. (1999). Some issues in the statistical analysis of completely randomized and repeated measures designs for speech, language, and hearing research. *Journal of Speech-Language-Hearing Research, 42,* 261–270. https://doi.org/10.1044/jslhr.4202.261

Meline, T., & Paradiso, T. (2003). Evidence-based practice in schools: Evaluating research and reducing barriers. *Language, Speech, and Hearing Services in Schools, 34,* 273–283. https://doi.org/10.1044/0161-1461(2003/023)

Newhart, M., & Patten, M. L. (2023). *Understanding research methods: An overview of the essentials* (11th ed.). Routledge Taylor & Francis Group.

Oh, D. M., & Pyrczak, F. (2023). *Making sense of statistics: A conceptual overview* (7th ed.). Routledge Taylor & Francis Group.

Oleson, J. J., Brown, G. D., & McCreery, R. (2019a). Essential statistical concepts for research in speech, language, and hearing sciences. *Journal of Speech, Language, and Hearing Research, 62,* 489–497. https://doi.org/10.1044/2018_JSLHR-S-ASTM-18-0239

Oleson, J. J., Brown, G. D., & McCreery, R. (2019b). The evolution of statistical methods in speech, language, and hearing sciences. *Journal of Speech, Language, and Hearing Research, 62,* 498–506. https://doi.org/10.1044/2018_JSLHR-H-ASTM-18-0378

Ottenbacher, K. J. (1986). A quantitative analysis of experimentwise error rates in applied behavioral science research. *Journal of Applied Behavioral Science, 22,* 495–501.

Pagano, R. T. (2013). *Understanding statistics in the behavioral sciences* (10th ed.). Cengage Learning.

Rosenthal, R., & Rosnow, R. L. (2008). *Essentials of behavioral research: Methods and data analysis* (3rd ed.). McGraw-Hill.

Satake, E. (2015). *Statistical methods and reasoning for the clinical sciences: Evidence-based practice.* Plural Publishing.

Soper, D. (2006–2020). *Free statistics calculators: Version 4.0.* https://www.danielsoper.com/statcalc/calculator.aspx?id=44

Trochim, W. M. K., Donnelly, J. P., & Arora, K. (2016). *Research methods: The essential knowledge base* (2nd ed.). Cengage Learning.

Velleman, P. F. (1997). *DataDesk version 6.0 statistics guide.* Data Description.

Wasserstein, R. L., & Lazar, N. A. (2016). The ASA statement on p-values: Context, process, and purpose. *The American Statistician, 70*(2),

129–133. https://doi.org/10.1080/00031305.2016.1154108

Wilson, D. B. (n.d.). *Practical meta-analysis effect size calculator* [Online calculator]. https://www.campbellcollaboration.org/research-resources/effect-size-calculator.html

Yampolsky, S. A., & Matthies, M. L. (2002). Evidence-based practice in speech-language pathology. *Perspectives on Language Learning and Education, 9*(1), 14–20. https://doi.org/10.1044/lle9.1.14

APPENDIX 11–1

Examples of Data Analysis Procedures

Nonexperimental Research

Archibald, L. M. D., & Gathercole, S. E. (2006). Visuospatial immediate memory in specific language impairment. *Journal of Speech, Language, and Hearing Research, 49*, 265–277. https://doi.org/10.1044/1092-4388(2006/022)

Bajaj, A. (2007). Analysis of oral narratives of children who stutter and their fluent peers: Kindergarten through second grade. *Clinical Linguistics and Phonetics, 21*(3), 227–245.

Fausto, B. A., Badana, A. N. S., Arnold, M. L., Lister, J. J., & Edwards, J. D. (2018). Comparison of subjective and objective measures of hearing, auditory processing, and cognition among older adults with and without mild cognitive impairment. *Journal of Speech, Language, and Hearing Research, 61*, 945–956. https://doi.org/10.1044/2017_JSLHR-H-17-0263

Hicks, C. B., & Tharpe, A. M. (2002). Listening effort and fatigue in school-age children with and without hearing loss. *Journal of Speech, Language, and Hearing Research, 45*, 573–584. https://doi.org/10.1044/1092-4388(2002/046)

Janky, K. L., Thomas, M. L. A., High, R. R., Schmid, K. K., & Ogun, O. A. (2018). Predictive factors for vestibular loss in children with hearing loss. *American Journal of Audiology, 27*, 137–146. https://doi.org/10.1044/2017_AJA-17-0058

Leigh, J., Farrell, R., Courtenay, D., Dowell, R., & Briggs, R. (2019). Relationship between objective and behavioral audiology for young children being assessed for cochlear implantation: Implications for CI candidacy assessment. *Otology & Neurotology, 40*, e252–e259. https://doi.org/10.1097/MAO.0000000000002125

Moeller, M. P., Hoover, B., Putnam, C., Arbataitis, K., Bohnenkamp, G., Petersen, B., Wood, S., Lewis, D., Pittman, A., & Stelmachowicz, P. (2007). Vocalizations of infants with hearing loss compared with infants with normal hearing: Part I. Phonetic development. *Ear and Hearing, 28*, 605–627.

Experimental Research

Arnott, S., Onslow, M., O'Brian, S., Packman, A., Jones, M., & Block, S. (2014). Group Lidcombe program treatment for early stuttering: A randomized controlled trial. *Journal of Speech, Language, and Hearing Research, 57*, 1606–1618. https://doi.org/10.1044/2014_JSLHR-S-13-0090

Brennan, M. A., McCreery, R., Kopun, J., Hoover, B., Alexander, J., Lewis, D., & Stelmachowicz, P. G. (2014). Paired comparisons of nonlinear frequency compression, extended bandwidth, and restricted bandwidth hearing-aid processing for children and adults with hearing loss. *Journal of the American Academy of Audiology, 25*(10), 983–998. https://doi.org/10.3766/jaaa.25.10.7

Brody, L., Yu-Hsiang, W., & Stangl, E. (2018). A comparison of personal sound amplification products and hearing aids in ecologically relevant test environments. *American Journal of Audiology, 27*, 581–593. https://doi.org/10.1044/2018_AJA-18-0027

Chisolm, T. H., Abrams, H. B., & McArdle, R. (2004). Short and long-term outcomes of adult audiological rehabilitation. *Ear and Hearing, 25*(5), 464–477.

Cohen, W., Hodson, A., O'Hare, A., Boyle, J., Durrani, T., McCartney, E., Mattey, M., Naftalin, L., Watson, J. (2005). Effects of computer-based intervention through acoustically modified speech (Fast ForWord) in severe mixed receptive-expressive language impairment:

Outcomes from a randomized controlled trial. *Journal of Speech, Language, and Hearing Research, 48,* 715–729. https://doi.org/10.1044/1092-4388(2005/049)

Doesborgh, S. J., van de Sandt-Koenderman, M. W., Dippel, D. W., van Harskamp, F., Koudstaal, P. J., & Visch-Brink, E. G. (2003). Effects of semantic treatment on verbal communication and linguistic processing in aphasia after stroke: A randomized controlled trial. *Stroke, 35*(1), 141–146.

Ebbels, S. H., van der Lely, H. K., & Dockrell, J. E. (2007). Intervention for verb argument structure in children with persistent SLI: A randomized control trial. *Journal of Speech, Language, and Hearing Research, 50,* 1330–1349. https://doi.org/10.1044/1092-4388(2007/093)

Harris, V., Onslow, M., Packman, A., Harrison, E., & Menzies, R. (2002). An experimental investigation of the impact of the Lidcombe Program on early stuttering. *Journal of Fluency Disorders, 27*(3), 203–213.

Hesketh, A., Dima, E., & Nelson, V. (2007). Teaching phoneme awareness to preliterate children with speech disorder: A randomized controlled trial. *International Journal of Language and Communication Disorders, 42,* 251–271.

Lau, M. K., Hicks, C., Kroll, T., & Zupancic, S. (2019). Effect of auditory task type on physiological and subjective measures of listening effort in individuals with normal hearing. *Journal of Speech, Language, and Hearing Research, 62,* 1549–1560. https://doi.org/10.1044/2018_JSLHR-H-17-0473

Mendel, L. L., Roberts, R. A., & Walton, J. H. (2003). Speech perception benefits from sound field FM amplification. *American Journal of Audiology, 12*(2), 114–124. https://doi.org/10.1044/1059-0889(2003/019)

Rvachew, S., Nowak, M., & Cloutier, G. (2004). Effect of phonemic perception training on the speech production and phonological awareness skills of children with expressive phonological delay. *American Journal of Speech-Language Pathology, 13,* 250–263. https://doi.org/10.1044/1058-0360(2004/026)

Sapir, S., Spielman, J. L., Ramig, L. O., Story, B. H., & Fox, C. (2007). Effects of intensive voice treatment (the Lee Silverman Voice Treatment [LSVT]) on vowel articulation in dysarthric individuals with idiopathic Parkinson disease: Acoustic and perceptual findings. *Journal of Speech, Language, and Hearing Research, 50,* 899–912. https://doi.org/10.1044/1092-4388(2007/064)

van Kleeck, A., Vander Woude, J., & Hammett, L. (2006). Fostering literal and inferential language skills in Head Start preschoolers with language impairment using scripted book-sharing discussions. *American Journal of Speech-Language Pathology, 15,* 85–95. https://doi.org/10.1044/1058-0360(2006/009)

12

Research Outcomes: Clinical Guidance, Research Reports

Main Points

- It is important to critically appraise research: evaluate the question, sample, design, procedures, analysis, and ethics to help you decide if you trust the study conclusions and will apply them in your own clinical practice.
- When writing up a completed study, the discussion section must reflect on how the results and conclusions compare, fit in, or add to other research, for example, to the research referenced in the literature review.
- Research should be shared—this can take the form of publications, conference presentations, self-published, or community presentations.

Perhaps the primary reason for professionals in communication sciences and disorders to engage in research is to make certain that their clients receive the best possible audiology and speech-language pathology services (Johnson, 2006). This research might fall under the category of evidence-based practice (EBP) and include a careful search and evaluation of existing research reports to uncover information to guide clinical decisions. Alternatively, this research might fall under the category of original, empirical research and involve gathering new data to answer previously unanswered questions. As discussed in earlier chapters, the knowledge and skills needed to engage in evidence-based practice and empirical research overlap to a great extent; however, the two forms of research lead to different final products. In EBP research, the culminating phases of the investigation include critically evaluating the existing research and considering its appropriateness for your clients and setting (Gallagher, 2002; Johnson, 2006).

The research outcome is a clinical decision guided by the best available evidence (American Speech-Language-Hearing Association [ASHA], 2004; Gallagher, 2002), as well as by the clinician's expertise and client/family values (Gallagher, 2002; Johnson, 2006). In empirical research, the final phase is preparation of a research report with the goal of presenting that report at a national or international conference and/or publishing it in a professional journal.

Knowledge Base for Evaluating Clinical Research

EBP is an approach to providing professional service that emerged in the field of medicine but subsequently has been incorporated into many areas of professional service, including audiology and speech-language pathology (ASHA, 2004). In previous chapters, EBP was summarized in a series of research steps beginning with formulation of a clinical question (e.g., the Population, Intervention, Comparison, and Outcome or PICO question), completing a thorough search of professional literature, reviewing and critiquing the identified research, and, finally, deciding how to apply the information in your clinical practice and how to evaluate and document your outcomes (Gallagher, 2002; Johnson, 2006). The topic of reviewing and critiquing studies was part of the chapters on writing a literature review (Chapter 5) and experimental research design (Chapter 8), and we expand on how to critique a study in this chapter.

The goal of EBP is to improve our clinical decision-making by reducing overreliance on expert opinion, increasing use of the best available evidence, and integrating use of evidence with clinical expertise and client/family desires and values (ASHA, 2004; Gallagher, 2002). For audiologists and speech-language pathologists to be competent in the process of EBP, they need knowledge of research design to judge the value of the available evidence and information literacy skills to find relevant studies quickly and efficiently (Nail-Chiwetalu & Ratner, 2006; Ratner, 2006). Additionally, they need to include the persons and families who receive services in the decision-making process. This means being able to communicate about "best practice" evidence in language clients and families will understand and having skills to facilitate decision-making by consensus and resolving conflicts.

Critical Appraisal

One of the concluding phases in the EBP process involves reading and appraising the identified research. If you were fortunate enough to identify a systematic review or meta-analysis on your topic, you have a single document that lists much of the available research on a topic, includes a review and evaluation of the available studies, and may include a statistical analysis or meta-analysis of the aggregated results across several studies (ASHA, 1997–2024; Cohen et al., 2018; Johnson, 2006; Trochim et al., 2016). However, you need to judge the value of even this type of document. First you should consider whether the document actually addresses the topic of interest. Search terms, such as *adult, child, speech, language, hearing, treatment, aphasia, voice, fluency or stuttering, phonology, perception*, and so forth, will lead to highly relevant articles as well as to less relevant articles on related topics. For example, if searching for research on treatment of phonological disorders in children, you might need to eliminate studies that addressed phonological or phonemic awareness and literacy skills; similarly, if searching for research on speech perception, the term *speech recognition* might lead to many studies of computer-based speech recognition. An EBP question usually has a specific clinical focus, and you need to read and review articles that pertain to that focus (Johnson, 2006).

If a systematic review fits your topic, the next step is to determine the quality of that review. The Centre for Evidence-Based Medicine (CEBM, 2024) developed a critical appraisal worksheet that provides guidance for evaluating a systematic review. Some of the criteria for you to consider as you read the review are a clearly identified question, thorough description of literature search strategies and procedures for inclusion or exclusion of articles, and the consistency of the findings across studies (CEBM, 2024).

Another consideration is the source of the review. Some sources are highly regarded professional organizations (ASHA, 1997–2024; Higgins et al., 2023). Other highly regarded sources are peer-reviewed professional journals. Such journals have editorial and review policies and procedures designed to ensure that published articles are accurate, complete, and well written. Peer review means submitted manuscripts are carefully read and evaluated by persons who are recognized experts on a topic (Nail-Chiwetalu & Ratner, 2006). Through this process, authors often have an opportunity to make corrections and resubmit their manuscripts. Ideally, the final, published article in a peer-reviewed journal should provide valuable information. Information about the review procedures for a particular journal may be included on an editorial page published in each issue of the journal or on the publisher's website (e.g., ASHA Journals Academy, 1997–2024).

A final factor to consider is the date of the review. A review may be well written and published in a credible source but have less value if it is several years old. Research completed and published after the review was finished, often a year or more before its actual publication, would not be included. If you find a relevant but dated systematic review, consider one of the search approaches described in Chapter 4 that allow you to search for articles that cite the report you identified. That way, you would be able to find more recent articles, usually on a similar topic, that cite the older review.

If the available evidence on a topic is insufficient for a systematic review, you might have uncovered a few or several studies to read and review yourself. A critical appraisal of research reports often starts with judging the strength of the research design and level of evidence. Thus, knowing what constitutes a strong research design is essential in the EBP process. The information in Chapters 6, 7, and 8, and in particular Table 8–7, should be useful in identifying research designs and levels of evidence. In a well-written research report, the authors should state the type of research design they employed. For treatment studies, the strongest designs are variations of randomized group designs such as a pretest-posttest randomized control group design. In this kind of research, the groups are usually experimental treatment and no-treatment control groups or experimental treatment and traditional treatment groups. A single-group pretest-posttest design is a weak design and inappropriate for establishing treatment effectiveness. Ideally, peer-reviewed journals would not publish such studies, although you may find this kind of information presented at some professional conferences or included in self-published reports.

Although determining the research design and level of evidence for a research report is a crucial and often the beginning step in critical appraisal (CEBM, 2011), additional factors are important as well. Even in randomized control studies, some additional characteristics may strengthen the validity of the evidence. One of these characteristics is whether or not those who made observations, completed assessments, and analyzed the data knew the group membership. When researchers who obtain measurements and analyze data know whether or not participants received the experimental or control treatment, they might even inadvertently bias the measurement and analysis process. When those involved in measurement and analysis do not know who was in the experimental and control groups, they are "blinded" to group membership (ASHA, 2004; Gillam & Gillam, 2006).

Another factor to consider is how participants were recruited for the study. In a randomized control study, assignment to groups obviously is random, but the sample might or might not be a random sample. The evidence is stronger if the researchers had many possible participants and randomly selected the groups from this larger set. Sample size is an important consideration as well. Davidow et al. (2006) suggested 10 participants per group as a minimum sample size for research in fluency disorders. If the expected difference is small but important, however, even 10 persons per group would be inadequate (Rosenthal & Rosnow, 2008). Other factors being equal, a large sample is more representative of a population than a small sample (Newhart & Patten, 2023), and researchers should consider sample size and the issue of statistical power before starting a study.

Another issue to consider is whether or not any participants dropped out over the course of the study (Davidow et al., 2006). The loss of participants could affect the results of a study if the loss occurred due to systematic rather than random factors. For example, if some participants experienced little or no benefit from an experimental treatment, they might drop out of the study. This would leave mostly those persons who experienced positive outcomes for the posttest measurement and data analysis and would make the treatment look more effective than it actually was. Usually, when loss of participants occurs, researchers include some explanation of this and even a follow-up analysis to determine if those who dropped out differed from those who finished the study in some systematic way. In addition to providing information about sample size, recruitment, and loss of participants, researchers should include a thorough description of the participants, such as presence or absence of a disorder, age range, general health or development, native language, criteria for excluding participants, and so forth.

Another question to consider when evaluating an experimental treatment study relates to the precision and fidelity of treatment (Kaderavek & Justice, 2010). Did the investigators take steps to make sure a treatment or diagnostic procedure was executed as intended and report these steps in their research report? For readers to judge the procedural integrity of a study, the researchers need to report their procedures in a detailed way that would allow other researchers to replicate the study. One way that investigators might address the issue of quality and consistency of the treatment would be to monitor and analyze treatment delivery, and then include that information in the research report. Additionally, they might recruit one or more highly qualified clinicians to deliver the treatment and provide thorough training in the experimental procedures (Davidow et al., 2006). If only one audiologist or speech-language pathologist provided the treatment and it appeared to be effective, that result might be due to the qualities of a uniquely talented clinician. On the other hand, if a promising treatment approach proved to be ineffective, that result also could have occurred because of some limitation in the clinician's skills. A study in which several well-trained clinicians provided the treatment would be stronger than one in which a single, perhaps inexperienced clinician provided the treatment.

The adequacy of the dependent variables or outcome measures is another consideration (Baker & McLeod, 2011; Gillam & Gillam, 2006). Audiologists and speech-language pathologists, through their clinical training and experience, are well qualified to evaluate formal and informal measures of treatment progress. The expectation is that researchers will select outcome measures that have demonstrated reliability and validity. Alternatively, if the researchers use a novel measure that has not been well studied, they should include information about reliability and validity in the research report. Another question about outcome measures concerns the extent to which the researchers assessed generalization outside the experimental setting or included measures that addressed improvement in social participation (Baker & McLeod, 2011). A final consideration is whether the researchers obtained both short-term and long-term outcome measures or only short-term outcome measures (Davidow et al., 2006). Many otherwise well-designed studies have limited outcome data consisting of treatment probes obtained in the experimental setting shortly after the conclusion of treatment.

Although randomized group designs provide the strongest evidence, practical limitations sometimes force researchers to use quasi-experimental or single-participant research designs. When the design is a quasi-experimental, nonrandom control group design, including a pretest is essential to establish that treatment and control groups were similar at the start of the study (Trochim et al., 2016). Otherwise, the researchers will not know whether to attribute differences observed at the end of the study to treatment effects or preexisting group differences. In single-participant research, we need to consider the strength of the design as well. The simplest single-participant design is a baseline and treatment design. Such a design is seldom adequate for experimental purposes, and researchers usually adopt a stronger design, such as a treatment replication design and/or a multiple baseline across participants design. If the single-participant research involves comparing more than one treatment, the researchers need to consider the possibility of order of treatment effects. Recruiting four or more participants and randomly assigning them to different treatment orders is one way for researchers to address the issue of order in single-participant designs.

For studies of diagnostic procedures, the research design will be nonexperimental. Thus, the best levels of evidence for diagnostic studies are different from those for treatment-control studies. One expectation for diagnostic studies is a comparison between the experimental diagnostic measure and some well-established diagnostic measure as the reference standard (CEBM, 2024; Dollaghan, 2004). In analyzing the accuracy of the new diagnostic tool, researchers should report the sensitivity and specificity of their experimental measure compared to the reference standard.

A well-written research article also follows established guidelines for reporting results (Enhancing the QUAlity and Transparency Of health Research [Equator], 2024). In older literature, authors of quantitative research reports commonly reported descriptive statistics and the results of their inferential tests, such as t-test or ANOVA results. Many publishers of research reports now require, or at least strongly encourage, authors to include measures of the practical importance and precision of their findings. Thus, a well-written report should include effect size measures (e.g., Cohen's *d* or number needed to treat) and confidence intervals whenever applicable.

The source of a research report is an important consideration as well. If you found an unpublished research report on the Internet, you should question why the authors never published the study. Certainly, authors have good reasons for generating a self-published report and not submitting it for peer review. Examining unpublished reports would be a way to identify negative evidence; however, some self-published reports are of low quality. Generally, reports from peer-reviewed sources are more trustworthy than those from personal websites or nonreviewed publications (Nail-Chiwetalu & Ratner, 2006). Some additional factors to consider in evaluating a study are the breadth of evidence and the source of the evidence. Recall that the highest level of evidence is a meta-analysis or systematic review and that you need several studies on the same topic to prepare this type of document. When evaluating the body of evidence for a particular treatment, you need to consider how many studies are available, whether these studies provide conflicting or converging evidence (ASHA, 2004), and who conducted the study and wrote the research report. A body of evidence from multiple researchers, persons other than those who first developed an approach, and multiple treatment sites would be much stronger than evidence from a single research group (Nail-Chiwetalu & Ratner, 2006; Ratner, 2006).

The various criteria for appraising clinical research are summarized in Table 12–1. Researchers might use criteria such as those in the table when evaluating studies for evidence-based practice or when writing a review of literature for an original research report. You also might consider other sources like the critical appraisal worksheets provided by the Centre for Evidence-Based Medicine (CEBM, 2024), the PEDro-Scale (Speech Pathology Database for Best Interventions and Treatment Efficacy [SpeechBITE], n.d.), or the criteria used in recent systematic reviews and meta-analyses (e.g., Gerber et al., 2012; McCauley et al., 2009). If the research article is a single-subject design study, many of the criteria in Table 12–1 are still applicable, such as the type of design, blinding, long-term posttest, detailed description of participants, evidence of treatment fidelity, quality of the outcome measures, and source of the report. Published appraisal tools intended specifically for single-subject research designs are a good option as well. Examples of these include the "*Evaluative Method*" from Reichow et al. (2008), the revised *Risk of Bias in N-of-1 Trials* (RoBiNT) scale (Tate et al., 2013), or the *What Works Clearinghouse* standards (Kratochwill et al., 2010). Informally, you might consider the questions listed below when appraising single-subject studies (Wendt & Miller, 2012).

1. Did the study include a sufficient number of baseline observations (at least five), and were the baseline observations relatively stable over time?
2. Did the researchers provide detailed, operational descriptions of the dependent measure(s), did they obtain repeated measurements in both baseline and experimental phases, and was the interobserver agreement for these measurements sufficiently strong?

Table 12–1. Summary of Criteria for Critical Appraisal of a Research Report

1. Purpose or focus of the study		
2. Basic research design	Randomized group design	If yes, what type?
	Quasi-experimental group design	If yes, what type?
	Single participant design	If yes, what type?
	Case study	If yes, what type?
	Other	Specify
3. Other design features	Pretest	If yes, were participants similar?
	Long-term posttest	Briefly describe
	Blinding for outcome measurement	
4. Participants	Age	Briefly describe
	Diagnosis, if relevant	Briefly describe
	Gender	Briefly describe
	Cultural and linguistic background	Briefly describe
	Random assignment to groups	
	Random selection	If not randomly selected, briefly describe participant recruitment
	Number of participants in each group	
	Participant loss	If yes, did the authors include an explanation?
5. Treatment dependability/ fidelity	One or several clinicians	
	Qualifications of the clinician(s)	
	Procedures to monitor treatment fidelity	Briefly describe
6. Outcome measures	Tests with known reliability and validity	
	Informal or unique measures	If yes, did the authors include information about reliability and validity?
	Generalization measures	Briefly describe
	Measures of social importance (e.g., activity and participation)	Briefly describe

continues

Table 12–1. *continued*

7. Source of the report	Peer-reviewed	
	Publication but not peer-reviewed	
	Presentation at peer-reviewed conference	
	Presentation at conference but not peer-reviewed	
	Website	If yes, is it a reputable source?
	Other	
8. Body of evidence	Multiple studies	If yes, are findings similar or conflicting?
	Multiple treatment centers	
	Researchers other than originators	

3. Did the researchers provide detailed descriptions of the independent variable or experimental manipulation, and did they take steps to determine treatment fidelity and include that information in the research report?
4. Did the researchers demonstrate experimental control by showing a clearly identifiable change in behavior that occurred near the onset of treatment, and did they demonstrate this behavior change through repeated baseline and experimental phases?
5. For multiple baseline studies, did the researchers stagger the onset of treatment phases for new behaviors, participants, or settings?
6. Did the data analysis include graphs showing measurements in the baseline and experimental phases for visual inspection and also include statistical analysis to supplement visual inspection?

How Applicable Are the Findings?

Audiologists and speech-language pathologists ultimately must decide whether or not research findings apply to their clients and clinical settings. Even information from a well-designed study may have limited value if the participants in the study and your clients have different characteristics. Similarly, the findings may have little practical importance if the intensity of treatment, type of treatment, or required equipment is unique to the research setting. Researchers should report detailed information about their participants, including information about ages; gender; type and severity of disorder; cultural, ethnic, and linguistic background; educational level; family incomes; and so forth (Equator, 2024; Gillam & Gillam, 2006). Some of this information will be more important for certain types of experimental treatments than others, but having a detailed description of participants is a crucial section in any research report. Similarly, professionals conducting EBP research need detailed descriptions of the treatment procedures and settings in order to judge how similar the research setting was to their clinical setting.

After completing a literature search and reading and evaluating several research reports, audiologists and speech-language pathologists need to make a decision about adopting a particular treatment approach. One aspect of this decision is weighing the costs and potential benefits of the new treatment (Johnson, 2006). Costs might include greater demands on the clinicians' time to prepare and provide the new treatment. Other costs are more direct, such as paying for specialized training required to deliver the new treatment. A treatment with high costs would need to show substantial benefit to justify its adoption.

Additional factors in deciding how to apply findings from EBP research are the client's and family's opinions and values. Families sometimes hear about and desire certain treatment approaches because of information they obtained from friends and acquaintances or from nonreviewed information sources such as the Internet. Audiologists and speech-language pathologists need to weigh the desires of the client and family against the strength of the empirical evidence. If strong evidence is available that is consistent with client and family desires, then no conflict exists. However, if strong evidence is available that goes counter to the family's choices, professionals ethically need to recommend and implement the most effective treatment. In this case, the audiologist or speech-language pathologist needs to communicate with the client and family about what the evidence shows and facilitate resolution of any conflicts that may arise. Although the audiologists' or speech-language pathologists' expertise is always an important factor in clinical decision-making, this expertise is even more important when the evidence is unclear. Clinicians still need to decide how best to serve a client even in the face of limited or conflicting evidence. In such cases, they need to choose based on their own expertise, carefully monitor the client's progress, and make adjustments to the treatment approach as needed.

Given the level of knowledge and skills needed to participate in EBP research, many might wonder why this concept has become firmly established across many professions. The answer involves weighing the costs in terms of training and time against the benefits. A few of the many benefits of evidence-based practice include (a) improved services for the persons audiologists and speech-language pathologists serve professionally (ASHA, 2004), (b) increased opportunities for research funding by improving our professions' standing in the research community, (c) increased public and private support for our services by using evidence that documents its effectiveness, and (d) enhanced ability to respond to questions about the cost and effectiveness of our services. Although individual audiologists and speech-language pathologists need knowledge and skills to participate in EBP research, this type of research is not ideally an individual effort. The quality and availability of EBP research will be greater through collective and collaborative efforts (Equator, 2024; Johnson, 2006).

Reporting Research Findings

In empirical research, the final phase is preparation and dissemination of a research report. Most research reports follow a similar structure with regard to content. A well-written report includes the following: (a) a title that reflects the subject matter of the study; (b) a brief abstract that summarizes the purpose, methods, and results of the study; (c) an introduction and review of previous literature; (d) a methods section with information about participants, instrumentation and procedures, and data analysis; (e) a results section; (f) a discussion section; and (g) references (American Psychological Association [APA], 2020; Newhart & Patten, 2023; Trochim et al., 2016). Several of these sections are relevant for preparing an evidence-based course paper, including the title, introduction and review of literature, and references.

Components of a Research Report

The *title* of a research report might be approximately 10 to 15 words long and conveys the essence of the study. A good title usually conveys what actions occurred during the study, such as investigating a relationship, identifying characteristics, or comparing treatments; what the major variables were; and who participated in the study. The *abstract* for a research report is a short synopsis of the content of the entire article. An abstract might range from 100 to 150 words; some publications have specific guidelines regarding the length of an abstract. The content of the abstract usually includes a statement of purpose, a brief description of the participants, the most important information about instrumentation and procedures, and a brief summary of the most important findings (Newhart & Patten, 2023; Trochim et al., 2016). Recently, some journals have adopted a *structured abstract* as a requirement for published articles. Structured abstracts are easy to recognize because you see headings associated with the major parts of the abstract such as Objective, Methods, Results, and Conclusions (Bayley & Eldredge, 2003).[1]

The first section in the main body of a research report is the *Introduction* and *Review of Literature*. This section seldom has a section heading, except in longer documents like theses and dissertations. Often researchers begin a paper with a general statement of purpose or the issue under investigation. The major portion of this first section is a review of important prior work on the topic (APA, 2020). This prior work might take the form of discussions of the theory that is being tested, brief summaries of previous related research, and a critique of previous research focusing on conflicting evidence and missing information. This critique might employ many of the criteria discussed in the previous section on evidence-based practice. The literature review typically ends with the authors' reasons for conducting their research, along with an explicit statement of purpose or a set of research questions (Newhart & Patten, 2023). In most published research reports, the review of literature has a relatively narrow focus and does not include general background information that most persons in the field would know. At the same time, the review of literature must be up to date and cover the primary topics in a thorough manner. Because an introduction and review of literature are important for many types of writing, we cover this section in more detail in Chapter 5.

The *Methods* section follows the review of literature and statement of research questions. This section has subsections such as

---

[1] For examples of structured abstracts, you might examine research reports published in recent issues of journals like the *American Journal of Speech-Language Pathology, American Journal of Audiology, Journal of Speech-Language Hearing Research, Journal of the American Academy of Audiology, Journal of Fluency Disorders*, and *Journal of Voice*.

participants, instrumentation, procedures, and data analysis. The participants section should include a detailed description of participants with relevant information: age, speech, language, and hearing abilities; educational status; cultural and linguistic background; native language; and so forth. This section also should include information about how the researchers recruited their participants and procedures for selecting the samples and for assigning participants to groups. The instrumentation section includes a description of measurement tools such as formal tests, questionnaires, and laboratory equipment. If available for the measurement tools used in the study, the instrumentation section would include information about the reliability and validity of the measures as well. The procedures section might also be called design and procedures (Trochim et al., 2016). This section will include information about the basic design, such as pretest-posttest randomized control group design, multiple baseline across subjects design, or nonexperimental qualitative case study. In addition, the researchers should include information about how frequently they saw the participants, how long the sessions were, who actually administered the treatments or other experimental procedures, and a detailed description of the treatments. The final subsection under methods is often a data analysis and reliability section.

The next section in a research report is a *Results* section. In quantitative research, this section presents both descriptive and inferential statistics. The results reported typically relate directly to the research questions and research design. Thus, if the investigation involved a comparison of two measures, readers will expect to see some type of correlation analysis in the results. On the other hand, if the investigation involved determining differences between three or more groups, readers will expect to see some type of analysis of variance. Newhart and Patten (2023) recommended reporting descriptive information first and then the results of any inferential statistical tests. When a study has several groups, researchers often present their findings in tables. However, when reporting the results, just stating that the results are shown in Table X is insufficient. Writers should also provide a brief verbal description of the main points shown in the table (Newhart & Patten, 2023).

The results section in a qualitative research report often begins with a statement of the method of data analysis. The content generally is verbal in nature with few if any numbers. The nature of the data in qualitative research might be a series of themes that emerged from the researchers' analysis (Cohen et al., 2018). In addition to these themes, researchers usually include verbatim quotes from interview transcripts and/or detailed descriptions of events and situations that represent the themes.

The fourth section in a research report is the *Discussion* section, which sometimes is called *Discussion and Conclusions*, or *Discussion and Summary*. The discussion usually includes a restatement of the findings without the numerical data. One way to structure a discussion is to include sections that address each of the research questions, either providing an answer to the question or, if the results were ambiguous, explaining that aspect. Authors usually describe how their findings related to previous, similar research on the topic. This might include explicitly noting when findings agree and when they conflict with prior research. If the researchers uncovered conflicting evidence, they usually consider possible explanations for the difference. If the authors presented possible theoretical implications in their review of literature, the discussion section should include an explanation of how the findings relate to theory as well. Usually toward the end of a discussion section, authors include information about possible weaknesses in their research, either because of design limitations or because of unanticipated factors that emerged over the course of the study (Newhart & Patten, 2023). They also consider possible avenues for future research on the topic.

The final section of the research report is the *References* section. This section includes all the works cited in the paper, including previous research reports, books, chapters in books, documents from websites, and so forth. The list of references should only include works actually cited in the paper and no additional items. The list is organized by authors' last names and date of publication. Some research reports include an appendix, which is an optional section. Authors might decide to include an appendix to provide a lengthy document that might disrupt the flow of ideas in the main body of the manuscript. An appendix might include items like a questionnaire, a detailed treatment protocol, or a verbatim transcript of an interview.

Writing Guidelines and Writing Style

Most journal publications have editorial guidelines regarding the content, style, and format of manuscripts. In the field of communication sciences and disorders, many publications have adopted American Psychological Association (APA) publication guidelines. These content and style guidelines are presented in depth in the *Publication Manual of the American Psychological Association, Seventh Edition* (APA, 2020).

The APA style manual provides guidance on topics such as how to write in a clear and concise manner, how to cite sources in the body of your paper, how to organize information in tables and figures, how to report statistical and other numerical information, and how to format entries in a reference list.

When writing a research report, a good strategy is to focus on communicating about the research rather than on writing in an impressive and entertaining way. Highly regarded research writing is clear, concise, and to the point (Meline & Paradiso, 2003).

The APA (2020) publication manual provides considerable writing guidance. When the emphasis is on communication, writers strive to present information in a parallel and consistent way to facilitate comprehension. Understanding information in a list is easier if all of the items start with the same syntactic form. For example, if authors wanted to list a series of actions, they might adopt an infinitive form and begin each item in the list with *to + verb* (e.g., to identify, to select, to evaluate, to decide, and so forth). Similarly, authors should use a single tense throughout certain sections of the paper. APA guidelines suggest staying in past tense for the review of literature, methods, and results section, all of which report completed phases of the research. On the other hand, authors should use present tense in the discussion and conclusions as a way to encourage readers to reflect on the findings with them.

Authors also should use language that ties related ideas together but need to be careful to choose the appropriate linking words (APA, 2020). Many of us have written sentences such as, "Persons with communication disorders performed better on Task A, *while* persons with normal communication performed better on Task B." The intent of this sentence is to contrast the performance of the two groups. However, the transition word *while* has a temporal meaning and literally means doing something at the same time. A better choice of transition word when trying to communicate a contrast is *whereas* or *however*. Similarly, writers sometimes use the word *since* in place of *because*. However, these two words have specific alternative uses. The word *since* conveys a temporal relationship, whereas the word *because* conveys a causal relationship.

In research writing, straightforward, relatively short sentences are preferable to lengthy sentences that incorporate many modifiers or link too many ideas together. Similarly, active voice is preferable to passive voice. Many of us adopt a passive voice to avoid talking about ourselves when we write. For example, one might write, "The participants were tested three times during the study." However, APA guidelines advise using first person to improve the strength and clarity of writing. Therefore, we should write, "We tested the participants three times during the study" (or "I tested . . . " if the research was conducted by one person). Other important guidelines in the APA style manual address how to refer to persons. One key point is to refer to persons in a specific rather than abstract way (e.g., write about infants, children, persons age 20 to 25, or women age 50 to 65, rather than the "subjects"). The APA manual also is useful for those who are uncertain about punctuation and grammatical usage.

Authors who want guidance regarding the recommended content for research reports have several sources to consult. A few group initiatives have resulted in reporting guidelines for randomized clinical trials, nonrandomized research designs, and studies of diagnostic tests (Bossuyt et al., 2015; Equator, 2024; Des Jarlais et al., 2004). Each of these documents includes information about recommended content for various sections of research reports, including background information, methods and participants, results and data analysis, and discussion.

Disseminating Research Findings

When authors prepare a research report, they usually have a plan for disseminating the information. Their options include publication in a peer-reviewed journal, a presentation at a professional conference, and self-published reports. Generally, articles in peer-reviewed journals have higher status because these articles have met standards set by the journal editorial board. Peer review includes reading and evaluation of manuscripts prior to publication by persons with expertise on the topic. The field of communication sciences and disorders has many peer-reviewed journals, some published by professional organizations such as the American Speech-Language-Hearing Association and the American Academy of Audiology (AAA), and others from private publishers. In some fields of study, including communication sciences and disorders, web-based journals are expanding as an alternative to traditional print media. Some of these historically were print-based journals, and others were web-based journals from their onset. Web-based publications have the same status as a print publication as long as they have editorial policies that require peer review prior to publication and high standards for article content. The publication policies of a journal are more important than its manner of dissemination for determining the trustworthiness of articles.

Another option for disseminating information is a presentation at a professional conference. Some conference presentations are poster sessions or visual presentations of a research report, with large type designed to be read at a distance, extensive use of charts and graphs, and limited text (e.g., bulleted points or brief figure captions). The poster usually includes all components of a research report, including introduction and research questions, methods and participants, results, and discussion. However, the introduction and discussion tend to be brief and authors emphasize their methods and results.

Some conference programs also include technical sessions and technical papers. A technical paper is a relatively brief oral presentation, often accompanied by a few visual supports depicting key information. Like poster sessions, researchers making oral presentations usually include a brief introduction, spend most of their time explaining the methods and results, and end with a brief discussion. Typically, a technical session groups together several papers on related topics.

Some professional conferences also include research seminars in their schedule. Seminars are longer sessions often lasting 1.5 to 2 hours. Researchers who present during a research seminar often have conducted several related studies on a topic and present the aggregated findings of this research. The longer format of a research seminar allows the presenters to spend more time discussing theoretical issues and the implications of their findings.

Students in master's and doctoral-level graduate programs often conduct empirical research and prepare a thesis or dissertation. Theses and dissertations have an alternate distribution model. Most are housed in the libraries of the universities where they were produced. Doctoral dissertations and many master's theses also are distributed via the ProQuest Dissertations and Theses database (ProQuest, n.d.). The ProQuest databases are searchable, allow general access to abstracts, and provide a purchase option for most of the documents in the database. Dissertations and theses undergo a review process that is similar to peer review. Graduate students who are completing a dissertation or thesis have a committee of faculty who have expertise related to the topic of the research. This faculty committee must approve the document before it is distributed.

A final option for disseminating a research report is to generate and distribute a self-published report. With an increase in Internet usage, the usual way to distribute a self-published report is via a website. Some of these reports are distributed as a requirement of a research grant. The individuals who received a government grant to fund their research sometimes are obligated to prepare and disseminate a report in a way that makes it generally available with no fee. Another reason for disseminating a self-published report is that the authors were unable to find a professional journal that would publish the study. Ratner (2006) noted that research journals often have a bias toward publishing only studies with significant findings. Researchers could conduct a well-designed study and prepare a clearly written report but find that they cannot publish it because their findings were not statistically significant. Ratner noted clinicians need to know about treatment approaches that did not work as well as those that did. Thus, researchers who distribute self-published reports may be providing important information. Self-published reports usually have not gone through a formal review process, however, and clinicians and researchers need to be careful when using the information from such sources.

Summary

Research in the field of communication sciences and disorders encompasses both investigation of the existing research base to find answers to clinical questions, called evidence-based practice, and original empirical research to investigate unanswered questions that are theoretical and/or clinical in nature. EBP begins with formulation of a focused clinical question and progresses to a search of professional literature, to review and critical appraisal of the identified research, and finally to a decision about how to apply the information in professional practice. The process of critical appraisal requires knowledge of research design, the ability to judge the credibility of a source, knowledge of reliable and valid approaches to assessing outcomes, the ability to discuss evidence with clients and families, and the ability to determine if the available evidence applies to one's clients and setting.

When reading research reports, audiologists and speech-language pathologists need to consider the practical significance of the findings. A difference between groups can be statistically significant without being practically important. One way to determine practical significance is to apply a measure of effect size. Ideally, authors should include effect size measures and confidence intervals along with other statistical information in the results section of a research report.

In empirical research, the final phase is preparation and dissemination of a research report. Authors might publish their findings in a peer-reviewed journal or present a paper at a professional conference. Although the forms of information dissemination differ, the various report types usually have similar sections: a title, abstract, introduction and review of literature, methods, results, discussion and conclusions, and references. Usually, peer-reviewed journals contain the highest quality research reports because these journals have a process in which all manuscripts are read and evaluated by persons with expertise on the topic prior to publication.

Review Questions

1. What step comes first in evidence-based practice research?
   a. Completing a thorough literature search
   b. Deciding how to use your findings
   c. Formulating a focused clinical question
   d. Reading and evaluating research reports

2. What phase in evidence-based practice research involves reading existing research reports and using your knowledge of research design, measurement, and so on, to evaluate those reports?

3. Explain why articles published in peer-reviewed journals have higher status than self-published reports.

4. Explain why blinding is a desirable feature in treatment studies.

5. Identify two reasons why statistically significant differences might not be practically important in a clinical setting.

6. How does a critical appraisal of a diagnostic study differ from a critical appraisal of a treatment study?

7. Explain why a body of evidence from different researchers and different clinical settings is stronger than a single randomized clinical trial.

8. List seven sections that are included in most research reports.

9. What is a structured abstract?

10. Where will you find the formal statement of purpose and/or research questions in most research reports?

11. For each of the sentence pairs below, identify the one that best meets the writing guideline.

    Presents information in a parallel form:
    a. The participants most often reported writing for program information, the websites for each program, contacts with previous graduates, and receiving information from a professional organization website.
    b. The participants most often reported receiving information from written contacts with each program, the websites for each program, their contacts with previous graduates, and a professional organization website.

    Uses affect/effect correctly:
    a. The high-frequency distractor signal effected the results for both children and adults.
    b. The high-frequency distractor signal affected the results for both children and adults.

    Uses the most appropriate linking term:
    a. The 6-year-old children performed significantly better under Condition A, whereas the 9-year-old children performed significantly better under Condition B.
    b. The 6-year-old children performed significantly better under Condition A, while the 9-year-old children performed significantly better under Condition B.

    Uses active voice:
    a. Smith and Jones (2001) conducted a study to validate the new test procedure.
    b. A study was conducted by Smith and Jones (2001) to validate the new test procedure.

12. Many journals in the field of communication sciences and disorders use the same writing and style guidelines. What is the source of these guidelines?

Learning Activities

1. Identify a research report on a topic of interest. Read this article and prepare a brief summary like the ones you have read in the professional literature. You might find the following websites helpful in preparing your summary.

    The Purdue Online Writing Lab. (1995–2020). *Quoting, paraphrasing, and sum-*

marizing. https://owl.purdue.edu/owl/research_and_citation/using_research/quoting_paraphrasing_and_summarizing/index.html

The Writing Center @ The University of Wisconsin–Madison. (2020). *The writer's handbook.* https://writing.wisc.edu/handbook/

2. Use the information in Table 12–1 to complete a critical appraisal of a research report on a treatment topic. If you read a treatment-related report for Activity 1, you could use the same report. Otherwise, you could identify another report that covers a treatment approach that you find interesting.

References

American Psychological Association. (2020). *Publication manual of the American Psychological Association* (7th ed.).

American Speech-Language-Hearing Association. (1997–2024). *Evidence maps.* https://apps.asha.org/EvidenceMaps/

American Speech-Language-Hearing Association. (2004). *Evidence-based practice in communication disorders: An introduction* [Technical report]. https://www.asha.org/policy/tr2004-00001/

ASHA Journals Academy. (1997–2024). *Publishing and applying research in CSD.* https://academy.pubs.asha.org/

Baker, E., & McLeod, S. (2011). Evidence-based practice for children with speech sound disorders: Part 1 narrative review. *Language, Speech, and Hearing Services in Schools, 42,* 102–139. https://doi.org/10.1044/0161-1461(2010/09-0075)

Bayley, L., & Eldredge, J. D. (2003). The structured abstract: An essential tool for researchers. *Hypothesis, 17*(1), 11–13. https://www.mlanet.org/p/cm/ld/fid=517

Bossuyt, P. M., Reitsma, J. B., Bruns, D. E., Gatsonis, C. A., Glasziou, P. P., Irwig, L., Lijmer, J. G., Moher, D., Rennie, D., de Vet, H. C. W., Kressel, H. Y., Rifai, N., Golub, R. M., Altman, D. G., Hooft, L., Korevaar, D., A., & Cohen, J. F., for the STARD Group. (2015). STARD 2015: An updated list of essential items for reporting diagnostic accuracy studies. *Clinical Chemistry, 61,* 1446–1452. https://doi.org/10.1373/clinchem.2015.246280

Centre for Evidence-Based Medicine. (2011). *Oxford Centre for Evidence-Based Medicine 2011 levels of evidence.* https://www.cebm.net/2016/05/ocebm-levels-of-evidence/

Centre for Evidence-Based Medicine. (2024). *Critical appraisal tools.* https://www.cebm.ox.ac.uk/resources/ebm-tools/critical-appraisal-tools

Cohen, L., Manion, L., & Morrison, K. (2018). *Research methods in education* (8th ed.). Routledge.

Davidow, J. H., Bothe, A. K., & Bramlett, R. E. (2006). The Stuttering Treatment Research Evaluation and Assessment Tool (STREAT): Evaluating treatment research as part of evidence-based practice. *American Journal of Speech-Language Pathology, 15,* 126–141. https://doi.org/10.1044/1058-0360(2006/013)

Des Jarlais, D. C., Lyles, C., Crepaz, N., & the TREND Group. (2004). Improving the reporting quality of nonrandomized evaluations of behavioral and public health interventions: The TREND statement. *American Journal of Public Health, 94*(3), 361–366. https://doi.org/0.2105/ajph.94.3.361

Dollaghan, C. A. (2004). Evidence-based practice in communication disorders: What do we know and when do we know it? *Journal of Communication Disorders, 37,* 391–400. https://doi.org/10.1016/j.jcomdis.2004.04.002

Enhancing the QUAlity and Transparency Of health Research. (2024, January). *CONSORT 2010 statement: Updated guidelines for reporting parallel group randomised trials.* Equator network. https://www.equator-network.org/reporting-guidelines/consort/

Gallagher, T. M. (2002). Evidence-based practice: Applications to speech-language pathology. *Perspectives on Language Learning and Education*, *9*(1), 2–5. https://doi.org/10.1044/lle9.1.2

Gerber, S., Brice, A., Capone, N., Fujiki, M., & Timler, G. (2012). Language use in social interactions of school-age children with language impairments: An evidence-based systematic review of treatment. *Language, Speech & Hearing Services in Schools*, *43*, 235–249. https://doi.org/10.1044/0161-1461(2011/10-0047).

Gillam, S. L., & Gillam, R. B. (2006). Making evidence-based decisions about child language intervention in schools. *Language, Speech, and Hearing Services in Schools*, *37*, 304–315. https://doi.org/10.1044/0161-1461(2006/035)

Higgins, J. P. T., Thomas, J., Chandler, J., Cumpston, M., Li, T., Page, M. J., & Welch, V. A. (Eds.). (2023). *Cochrane Handbook for Systematic Reviews of Interventions* (Version 6.3). https://training.cochrane.org/handbook/current

Johnson, C. J. (2006). Getting started in evidence-based practice for childhood speech-language disorders. *American Journal of Speech-Language Pathology*, *15*, 20–35. https://doi.org/10.1044/1058-0360(2006/004)

Kaderavek, J. N., & Justice, L. M. (2010). Fidelity: An essential component of evidence-based practice in speech-language pathology. *American Journal of Speech-Language Pathology*, *19*, 369–379. https://doi.org/10.1044/1058-0360(2010/09-0097)

Kratochwill, T. R., Hitchcock, J., Horner, R. H., Levin, J. R., Odom, S. L., Rindskopf, D. M., & Shadish, W. R. (2010). *Single-case designs technical documentation*. What Works Clearinghouse. https://ies.ed.gov/ncee/wwc/Document/229

McCauley, R. J., Strand, E., Lof, G. L., Schooling, T., & Frymark, T. (2009). Evidence-based systematic review: Effects of nonspeech oral motor exercises on speech. *American Journal of Speech-Language Pathology*, *18*, 343–360. https://doi.org/10.1044/1058-0360(2009/09-0006)

Meline, T., & Paradiso, T. (2003). Evidence-based practice in schools: Evaluating research and reducing barriers. *Language, Speech, and Hearing Services in Schools*, *34*, 273–283.

Nail-Chiwetalu, B. J., & Ratner, N. B. (2006). Information literacy for speech-language pathologists: A key to evidence-based practice. *Language, Speech, and Hearing Services in Schools*, *37*, 157–167.

Newhart, M., & Patten, M. L. (2023). *Understanding research methods: An overview of the essentials* (11th ed.). Routledge Taylor & Francis Group.

ProQuest. (n.d.). *ProQuest dissertations and theses global*. https://www.proquest.com/products-services/pqdtglobal.html

Ratner, N. B. (2006). Evidence-based practice: An examination of its ramifications for the practice of speech-language pathology. *Language, Speech, and Hearing Services in Schools*, *37*, 257–267. https://doi.org/10.1044/0161-1461(2006/029)

Reichow, B., Volkmar, F. R., & Cicchetti, D. V. (2008). Development of the evaluative method for evaluating and determining evidence-based practices in autism. *Journal of Autism and Developmental Disorders*, *38*, 1311–1319. https://doi.org/10.1007/s10803-007-0517-7

Rosenthal, R., & Rosnow, R. L. (2008). *Essentials of behavioral research: Methods and data analysis* (3rd ed.). McGraw-Hill.

Speech Pathology Database for Best Interventions and Treatment Efficacy. (n.d.). *Group comparison studies*. https://speechbite.com/group-comparison-studies/

Tate, R. L., Perdices, M., Rosenkoetter, U., Wakim, D., Godbee, K., Togher, L, & McDonald, S. (2013). Revision of a method quality rating scale for single-case experimental designs and n-of-1 trials: The 15-item Risk of Bias in N-of-1 Trials (RoBiNT) scale. *Neuropsychological Rehabilitation*, *23*, 619–638. https://doi.org/10.1080/09602011.2013.824383

Trochim, W. M. K., Donnelly, J. P., & Arora, K. (2016). *Research methods: The essential knowledge base* (2nd ed.). Cengage Learning.

Wendt, O., & Miller, B. (2012). Quality appraisal of single-subject experimental designs: An overview and comparison of different appraisal tools. *Education and Treatment of Children, 35,* 235–268. https://doi.org/10.1353/etc.2012.0010

INDEX

Note: Page numbers in **bold** reference non-text material.

A

AAA. *See* American Academy of Audiology
Abstract, 10, 286
Academy of Doctors of Audiology, 70
Accuracy
   in information reporting, 32–33
   of measurement, 139–146
Adequacy
   descriptive, 122
   interpretive, 123
Adverse effects, 20
AERA. *See* American Educational Research Association
Alternate forms reliability, 148–149
American Academy of Audiology, 69–70, 289
American Auditory Society, 70
American Educational Research Association, 139
American Psychological Association, 69
   publication guidelines, 288–289
   publication manual, 243
   on research participants, 200
   style manual, 94–96
American Speech-Language-Hearing Association
   Code of Ethics, 20
   description of, 69–70, 105, 289
   evidence reviews, 4
   web-based tutorials, 56
Analysis
   qualitative, 4
   quantitative, 4
Analysis of variance, 258
AND operator, 74
ANOVA. *See* Analysis of variance
APA. *See* American Psychological Association
ASHA. *See* American Speech-Language-Hearing Association
Assessments
   learning activities, 156
   reliability of. *See* Reliability
   review questions, 155–156
   validity of. *See* Validity
Assignment, random, 206–207
Association for Research in Otolaryngology, 70
Audiologists
   Automatic term mapping, 69
   evidence-based practice and, 4
   treatment approaches and, 19–20
Average, described, 224
Axial coding, 118

B

Bar graphs, 220, **220**
Behavior Research Methods, 67
Belmont Report, 18
Beneficence, 19, 22–23, 27–28
Between-subjects factor, 163
Bias
   researcher, 122
   sample, 202
Bimodal, described, 224
Bing™, 68
Bonferroni correction, 261
Books, information from, 72–73
Boolean logic, 74

C

CA. *See* Conversation analysis
Case control, 111
Case studies, 119–120
   design examples, 133
   inspiration for research from, 46
   nonexperimental research, 105–108, 119–120
Casual-comparative research
   description of, 111–114
   design examples, 134–135
CDaCI study. *See* Childhood Development after Cochlear Implantation study
CEBM. *See* Centre for Evidence-Based Medicine
Census, 201
Central tendency, measures of, 224–226
Centre for Evidence-Based Medicine, 96, 279
Charts, 218
Child Development, 67
Childhood Development after Cochlear Implantation study, 109
Children, protection from exploitation, 21
Chi-square, 246–247
Chronological order, 89
Citation search, 72
Classical test theory
   description of, 138, 150
   studies within, **153–154**
Client-specific EBP question, 58
Clinical trial
   nonrandomized control study, **188**
   participant protections in, 28
   randomized, levels of evidence, **188**
   research strategy and, 74
Clinicians, evidence-based practice and, 4
Clinician-scientist, 3–4
Cluster sampling, 205–206
Code of Ethics, of the American Speech-Language-Hearing Association, 20
Codes, 116
Coding, open, 118
Coefficient
   contingency, 246–247
   of determination, 245
Coercive influence, 23
Cognition, 67

Cognitive Psychology, 67
Cohen's *d*, 266
Cohen's kappa statistic, 147
Cohort study, 108
Collective case study, 119
Column graphs, **220**
   data analysis and, 220
ComDisDome, 68, 71
"Common Rule," 18
Communication Sciences and Disorders Dome, 71
Concurrent validity, 141
Conditional statement, 55
Confidence intervals, 227, 255
Confidence levels, 254–256
Confidentiality, ethics and, 34
Confirmatory factor analysis, 145
Conflict of interest, 29–30
Consonant-vowel ratio, 50
Construct(s)
   behavioral, 145
   definition of, 138
Construct validity, 144–146
Content validity, 139–141
Content validity index, 141
Content validity ratio, 141
Contingency coefficient (C), 246–247
Control, experimental, 169–173
Control group
   nonequivalent designs of, 174–175
   no-treatment, 161
   posttest-only randomized, 161–162
   pretest-posttest randomized, 162–163
Control study, nonrandomized, 189
Convergence, 144–145
Conversational speech intelligibility index, 53–54
Conversation analysis
   description of, 120–122
   design examples, 136
Correlation
   design examples, 134
   negative, 240
   positive, 240
   research, 109–110
Correlation analysis
   description of, 109–110
   design examples, 133

Correlation coefficient, 142
Cost-benefit research, 4–5
Credit, for intellectual effort, 30–31
Criterion validity, 141–144
Cronbach's alpha, 150
CSII. *See* Conversational speech intelligibility index
CVI. *See* Content validity index
CVR. *See* Content validity ratio
CV ratio. *See* Consonant-vowel ratio

D

Data, 215
Data analysis
 inferential statistics, described, 237
 learning activities, 234
 measures of central tendency, 224–226
 measures of variability, 226–227
 review questions, 233–234
 shapes of distributions, 229–232
 variability estimates, 227–229
 visual representation of, 218–222
Data management, 33–34
Data sharing, 34
Data triangulation, 123
Datum, 215
Deductive reasoning, 114
Degrees of freedom, 242–243
Dependent variables, 9, 49, 160, 281
Depth of evidence, **187**
Description, thick, 123
Descriptive adequacy, 122
Descriptive statistics, 222–224
Descriptive studies, **50**
Designs
 experimental. *See* Experimental designs
 factorial, 164–169
  home program provision, **167**
  intervention types, **168**
  type of intervention, **165**
  type of orientation program, **166**
 true experimental, 160
Difference studies
 experimental, **50**
  directional hypothesis for, **53**
  hypothesis, **52**
 nonexperimental, **50**
  directional hypothesis for, **53**
  hypothesis, **52**
Directional hypothesis, 52, **53**
Direct quote, 32, 91
Direct relationship, 240
Discussion section
 of article, 10
 of research report, 287–288
Dissemination, of research results, 290
Dissertations & Theses, ProQuest, 69, 71, 290
Distributions
 data analysis, shapes of, 229–232
 sampling, 227
Divergence, 144–145
Divergent relationship, 144
Double pretest design, 175
DuckDuckGo, 68
Dysphagia Research Society, 70

E

EBP. *See* Evidence-based practice
Educational Audiology Association, 70
Education Resources Information Center database
 description of, 69, 72, 76
 search of, 80–82
Effect size, 266
Electronic literature search, 79–86
 ERIC database, 80–82
 Google Scholar, 84–86
 key terms/synonyms identification, 79–80
 PubMed, 82–84
Empirical research
 description of, 7
 goal of, 66
 review questions, 12–13
Engagement, prolonged, 122–123
ERIC database. *See* Education Resources Information Center database
Error
 margin of, 227
 sampling, 227
 type I, 239
 type II, 239, 268
Error bars, **221**
Estimates, means as, 227–229

Ethics
  accuracy in information reporting, 32–33
  attribution of ideas and, 31–32
  Code of, 20
  confidentiality and, 34
  conflict of interest, 29–30
  data management, 33–34
  exploitation and, 21
  historical perspective, 22–26
  human participants, protection of, 18–21
  intellectual effort credit and, 30
  learning activities, 37–38
  privacy and, 34
  review questions, 36–37
  violations of, 28
Ethnographic research, 117, 135
"Evaluative Method," 282
Evidence
  depth of, **187**
  levels of, 184–188
    experimental research, 189–190
    learning activities, 190–192
    research scenario, 196–197
    review questions, 190–192
  reviews, 4
Evidence-based practice
  description of, 4, 184–188
  literacy skills and, 65
Evidence-based questions, 55–58
Experiment, true, 7
Experimental designs, 160, 161–169
  factorial designs, 164–169
  importance of control, 169–173
  levels of evidence, 184–188, 189–192
  posttest-only, 161–162
  pretest-posttest randomized, 162–163
  quasi, 160–161
  Solomon randomized four-group design, 163–164
  switching replications design, 164
  true, 160–161
Experimental research
  data analysis procedures, 274–275
  description of, 7–8, 49
  difference study, **50**
  quasi-experimental study, **188**
  review questions, 189–190
  scenario, 196–197
  single-subject, **185**

Expert opinion, **188**
Exploitation, protection from, 21
Exploratory factor analysis, 145

F

Face validity, 139–141, 153
Factor analysis, 145
Factorial designs, 164–169
  home program provision, **167**
  intervention types, **168**
  statistical analysis and, 258–262
  type of, intervention, **165**
  types of, orientation program, **166**
"Federal Policy for the Protection of Human Subjects," 18
Feedback, participant, 123
Fetuses, protection from exploitation, 21
Findings
  applicability of, 284–285
  reporting, 285–286
Formal hypotheses, 51
Four-group design, 163–164
F ratio, 262
Frequencies, data analysis and, 222–224
Frequency polygon, 230, **231**, **259**
Friedman's two-way analysis of variance, 262
F test, 260

G

Google, 68
Google Books, 68
Google Scholar
  description of, 68, 70, 76
  search of, 84–86
Graphs, 218, 220, **221**
Grounded theory
  description of, 117–118
  design examples, 135
Group comparisons, 111, 134
Group design, repeated-measures, 175–177
Group research, 8

H

Health Insurance Portability and Accountability Act, 34–36

Hepatitis study, at Willowbrook State School, 22–23, 23–24
HIPPA. *See* Health Insurance Portability and Accountability Act
Hippocratic Oath, 19
Historical responses, 7
Hypotheses
  defined, 51
  directional, 52, **53**
  formal, 51
  nondirectional, 52
  null, 51, **52**
  research, 51

I

Ideas, attribution of, 31–32
If-then statements, 51, 55
Impaired people, protection from exploitation, 21
Independent *t*-tests, 251–254
Independent variables
  description of, 9, 49
  levels of, 160
Inductive reasoning, 114, 124
Inferences, defined, 201
Inferential statistics
  described, 237–240
  factorial designs for, 258–262
  learning activities, 270–271
  measures of association, 240–250
  references
    experimental, 274–275
    nonexperimental, 274
  review questions, 269–270
  testing differences
    among three or more samples, 258–262
    between two samples, 250–258
Information
  accuracy of, in reporting, 32–33
  from books, 72–73
Information literacy, 65, 75
Informed consent
  data sharing and, 34
  description of, 18, 27, 202
  HIPPA and, 35
  principles of, 30
  third party management of, 29
  Willowbrook hepatitis studies and, 23

Informed decision-making, 21
Inquiry, systematic, 2
Inspiration, 46
Institute of Education Sciences, 69
Institutional review boards, 26–27
Instrumental case study, 119
Instrumentation, pretest–posttest design, 172
Integrity, of research, 28–29
Intellectual effort, credit for, 30–31
Interaction effects, 166, 263
Internal consistency reliability, 149–150
Internal validity, threats to, 169
International Association of Logopedics and Phoniatrics, 70
International Society of Augmentative and Alternative Communication, 70
Interpretive adequacy, 123
Interquartile range, 226
Interrater reliability, 146
Interval level of measurement, 217
Intrarater reliability, 146
Intrinsic case study, 119
Introduction section
  of article, 10
  of research report, 286
Inverse relationship, 240
Iowa Soldiers and Sailors Orphans' Home, Tudor study at, 24
IRB. *See* Institutional review boards
IRT. *See* Item response theory
Item characteristic curve, 151
Item response theory
  description of, 138–139, 150–153
  studies within, **153–154**

J

Johnson, Wendell, University of Iowa Tudor study by, 25–26
Journal of Cognitive Neuroscience, 67
Journal of Epidemiology and Community Health, 67
Journal of Fluency Disorders, 25
Journal of Medical Speech-Language Pathology, 71
Journal of Memory and Language, 67
Journal of Speech-Language-Hearing Research, 10, 61–62

Journal of the Acoustical Society of America, 67
Journal of Verbal Learning and Verbal Behavior, 67
Justice, 20–24

K

Kruskal-Wallis test, 262
Kuder-Richardson 20 procedure, 150

L

Learning activities
  assessments, 156
  data analysis, 234
  ethics, 37–38
  experimental research, 190–192
  inferential statistics, 270–271
  levels of evidence, 189–192
  literature search, 76–77
  nonexperimental research, 125
  research reports, 292–293
  sampling, 212
  writing literature review, 99–100
Levels of evidence, 184–188
  experimental research, 189–190
  learning activities, 190–192
  research scenario, 196–197
  review questions, 189–190
Line graph, 220, **221**
Literacy skills, evidence-based practice and, 65
Literature reviews
  described, 96
  description of, 7
  narrative, 88
  in research proposal, 97
  search tools, 68–72
  strategies, 89
  topics, strategies for introducing, **90**
  writing of, 92
    citations, 94–96
    example of outline, 92–93
    introducing topic, 88
    learning activities, 99–100
    note taking, 91–92
    organization of, 88–91
    purposes of, 88
    references, 94–96
    research phase, 87–88
    review checklist, 96
    review questions, 99
    summary/conclusions section, 93–94
    types of, 96
Literature search
  designing strategy for, 73–75
  documenting, 75
  electronic, 79–86
    ERIC database, 80–82
    Google Scholar, 84–86
    key terms/synonyms identification, 79–80
    PubMed, 82–84
  organizing, 75
  purposes of, 66–68
Lived experience, 118
Longitudinal research, 108–109

M

Main effects, 166, 263
Mann-Whitney *U*, 256–257
Margin of error, 227
Maturation, 171
Maximum scores, variability and, 226
Mean
  described, 225
  as estimates, 227–229
  sample size and, 255
Measurement
  accuracy of, 139–146
  consistency of, 146–150
  key concepts in, 137–139
  levels of, 215–218
Measures of association, 240–250
  chi-square, 246–247
  coefficient of determination, 245
  contingency coefficient, 246–247
  Pearson product-moment correlation coefficient, 240–245
  regression, simple/multiple, 247–250
  Spearman rank-order correlation (Spearman *Rho*), 245–246
Median, described, 225
Memory and Cognition, 67

Mentor, 46
Meta-analysis
  critical appraisal and, 278
  definition of, 186
  description of, 4, 282
  levels of evidence, 186, 189
  research strategy and, 74
  review, 96
Methods section
  of article, 10
  of literature review, 89
  of research report, 286–287
Methods triangulation, 116, 123
Minimum scores, variability and, 226
Mixed model designs, 163
Mode, 224
Mortality threat, 173
Multiple baseline across behaviors design, 181
Multiple baseline design, 181
Multiple regression, 247–250
Multiple treatment design, 179–180
Multistage sampling, 205

N

Narrative review
  description of, 96
  of literature, 88
National Institutes of Health, 69
National Library of Medicine, 69
Nature Neuroscience, 67
Negative case sampling, 122
Negative correlation, 240
Negative predictive value, 143
Negative skew, 230
Noise and Health, 67
Nominal level of measurement, 216
Nondirectional hypothesis, 52
Nonempirical research, 7
Nonexperimental research
  case studies, 105–108, 119–120
  casual-comparative, 111–114
  conversation analysis, 120–122
  correlative, 109–110
  description of, 7–8, 49
  design, 104
  difference study, **50**
  ethnographic research, 117
  grounded theory, 117–118
  group comparisons, 111
  hypothesis, **52**
  inferential statistics, 274
  learning activities, 125
  longitudinal research, 108–109
  phenomenology, 118–119
  qualitative research, 114–117
  regression, 109–110
  review questions, 12–13, 124–125
  survey research, 104–105
Nonrandomized control study, **188**
Note taking, 91–92
NOT operator, 74
No-treatment control group, 161
Null hypothesis, 51, **52**
Number needed to treat, 266–267

O

OCHL. *See* Outcomes of Children with Hearing Loss
Office of Research Integrity, 29
One-way ANOVA, 259
One-way repeated-measures ANOVA, 261
Open coding, 118
Operationalize, 58–59, 60
Ordinal level of measurement, 216–217
OR operator, 74
Otoacoustic emissions, 7
Outcomes of Children with Hearing Loss, 109
Outliers, 230
Outline, 92–93
Oxford Centre for Evidence-Based Medicine, 187

P

Paired *t*-tests, 251–254
Parameters, 201
Paraphrase, 32, 94
Participants
  feedback from, 123
  protection of, 18–21
  recruitment of, 280

Patient/Population, Intervention, Comparison, and Outcome question, 56, **57**
Peabody Picture Vocabulary Test--Fourth Edition, 144
Pearson correlation coefficient, 147, **148**
Pearson product-moment correlation coefficient, 240–245
Peer-reviewed journals, 279
Percentages, 222–224
Percent agreement, 147
Personal sound amplification products, 57
Phase I trial, 8
Phase II trial, 8
Phase III trial, 8
Phase IV research, 8
Phenomenology research
　description of, 118–119
　design examples, 135
PICO question. *See* Patient/Population, Intervention, Comparison, and Outcome question
Pie charts, 218, **219**
Pooled standard deviation, 266
Populations
　defined, 200
　samples and, 200–201
Positive correlation, 240
Positive predictive value, 143
Positive skew, 230
Posttest-only designs, 161–162
Precision, sample, 207
Predictive study, 110
Predictive validity, 141–142
Preferred Reporting Items for Systematic Reviews and Meta-Analyses, 4, 96
Pregnant women, protection from exploitation, 21
Pretest-posttest randomized control group design, 162–163
Pretest sensitization, 162
PRISMA. *See* Preferred Reporting Items for Systematic Reviews and Meta-Analyses
Prisoners, protection from exploitation, 21
Privacy, ethics and, 34
Probability of error, 238
Problems
　defining, 51
　research, formulating, 51–55
Professional associations, 69
Prolonged engagement, 122–123
Proportions, 223–224
ProQuest
　description of, 71
　Dissertations & Theses, 69, 71, 290
"Protecting Personal Health Information in Research: Understanding the HIPAA Privacy Rule," 36
Protection, from exploitation, 21
PSAPs. *See* Personal sound amplification products
Psychological Review, 67
Psychological Science, 67
Psychometrics, 138
Publication Manual of the American Psychological Association, 94–96, 288
Public policy, scientific research and, 5
PubMed
　description of, 68–69, 71–72, 76
　search of, 82–84
Purposive sampling, 206

Q

Qualitative analysis, 4
Qualitative research
　description of, 7, 114–117
　quantitative research versus, **115**
　scientific rigor in, 122–123
Qualitative researchers, 206
　grounded theory and, 117–118
　inductive reasoning and, 114
　participant feedback and, 123
　qualitative research and, 114–115
　scientific rigor and, 122–123
Quantitative analysis, 4
Quantitative research
　deductive reasoning and, 114
　description of, 7
　qualitative research versus, **115**
Quarterly Journal of Experimental Psychology: Human Experimental Psychology, The, 67
Quasi-experimental approaches, 173–184
Quasi-experimental designs, 160–161
Quasi-experimental research, 7
Quasi-experimental study, **188**

INDEX

Questions
  evidence-based, 55–58
  research. *See* Research questions
  review. *See* Review questions
  well-formed, 58–60

R

Random assignment, 206–207
Randomized clinical trial, 186, **188**
Randomized treatment-control group designs, **170**
Random sampling
  simple, 203
  spreadsheet generated list, **204**
  stratified, 204
Range
  defined, 226
  interquartile, 226
  variability and, 226–227
Rapid Spontaneous Speech Analysis, 125
Ratio level of measurement, 217
Reactive effect of testing, 162
Reasoning
  deductive, 114
  inductive, 114
Reference list, 96
References, 94–96, 288
Reference standard, 142
Reflexivity, 122
Regression
  design examples, 134
  research, 109–110
Regression analysis
  description of, 109–110
  simple/multiple, 247–250
Relational studies, **50**
  directional hypothesis for, **53**
  hypothesis, example of, **52**
Relationship
  direct, 240
  inverse, 240
Reliability
  across time, 148–149
  alternate forms, 148–149
  definition of, 146
  described, 60
  internal consistency, 149–150
  interrater, 146

intrarater, 146
rater, 146–148
split-half, 149–150
test-retest, 148–149
Repeated group design measures, 175–177, 184
Repeated-measures ANOVA, 261
Research
  case studies, 105–108
  correlative, 109–110
  cost-benefit, 5
  empirical
    description of, 7
    goal of, 66
    review questions, 12–13
  experimental. *See* Experimental research
  getting started with, 9–11
  group, 8
  integrity of, 28–29
  longitudinal, 108–109
  nature of, 19
  nonexperimental. *See* Nonexperimental research
  participants in
    American Psychological Association guidelines for describing, 200
    protection of, 18–21
  public policy and, 5
  qualitative. *See* Qualitative research
  quantitative. *See* Quantitative research
  quasi-experimental, 7
  reading tips, 16
  review questions, 12–13
  roles of, 2–6
  single subject, 8
  types of, **6,** 6–9
Research designs
  description of, 103–104
  examples of, 133–136
  experimental, 161–169
  nonexperimental, 104
    case studies, 105–108
    longitudinal research, 108–109
    survey research, 104–105
  posttest-only, 161–162
  qualitative versus quantitative, **115**
Researchers
  attribution of ideas and, 31–32
  bias, 122

Researchers *(continued)*
  ethics violations, 28
  intellectual effort credit and, 30
  triangulation, 122
Research findings
  applicability of, 285
  disseminating, 290
  reporting, 285–286
Research grants, 33
Research hypothesis, 51
Research laboratories, 28
Research problems, 51–55
Research processes, **3**
Research proposal, 97–98
Research questions
  descriptive studies, **50**
  differential studies, **50**
  formulating, 49–51
  identifying, 46–49
  learning activities, 61–62
  relational studies, **50**
  review questions, 60–61
  well-formed, 58–60
Research reports
  components of, 286–288
  critical appraisal criteria, **283–284**
  learning activities, 292–293
  review questions, 291–292
  writing guidelines/style, 288–289
Research scenario, 42–43
Research variables, 9, **59**
Respect of persons, 18, 21–23, 27
Results, applicability of, 284–285
Results section
  of article, 10
  of research report, 287
Review
  literature. *See* Literature reviews
  meta-analysis, 96
  systematic. *See* Systematic review
Review questions, 99
  assessments, 155–156
  data analysis, 233–234
  ethics, 36–37
  experimental research, 189–190
  inferential statistics, 269–270
  levels of evidence, 189–190
  literature search, 76

  nonexperimental research, 124–125
  research, 12–13
  research reports, 291–292
  sampling, 211–212
  writing literature review, 99
Rho (Spearman rank-order correlation), 245–246
Risk of Bias in N-of-1 Trials scale, 282
RoBiNT. *See Risk of Bias in N-of-1 Trials* scale
rs (Spearman rank-order correlation), 245–246

S

Sample
  biased, 202
  characteristics of, 201–202
  of convenience, 202
  populations and, 200–201
  precision, 207
  testing differences among three or more samples, 258–262
  testing differences between confidence levels, 254–256
    Mann-Whitney U, 256–257
    sign test, 257–258
    t-tests, 251–254
    Wilcoxon matched-pairs signed-ranks test, 257–258
Sample of behaviors, 138
Sample sized
  appropriate, 207–210
  description of, 207–210, 243, 258
  estimates of means and, 255
  normal distribution and, 230
  observations and, 223
  significant results and, 252
  type II error and, 268
  unbiased, 202
  volunteerism and, 202
Sampling
  cluster, 205–206
  distribution, 227
  error, 227
  methods, 203–210
  multistage, 205
  negative case, 122
  purposive, 206

random
  simple, 203
  spreadsheet generated list, **204**
  stratified, 204–205
  review questions, 211–212
  systematic, 203–204
San Jose Mercury News, University of Iowa Tudor Study and, 25
Scatterplot, 218, **219**
Scheffé test, 261, 264
ScienceDirect, 69, 71
Scientific method, 2
Scientific misconduct, 32–33
Scientific research, public policy and, 5
Scientist, clinician, 3–4
Scoping review, 96
Scores, variability and, 226
SD. *See* Standard deviation
Search engines, 68–70
Search terms, 74
Selection threat, 172–173
Selective coding, 118
Sensitivity, 143, 143t, 267
Sensitization, pretest, 162
Significance test, 243
Simple random sampling, 203
Simple regression, 247–250
Single-group pretest-posttest design, 279
Single subject
  designs, 177–184
    quality, 184
  experimental designs, samples of studies, **185**
  research, 8
Skew
  negative, 230
  positive, 230
Solomon randomized four-group design, 163–164
Spearman rank-order correlation (Spearman Rho), 147, 245–246
Special protections, 21
Specificity, 143, 143t, 267
SpeechBITE. *See* Speech Pathology Database for Best Interventions and Treatment Efficacy
Speech-language pathologists
  evidence-based practice and, 4
  treatment approaches and, 19–20
Speech Pathology Database for Best Interventions and Treatment Efficacy, 69, 72, 76
Split-half reliability, 149–150
Standard deviation
  description of, 227
  formula for, 229
Statement(s)
  conditional, 51, 55
  if-then, 51, 55
Statement of purpose, 51, 54, 97
Statistical analysis
  clinical data analysis and, 265–267
  factorial designs for, 258–262
Statistically not significant, 238
Statistically significant, 211
Statistical regression, 171–172
Statistics
  caution in use and reporting of, 267–268
  described, 201
  descriptive, 222–224
  inferential. *See* Inferential statistics
Strata, 205
Stratified, random sampling, 204–205
Structured abstracts, 286
Structured review, 89
Sum of squares, 227
Survey
  design examples, 133
  questions, **106**
  research, 104–105
  responses, 7
Switching replications design, 164
Syphilis study, Tuskegee, 22–23
Systematic inquiry, 2
Systematic review
  critical appraisal and, 279, 282
  definition of, 186
  described, 186
  description of, 4, 96
  research strategy and, 74
Systematic sampling, 203–204

T

Table, 218
Testing, reactive effect of, 162

Test-retest reliability, 148–149
Theory formation, inductive reasoning and, 114
Thick description, 123
Threats to internal validity, 169
Transcripts, 118
Treatment
 described, 160
 levels of, 160
Treatment fidelity, 33
Treatment replication design, 179
Treatment withdrawal design, 178
Triangulation
 data, 123
 methods, 123
 researcher, 122
Trip Database, 70
True experiment
 criteria for, 7
 designs, 160
t-test, 267
 independent/paired, 251–254
 testing differences between samples, 250–258
Tudor, Mary, University of Iowa study by, 25–26
Tudor study, at University of Iowa, 22, 24–26
Tukey's honest significant difference test, 261, 264
Tuskegee Syphilis Study, 22–23
Two-way ANOVA, 262–263
Type I error, 239
Type II error, 239, 268

U

Unbiased sample, 202
University of Iowa, Tudor study at, 22, 25–26
University of Washington, Health Sciences Library, 56
U.S. Department of Education, 69
U.S. Department of Health and Human Services
 Belmont Report, 18
 Office of Research Integrity, 27
 "Protecting Personal Health Information in Research: Understanding the HIPAA Privacy Rule," 36
U.S. National Institutes of Health, 69
U.S. Public Health Service, Tuskegee Syphilis Study by, 22–23

V

Validity
 concurrent, 141
 construct, 144–146
 content, 139–141
 criterion, 141–144
 definition of, 139
 demonstrating of, 145–146
 described, 59, 60
 face, 139–141, 153
 internal, threats to, 169
 predictive, 141–142
Validity coefficient, 142
Variability
 measures of, 226–227
 minimum and maximum scores and, 226
Variables
 defined, 49
 dependent, 9, 49, 160, 281
 independent, 9, 49, 160
Variance, 227
Verbal labeling, 24
Voice Foundation, The, 70
Volunteerism, sample and, 202

W

Web-based tutorials, American Speech-Language-Hearing Association, 56
Web of Science, 69, 72
Well-formed questions, 58–60
What Works Clearinghouse standards, 282
Wilcoxon matched-pairs signed-ranks test, 257–258
Willowbrook State School, hepatitis study at, 22–23, 23–24
Within-subjects factor, 163
WorldCat, 68
Writing
 guidelines/style, 288–289
 literature reviews, 92
  citations, 94–96
  example of outline, 92–93

introducing topic, 88
learning activities, 99–100
note taking, 91–92
organization of, 88–91
purposes of, 88
references, 94–96
research phase, 87–88
review checklist, 96
review questions, 99
summary/conclusions section, 93–94
types of, 96

Y

Yahoo! Search, 68